FLUORESCENT ANTIBODY METHODS

Morris Goldman

BIONETICS RESEARCH LABORATORIES, INCORPORATED
FALLS CHURCH, VIRGINIA

formerly
COMMUNICABLE DISEASE CENTER
ATLANTA, GEORGIA

WITH A FOREWORD BY
ALBERT H. COONS

1968

ACADEMIC PRESS   New York and London

ACADEMIC PRESS, INC.
111 Fifth Avenue, New York, New York 10003

United Kingdom Edition published by
ACADEMIC PRESS, INC. (LONDON) LTD.
Berkeley Square House, London W.1

LIBRARY OF CONGRESS CATALOG CARD NUMBER: 68-14660

Second Printing, 1969

PRINTED IN THE UNITED STATES OF AMERICA

*This book is lovingly dedicated
to my wife and family*

FOREWORD

The steady increase in the use of immunofluorescence suggests that a critical monograph on the subject, in addition to the excellent book by Nairn, would be welcomed by many investigators.

Dr. Goldman's work is the product of fifteen years' experience with the use of fluorescent antibody, and some five years of compilation. He has brought to his task a quiet and critical outlook and a deep understanding of both the strengths and the limitations of the methodology he describes. The result is a thoroughly documented and scholarly work containing both historical perspective and explicit technical detail.

ALBERT H. COONS

Boston, Massachusetts
December, 1967

PREFACE

In certain respects it is true to say that all the techniques one needs in order to do fluorescent antibody work are already available in current texts on immunology, microscopy, chemistry, and histology. The reason for this is that the fluorescent antibody procedure is fundamentally an eclectic technology based on the methods of classic scientific disciplines. However, it is the very richness of the parent disciplines which makes it so desirable to sift out and bring together in one book those procedures specifically applicable to immunocytochemistry. Thus, this monograph is intended to provide in a compact form the practical information needed to implement fluorescent antibody work in the research and diagnostic laboratory.

I have directed this book primarily to the technical level of professional biomedical investigators and senior laboratory assistants. In other words, it is assumed that basic, ancillary laboratory skills are known or can be acquired independently as needed. The contents have been arranged in what I consider to be a "natural" manner, starting with descriptions of equipment, going on to laboratory procedures, and ending with references to applications in specific areas. However, each chapter and section is essentially self-contained, so that one may discover how to label antiserum, for example, without the necessity of wading through methods for producing such serum.

The section on applications has been organized in the form of an annotated reference list based on the extensive bibliography to be found at the end of the book. In particular, I have attempted to include review articles written by specialists in the diverse areas to which fluorescent antibody methods have been applied. It is hoped that this approach will make it possible for the newcomer to acquaint himself rapidly with work already carried out on specific organisms or disease conditions. The short, special bibliographies attached to most of the chapters refer mainly to worthwhile texts and articles

ix

from which I drew heavily in writing those chapters. My debt to the authors of such publications is hereby cheerfully confessed with thanks.

All commercial sources of equipment and reagents which are mentioned specifically in the text are listed in Appendix A, together with their American and foreign addresses, if not of United States origin. In addition, commercial suppliers of labeled and unlabeled sera and of labeling compounds, are listed separately in the same Appendix. Recipes for preparing phosphate and carbonate buffers commonly used in fluorescent antibody work are given in Appendix B.

I am grateful to the National Library of Medicine for providing the greater number of bibliographic references since 1963 by means of the MEDLARS data retrieval system. Thanks are also due to the Histochemical Society, Williams and Wilkins Co., Blackwell Scientific Publications, American Society for Microbiology, and the University of Maryland for permission to reproduce figures which appeared originally in the *Journal of Histochemistry and Cytochemistry, Journal of Immunology, Immunology, Applied Microbiology,* and *Fluorescent Compounds Used in Protein Tracing,* respectively. To Dr. W. B. Cherry of the National Communicable Disease Center, I acknowledge my indebtedness for use of the figures depicting optical equipment and staining methods, prepared by the Medical Arts Section of the National Institutes of Health. Finally, preparation of the book was greatly facilitated by the patient efforts of my wife, Esther, in transcribing handwritten copy into typewritten manuscript.

MORRIS GOLDMAN

December, 1967

CONTENTS

Chapter 7. **Labeling Agents and Procedures for Conjugation**

Chapter 8. **Properties of Conjugated Sera**

Chapter 9. **Cytological and Histological Methods**

Chapter 10. **Staining Methods**

Appendix A

Appendix B—Buffers

References

INTRODUCTORY

Chapter One

INTRODUCTION

I. GENERAL COMMENTS

The early decades of this century saw classic microscopic morphology reach what appeared to be the apogee of its contribution to biological knowledge. Exquisitely detailed descriptions existed of important histological elements, of protozoans, and indeed of most objects of interest to microscopists. The future of microscopy appeared to consist of an uninspired cataloging of the morphology of less important structures stranded in the wake of the grand sweep of classic microscopists of previous decades.

This gloomy picture began to change in the 1930's with the development of microscopic techniques for localizing biochemicals by ultraviolet absorption and by chemically specific staining reactions. The same decade saw the invention of the phase microscope which returned the world of living cells to the biologist so long preoccupied with fixed, stained artifacts; and the opening lines of a new literature of ultramorphology began to be written with the first electron microscopes. In subsequent years the X-ray and interference microscopes and autoradiographic techniques extended further the reach of the microscope.

The fluorescent antibody technique is a major participant in this historic return to the microscope, welding together, as it were, the test-tube techniques of immunology with the microscopic methods of cytology. In broad terms, the rationale is as follows: Serum proteins may be labeled with fluorescent markers by means of firm chemical bonds to yield fluorescent solutions whose biological activity is essentially unaltered. If a few drops of such conjugated serum containing antibodies are layered over a smear or section containing homologous antigen, antibody will be precipitated and fixed in space. Unreacted and non-antibody proteins can then be rinsed away and the preparation examined under a fluorescence microscope. Sites of antibody deposition can then be seen by virtue of their fluorescence against the dark background of non-antigen-containing materials. Thus, the procedure is essentially a cytochemical staining method, based upon the ability of antigens to form insoluble reaction products with antibodies.

Staining with fluorescent antibody can be manipulated in accordance with classic immunological principles. For example, staining can be blocked by previous or simultaneous exposure of antigen to unlabeled antibody, and fluorescent antisera can be deprived of their staining capabilities by absorbing the antibodies with sufficient antigen. On the other hand, univalent antibodies, which are non-precipitating in conventional systems, can be fixed to antigens and visualized as readily as polyvalent antibodies.

Fluorescence microscopes are basically conventional microscopes fitted with color filters on the far side of the object to provide proper excitation light, and other, matching filters on the near side to permit observation of fluorescence. Since the amount of fluorescent protein bound to antigen on smears or sections is extremely small, high intensity light sources are necessary to provide sufficient energy for stimulating adequate fluorescence. Although the underlying mechanism for staining with labeled antibody is immunochemical in nature, the great majority of publications involving fluorescent antibodies have dealt with non-immunological problems, e.g., localization of infectious agents or specific proteins in tissues, and identification of microorganisms in cultures or pathologic exudates.

II. DEVELOPMENT OF THE FLUORESCENT ANTIBODY TECHNIQUE

The following pages provide a chronological review of the development of fluorescent antibody methodology. References are made to the first reported uses of important new techniques, and the first reported applications in new areas, as nearly as these facts can be ascertained. The reader may safely conclude that each new development was soon exploited by additional investigators. Since this chapter is *not* intended as a history of the fluorescent antibody technique in bacteriology, pathology, virology, etc., many excellent early papers will be passed over. Most of the earlier contributions will find their way into the bibliography at the end of this book by virtue of being mentioned in later chapters on techniques, or in Chapter 12.

The publication in 1941 by Coons, Creech, and Jones of a short paper on the "Immunological properties of an antibody containing a fluorescent group" marked the public debut of the fluorescent antibody technique (186). Although this was by no means the first paper to deal with antibodies carrying chemical markers, one major consideration set it apart from the others. Previous workers (273, 466, 687) had studied the effects of various radicals on the *immunological activity* of antibodies; Coons and his associates were interested in the marked antibody only as a *tracer* that would lead them to unmarked antigen. This difference in objectives underlay the important difference in labeling compounds used by Coons and by previous workers. Non-fluorescent dyes employed in the past were unsuitable as tracers at the microscopic level, since the minute quantities of material involved made detection by light absorption extremely difficult. On the other hand, fluorescent dyes, whose presence could be detected as bright spots on a dark background, represented as much as a thousandfold increase in detectability over the previously employed absorption systems.

The first marker used by Coons and his associates was β-anthracene, introduced into antipneumococcus Type III serum by reacting the latter with β-anthryl isocyanate. The highly fluorescent conjugate agglutinated Type III pneumococci, imparting a grossly visible blue fluorescence to washed clumps of bacteria. Individual cells of Type III organisms were readily visible in the fluorescence microscope after exposure to labeled antiserum for 30 min. On the other hand, Type II pneumococci remained non-fluorescent after exposure to Type III antiserum under the same conditions.

Coons was interested in demonstrating antigens in tissue sections which, however, themselves exhibited blue fluorescence under ultraviolet illumination. He turned therefore from blue-fluorescent anthracene to the green-fluorescent dye, fluorescein, again employing the isocyanate derivative for purposes of coupling. In 1942, Coons, Creech, Jones, and Berliner published a fairly detailed description of the preparation of fluorescein–protein conjugates, and of their use in detecting pneumococcal antigen in tissues of infected mice (187). The report was exemplary in its conservative claims, its emphasis on controls to demonstrate specificity of observed staining, and in the many valuable technical details which were presented. However, this was during the period of World War II and further work with the technique by Coons and others was suspended for the next few years.

Upon return to civilian life, Coons picked up the problem once more and in 1950 and 1951 a now-classic series of five papers appeared. In the first of these (188), improvements in the synthesis of fluorescein isocyanate and of its conjugation to antiserum were thoroughly described. In addition, preparation of frozen sections for staining, a suitable filter system for fluorescence microscopy, removal of non-specific staining by means of tissue powders, and immunological proofs of specificity of staining were all given in sufficient detail to allow anyone seriously interested in the method to repeat Coons' experiments successfully. For several years thereafter this paper served as a *vade mecum* for workers in the field. The other four papers (190, 191, 441, 519) described localization of injected soluble antigens and of injected rickettsial and viral agents in tissues of experimental animals. The sum total of these papers was to establish beyond question that the fluorescent antibody method represented an extremely versatile and valuable contribution to the art of microscopy. With the publication of these five papers, the first, introductory phase of fluorescent antibody methodology might be considered to have ended. What had been accomplished?

1. Antisera had been converted into specific cytochemical stains for antigens by introducing fluorescein into the serum proteins.

2. Fluorescent antisera were shown to be effective for staining soluble as well as particulate antigens. The method was sensitive enough to render single bacterial cells and aggregates of viral particles clearly visible in the fluorescence microscope.

3. Basic technical details had been worked out; carbon arc light source, ultraviolet filter system, bright-field illumination, conventional fixation and paraffin embedding for some antigens, frozen sections cut in a cryostat and fixed in ethanol or unfixed for others, suitable immunological controls for proving specificity and reduction of non-specific staining by treating conjugates with tissue powders.

During the next few years the bulk of publications dealing with fluorescent antibodies came from a rather limited number of laboratories. This was undoubtedly the result in part of the formidable technical problems implicit in the technique. The labeling compound, fluorescein isocyanate, was not available commercially, and its synthesis, involving catalytic hydrogenation and reaction with phosgene among other steps, presupposed a rather well-equipped chemical environment for its success. Furthermore, fluorescence microscopes were not available as such, but needed to be assembled independently. The intense light-source requirement was especially difficult to meet. Finally must be mentioned the lurking doubt, in spite of Coons' admirable publications, that the method might simply not work with some particular antigens.

In spite of these difficulties, significant practical and theoretical contributions began to appear almost at once. Marshall, stimulated by the 1942 report of Coons *et al.,* described the localization of a native protein (adrenocorticotropic hormone) in normal tissue (hog pituitary) (691). This paper was particularly important for being the first to demonstrate that fluorescent antisera were specific enough to distinguish differences among native antigens comprising normal tissues, and that "contaminant" antibodies, resulting from impure immunizing antigens, could be absorbed away from labeled antiserum without affecting the specific staining capacity of the serum. In addition, several technical points were made: freeze-drying of tissues followed by paraffin embedding for preservation of antigenicity; fixation of sections with methanol; and use of a dark-field substage condenser in order to improve the fluorescence image. A final observation which, unfortunately, went generally unnoticed for several years, was that fluorescein isocyanate in acetone solution could be stored for as much as a year if protected from moisture, light, and heat.

Marshall's prototype paper on tissue antigens was followed by other studies of this nature using the same straightforward technical approach: i.e., tissue antigens were isolated in as pure a condition as possible, antisera were prepared against them and labeled with fluorescein, and the labeled sera were then employed to stain tissue sections of the animal species under investigation. Thus, an *in vitro* localization of antigens was accomplished. In 1955, Mellors *et al.* described a more involved technique that made it possible to demonstrate *in vivo* localization of injected antibodies to native antigens (716, 724). Antibody (Ab_1) against rat kidney antigen (Ag_1) was prepared in rabbits and left in its original, unlabeled condition. Anti-

body (Ab$_2$) against rabbit serum acting as antigen (Ag$_2$) was prepared in chickens and labeled with fluorescein. The unlabeled rabbit
antiserum (Ab$_1$) was inoculated into rats which were killed after
a suitable period of time. Sections of rat kidney were then exposed
to labeled antirabbit (Ab$_2$) obtained from the chickens. Thus, rabbit
serum was made to play a dual role, being antibody (Ab$_1$) at one
end and antigen (Ag$_2$) at the other. This modification of the basic
staining procedure made possible *in vivo* studies of antigen–antibody
reactions with more relevance to certain disease states than the earlier
in vitro techniques.

Mellors' method was apparently an independent discovery of the
feasibility of the "indirect" staining technique reported in 1954 by
Weller and Coons (1114). (In the latter publication, B. K. Watson
and A. H. Coons were credited with having prepared the rabbit
antiserum against human globulin which was used in the study, and a
footnote acknowledged that Dr. David Gitlin had concurrently and
independently developed a similar technique.) In this method, a
preparation of tissue culture cells containing virus was rendered
fluorescent by first exposing the cells to unlabeled human antiserum
against the virus, and then to fluorescent rabbit antiserum directed
against human globulin. By this technique all antigens capable of
reacting with, say, human antibodies could be stained with a single
antihuman conjugate; conversely, all human sera containing antibodies to a particular antigen were capable of being used as staining
agents for that antigen without the necessity of labeling each one
separately with fluorescein. This "indirect" procedure later came to
play an exceedingly important role in the widespread application of
fluorescent antibody.

Another sophisticated modification of basic fluorescent antibody
staining procedure was a method for staining native antibody *in situ*
(189). Tissue sections suspected of containing antibody-synthesizing
cells were flooded with unlabeled, diluted homologous antigen. After
allowing a suitable period for the antigen to react with cellular antibodies, the sections were rinsed and flooded with fluorescent antiserum
directed against the homologous antigen. By this means, localization
of native antibody in tissue cells was accomplished.

Although Coons had demonstrated in 1941 that a labeled antiserum
against one bacterial type (Type III pneumococcus) would not stain
a closely related form (Type II pneumococcus), Goldman's papers

in 1953 and 1954 on the differentiation with fluorescent antibody of two intestinal protozoan parasites, *Entamoeba histolytica* and *Entamoeba coli,* represented the first attempt to apply the technique as a diagnostic procedure (363, 364). No technical innovations were introduced by these reports but their importance lay in the fact that they confirmed at that early date the utility of the procedure in yet another area, protozoology, and they pointed the way toward diagnostic applications of the fluorescent antibody technique.

This area of application was developed further when in 1956, Moody, Thomason, and Goldman published two papers on staining bacterial smears for the purpose of identifying the contained organisms, rather than for tracing their distribution (747, 1054). They demonstrated that the species studied, *Malleomyces pseudomallei,* could be seen and identified by its fluorescence when present in as few as 220 organisms per milliliter, and in the presence of as many as 10 million other bacteria. This degree of sensitivity, and the speed with which the staining and examination of smears could be carried out, less than 1 hr, left no doubt concerning the potential of the technique for diagnostic microbiology. The same year brought a report by Liu on rapid diagnosis of influenza as a result of staining nasal washings from suspected cases (638). The fluorescence method did not detect all positive cases found by the hemagglutination inhibition test, but the latter required a delay of 10–14 days before serum from convalescents could be collected, whereas the staining method gave an answer the day specimens were collected.

The diagnostic potential of the fluorescent antibody method was enlarged by the appearance in 1957 of four independent reports in which the method was employed for the first time as a serologic test to detect antibodies in *unlabeled* test sera. Of course, the basic staining technique could have been used for detecting antibodies by simply labeling each test serum and observing its staining reactions. It is obvious, however, that such a course would be entirely impractical in any but the most special diagnostic situation. On the other hand, in the indirect staining procedure and in the inhibition control for specificity, basic outlines existed for practical serological tests, since in both procedures unlabeled sera were used. In the case of the indirect method, substitution of normal serum for antiserum in the intermediate layer would result in antigen showing no fluorescence after the fluorescent reagent was applied; in the inhibition control the same substitution would result in full fluorescence of the antigen since no blocking effect would derive from the normal serum.

The indirect method served as a basis for demonstrating antibody against primary atypical pneumonia (639), *Treponema pallidum* (236), and herpes simplex (812); while the inhibition method was used for antibodies against *Toxoplasma gondii* (366). In 1958, Goldwasser and Shepard described a complement staining method that was similar to the indirect method but possessed a broader applicability (386). In this method unlabeled guinea pig complement was added to the unlabeled antiserum overlayered on the antigen. Complement incorporated into the resulting antigen–antibody complex could then be stained by a fluorescent antiserum directed against guinea pig complement. Thus a single labeled anticomplement conjugate became a specific staining reagent for all antigens capable of binding complement in the course of their reaction with antibody, regardless of the species source of antibody. Furthermore, the same modifications of the indirect method which converted it into a test for antibodies were applicable to the complement staining technique.

It is a tribute to the thoroughness of Coons' work as well as a testimonial to the difficulties inherent in the problem, that it was not until 1958 that significant progress was reported in two technical aspects of fluorescent antibody work which had presented problems from the very beginning. The first of these stemmed from the fact that fluorescein isocyanate was an unstable compound that soon deteriorated upon exposure to moisture. Thus, it was recommended that it be prepared from the last stable intermediate, fluorescein amine, immediately before conjugation with proteins. However, since conversion of amine to isocyanate involved reaction with phosgene, most biological laboratories were excluded from the pale because of their lack of equipment and experience in handling the toxic gas. The second problem was the fact that the fluorescein label provided only a single fluorescent color. Many workers felt that availability of a contrast fluorescence to fluorescein would be desirable when working with material containing blue, green, or yellow autofluorescence, or when it was necessary to demonstrate two different antigens simultaneously in the same preparation.

Actually, some steps had already been taken toward solution of these problems before 1958. As mentioned previously, Marshall, as early as 1951 (691), had pointed out that fluorescein isocyanate in acetone solution could be stored for at least a year when protected from moisture, heat, and light. Goldman and Carver in 1957 had shown that fluorescein isocyanate dried onto filter paper, and stored in a dessicator for 7 months, would still react effectively with protein (374). With regard to contrast fluorescence colors, Clayton (1954) in a one-page report referred to use of a yellow dye (1-dimethylamino-5-sulfonyl chloride-naphthalene), and a red dye (nuclear fast red), as well as to fluorescein isocyanate, in a study of the distribution of embryonic antigens (146). Because of the absence of technical details, however, this report did not materially advance the technology at the time.

In 1958, three papers appeared that described in completely adequate detail more effective solutions to these two problems than any proposed heretofore. The most important of these, judged in clear-eyed hindsight, by Riggs, Seiwald, Burckhalter, Downs, and Metcalf, described the synthesis and use of isothiocyanate derivatives of both fluorescein and tetraethylrhodamine B (908). Isothiocyanate derivatives were superior to isocyanates in two important respects: their preparation involved use of liquid thiophosgene, which was considerably easier to handle than gaseous phosgene, and the final products were stable powders which could be stored for months and used for labeling proteins with no further chemical manipulations. Rhodamine B was a magenta-colored dye whose protein conjugates exhibited bright orange-red fluorescence, providing excellent contrast to the yellow-green of fluorescein and the blue of autofluorescent tissues.

Another orange-fluorescing derivative of rhodamine B, the disulfonic acid, was successfully conjugated to proteins by Chadwick, McEntegart, and Nairn (123). This stable dye, lissamine rhodamine B 200, obtained commercially as the sodium salt, was converted to the sulfonyl chloride by reaction with PCl_5. Conjugation was accomplished by stirring the sulfonyl chloride into a buffered solution of the protein and allowing the reaction to proceed for about 30 min. Thus another fluorescent conjugate resulting from relatively simple chemical manipulations was provided.

The third important paper was by Mayersbach, who described in full detail synthesis and use of the yellow-fluorescing dye that Clayton had mentioned (697). The labeling of proteins with 1-dimethyl-aminonaphthalene-5-sulfonyl chloride (DANS) had been described as far back as 1952 by Weber (1109), and in 1957 by Laurence

(608), but neither of these workers had used their labeled proteins in tracer work. Mayersbach redescribed preparation of the dye and dye–protein conjugate, and also compared such conjugates with fluorescein-labeled proteins as immunohistochemical reagents. DANS, in the sulfonyl chloride form, was stable for months when kept dry and under refrigeration. Although the yellow fluorescence of DANS was not as generally desirable as the orange-red of rhodamine, it nevertheless provided another simple alternative to fluorescein isocyanate as a labeling agent.

For the sake of completeness, it should be mentioned that Redetzki also described labeling of antibodies with DANS in 1958 (895), although he did not use the conjugates as histochemical stains; and finally that Hiramoto, Engel, and Pressman described conjugates prepared with tetramethylrhodamine isocyanate that same year (447). The latter dye has never become available commercially and presumably suffered from the same disabilities as fluorescein isocyanate with regard to synthesis and keeping qualities.

With the development of protein-labeling dyes that were stable enough to be marketed commercially, and which could be employed with a minimum of chemical manipulations, a major difficulty of fluorescent antibody technology was laid to rest. In comparison with this accomplishment, improvements in most other technical aspects of the art are relatively trivial. However, one important problem which has persisted since introduction of the technique—non-specific staining—has been brought under more effective control in recent years and deserves to be mentioned here.

Coons and Kaplan (188) had determined empirically that tissue powders reduced non-specific staining of tissues to bearable levels, but there was no underlying basis of information to explain either the staining or its reduction. In 1958, Curtain showed that labeled globulins consisted of a spectrum of protein molecules carrying different amounts of fluorescein, and that the more heavily loaded protein possessed the greatest non-specific activity (212). He confirmed this finding in 1961, using column chromatography on diethylaminoethyl cellulose to fractionate his conjugates, and proposed a simple method for preparing fractions with high antibody and low non-specific activity (214). For all practical purposes, this was the same method described a year earlier by Riggs et al. (907) who, however, did not relate their results to the fluorescein–protein ratios of the various fractions. Goldstein *et al.,* in a thoroughly documented study, confirmed the essential findings of Curtain and Riggs that fractions with desirable staining properties could be separated from crude conjugates by chromatography on anion-exchange cellulose (381). The problems of non-specific staining were by no means completely solved, but these studies provided a sound underpinning for further research in this area.

No history of fluorescent antibody technique would be complete without mentioning the important contribution to proliferation of the method made by commercial interests. Until about 1955, when Leitz and Reichert began to provide fluorescence microscopes on the American market, individual assembly of such instruments was a major hurdle that often took months to overcome. The possibility of purchasing a completely assembled unit, utilizing the convenient mercury arc lamp, advanced a laboratory's program immeasurably. A similar stimulating effect resulted from entry into the market of firms supplying labeling dyes and labeled antisera. Although such contributions are anonymous, so far as individuals are concerned, their practical importance must be acknowledged in any survey of development of the field.

BIBLIOGRAPHY

Coons, A. H. (1961). The beginnings of immunofluorescence. *J. Immunol.* **87**: 499-503.
Coons, A. H. (1962). The urge to find out. *J. Am. Med. Assoc.* **181**: 892-893.
Spink, W. W. (1962). The young investigator and his fluorescent antibody. *J. Am. Med. Assoc.* **181**: 889-891.

Chapter Two

FLUORESCENCE GENERALITIES

I. THE NATURE OF FLUORESCENCE

A dilute, alkaline solution of fluorescein in water is golden yellow when observed with the light behind it. Examined from the same side as the illumination, or at right angles to it, it shows a lovely green hue. This difference in color between the transmitted and what appears to be (but in reality is not) the reflected beam is the most characteristic, superficial, property of a strongly fluorescent dye in solution. The true nature of this phenomenon was long misunderstood to be a result of the diffusion or scattering of incident light. However, in 1852, G. G. Stokes showed that fluorescent substances actually "generated" new light internally while being irradiated from an outside source, and that the color of the emitted light did not need to be contained in the incident beam. From Stokes' explanation can be derived a simple definition of fluorescence: it is the emission of light of one color during the time a substance is irradiated with light of another color.

The full scope of fluorescence phenomena is very extensive, involving, as it does, a considerable portion of the electromagnetic spectrum—from wavelengths of about 5×10^{-3} to 8×10^3 A—and substances ranging from elementary gases to organic compounds of the utmost complexity. On the other hand, practical fluorescent antibody technology involves only the near ultraviolet and visible light portions of the spectrum, and a relatively small group of organic dyes. The following discussion will therefore be limited to an oversimplified consideration of fluorescence phenomena in order to provide the biologist with an elementary framework of reference in this area. General sources for rigorous and detailed treatment of the physics of fluorescence will be found in the bibliography at the end of the chapter.

Before discussing fluorescence as such, it is necessary to review briefly certain concepts about the nature of light and of energy states in molecules. We need not be detained for our purposes by complications arising from considering light both according to classical theory as a wave motion, and according to quantum theory as a stream of discrete energy units. Both concepts are necessary in a consideration of the events involved in fluorescence.

A wave motion in its simplest form can be described in terms of its *velocity* (c), its *frequency* or number of vibrations per second (v), and its *wavelength* or distance between similar points on consecutive waves (λ). These are related to each other by the formula:

$$c = v \, \lambda$$

Light of all frequencies has a constant velocity in a vacuum of 3×10^{10} cm/sec (about 186,000 miles/sec); thus, the greater the frequency the shorter the wavelength. Its wavelength is measured in angstrom units (1 Å = 1×10^{-8} cm) or in millimicrons (1 mμ = 10 Å). Frequency is expressed in sec. $^{-1}$ from the formula $v = c/\lambda$, or in terms of the wave number $\tilde{v} = 1/\lambda$, the unit of which is cm^{-1}. Visible light, consisting of radiation with wavelengths of roughly 400–750 mμ, constitutes only a small portion of the entire spectrum of electromagnetic radiation. The subjective impression of color is related to wavelength, and ranges from blue–violet at the short end of the visible spectrum to red at the long end. Sensitivity of the human eye is greatest to light of green–yellow color. Figure 1 summarizes some of these data.

In addition to showing properties of a wave motion, light also behaves as if the energy carried by its motion comes in discrete packets called quanta or photons. The energy of a photon is given by the expression

$$E = hv$$

where h is Planck's constant, 6.62×10^{-27} erg sec and v is the frequency of the light wave involved. It is apparent from this expression that a quantum of light of greater frequency (and thus shorter wavelength) has more energy than one of lesser frequency or longer wavelength. Absorption and emission of light can only take place in whole units of quanta. Thus, if energy is lost in the course of an absorption and emission cycle of a fluorescent material, it will be manifest by the longer wavelength of the emitted photons and not by a reduced number of these units.

The atomic model of Niels Bohr assumes that molecules exist only in certain specific energy states. At ordinary temperatures most molecules are at a low or ground state of energy. Raising a molecule to a higher or excited state requires specific energy increments which can be provided by absorption of quanta of the precise energy needed.

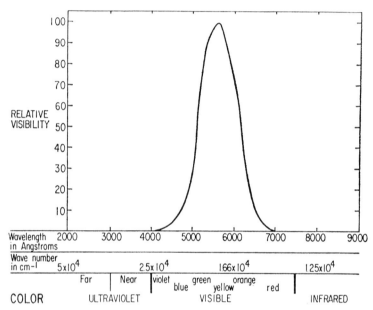

Fig. 1. Relative visibility and conventional subdivisions within the electromagnetic spectrum between 2000 and 9000 Å.

Conversely, return of a molecule from an excited to ground state or to some intermediate energy level requires loss of specific and discrete units of energy, either through non-radiative processes such as collisions with neighboring molecules or photochemical reactions, or by the radiative process of emitting photons.

The general term *luminescence* is applied to spontaneous emission of light occurring during the time molecules are returning to a lesser energy level from an excited state. When this reversion occurs within less than 10^{-8} sec of the time the molecules are excited by a stimulating light beam, the process is called *fluorescence*. Should reversion to ground state continue to take place for a longer time after the excitation beam has been removed, the process is called *phosphorescence*.

We may now describe the events that take place when a dilute solution of, say, fluorescein in water, is irradiated with a beam of natural white light or its equivalent. Photons of wavelength longer than 530 mμ, at the yellow and red end of the visible spectrum, will pass through unabsorbed by fluorescein molecules and only slightly absorbed by water molecules. For practical purposes the solution may be considered transparent to light of this color. On the other hand, blue and green light, in the range of 400–530 mμ, will be strongly absorbed by the fluorescein in the solution. In the case of about 15 out of every 100 photons absorbed, the energy imparted to the fluorescein molecules will be dissipated in the form of collisions with the other molecules and, to a lesser degree, in photochemical changes of the fluorescein. This will be recognized primarily by an increase in the temperature of the solution. The other 85 out of every 100 blue and green photons absorbed will stimulate radiation of fluorescent light: i.e., absorbing molecules will be raised to a higher energy level and will immediately revert to ground state by emission of the same number of photons of yellow–green light.

II. CHARACTERISTICS OF FLUORESCENCE

Fluorescence may be excited by any visible or ultraviolet radiation which is absorbed. Inasmuch as in the course of absorption and emission, excited molecules are likely to lose a certain amount of absorbed energy by collision before they return to ground state by emission of radiation, emitted photons will have less energy, and therefore longer wavelengths, than exciting photons. This phenomenon, known as Stokes' law, may be contravened in special situations in which cases absorption and emission spectra may overlap slightly, but for our purposes the law may be taken as absolute. Typically, the emission spectrum will adjoin the long wavelength end of the absorption spectrum, i.e. orange fluorescence will be stimulated by green–yellow light, yellow by blue–green, and green by violet–blue (Fig. 2).

Substances with absorption bands in the visible portion of the spectrum may absorb additionally in the ultraviolet. Although photons in the ultraviolet range carry more energy than those of longer wave-length, the spectrum of fluorescent light will be the same regardless of the wavelength of the excitation light. This results from the fact that part of the additional energy transmitted to the absorbing mole-cule by ultraviolet light will be lost by non-fluorescent perturbations. When the excitation level is finally degraded to the energy state provided by light of longer wavelength, the molecule will return to ground state by a fluorescence emission similar to that which would have been stimulated by long-wave excitation in the first place. In practical terms this means that the basic color of fluorescence emis-

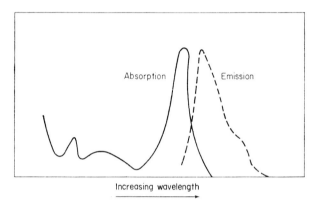

Increasing wavelength

FIG. 2.   Generalized absorption and emission spectrum of a fluorescent dye. Emission is always of longer wavelength than absorption (except for slight overlapping under some conditions), and is always the same, regardless of the wavelength which is absorbed.

sion cannot be altered by changing from blue to ultraviolet excitation. Nevertheless, the *effective* fluorescence color may be varied by use of different filter systems.

Brightness of fluorescence is influenced by three main considera-tions: (1) efficiency with which the substance converts incident into fluorescent radiation; (2) concentration of fluorescent material; and (3) intensity of exciting (= absorbed) radiation.

The most basic evaluation of fluorescence efficiency is quantum yield, Q, or ratio between number of quanta emitted to the number absorbed. Experimental determinations of absolute values for Q are subject to many technical difficulties and published values for the same material may differ significantly. For some dyes, values as high as 0.97 have been reported, but for most fluorescent dyes the quantum efficiency is considerably lower. Efficiency of a particular dye is independent of excitation wavelength as long as excitation is below the peak wavelength of the main absorption band. It is illusory, therefore, to expect that short wavelengths will stimulate brighter fluorescence because of their greater energy content. All other things being equal, the level of fluorescence will depend upon the degree of absorption of a particular spectral band and not upon its location in the long or short wavelength end of the spectrum. Quantum yield is influenced by such factors as concentration of dye, temperature, pH, viscosity, and chemical nature of the solvent. Much empirical data exist on the relationship of these conditions to emissions of specific substances, but dependable overall generalizations are few. For the restricted number of dyes utilized in fluorescent antibody work, a sufficient body of information has been accumulated to satisfy practical needs. Details will be found in the sections dealing with specific dyes.

At low dye concentrations, fluorescence intensity is directly proportional to concentration. At higher concentrations the increased probability of interactions between molecules of the same species results in a "self-quenching" effect, or a reduction in the quantum efficiency of the substance. Some limiting concentrations quoted by Pringsheim are 5×10^{-4} moles/liter for uranin (sodium fluorescein), 5×10^{-5} for rhodamine 6 G, and 3×10^{-3} for trypaflavine, all in aqueous solution.

In practical, qualitative fluorescent antibody work the possibility of self-quenching is more an academic than a real difficulty. There is ample experience to show that cells exposed to serial dilutions of the same specific conjugate show increasing brightness with increasing concentration up to very brilliant levels of fluorescence. Even if quantum efficiency is reduced at higher concentrations, the total fluorescence is still greater than at lower concentrations because of the greater number of fluorescent molecules that have been bound. But beyond this practical observation is the fact that data on self-quenching of solutions of free fluorescein do not necessarily reveal the behavior of fluorescein bound to protein which, in turn, is bound to an antigenic substrate. The problem is further complicated by the fact that fluorescence efficiency of fluorescein and rhodamine decreases with increasing numbers of fluorescent radicals attached per molecule of protein (see Chapter 8). Thus, in the present state of inadequate information one can only follow an empirical approach to the question of concentration vs. intensity in fluorescent antibody studies.

The third important factor that influences brightness is intensity of exciting radiation. Since the excitation lifetime of a fluorescent molecule is on the order of less than 10^{-8} sec, a fluorescent solution will always contain many more unexcited than excited molecules. Fluorescence will thus continue to increase up to the highest intensities of exciting radiation.

In gauging the intensity of a light source for stimulating fluorescence, it must be remembered that only *absorbed* light is effective for this purpose. No intensity level of red light, for example, will excite fluorescence in a solution of fluorescein, inasmuch as the latter does not absorb in those wavelengths. For substances absorbing primarily in the ultraviolet, the visual brightness of a light source whose ultraviolet component is unknown may be deceptive. However, the most important dyes used in fluorescent antibody procedures (fluorescein and rhodamine) show absorption maxima in the visible; for such dyes the brightness to the eye of a white light source will generally parallel its efficiency as an exciting source for fluorescence.

During photomicrography or other prolonged exposure of fluorescent preparations to bright light, it is frequently noted that the object has either faded considerably or changed color, or both. This results from the fact that a percentage of molecules raised to higher energy levels by absorption of light may undergo chemical changes. These may result in formation of nonfluorescent substances, or in substances with absorption and emission characteristics different from the parent material. Quanta of near ultraviolet and visible light (360–780 mμ) carry energy equivalent to from 35 to 80 kcal/mole. Chemical bonding energies of groups such as C—O, H—I, C—C, C—Cl, C—N, N—N, O—O, O—Cl, and C—Br fall within this range. It is not surprising, therefore, that photochemical changes may be induced by irradiation intended to stimulate fluorescence.

BIBLIOGRAPHY

Bowen, E. J., and Wokes, F. (1953). "Fluorescence of Solutions." Longmans, Green, New York.
Hirschlaff, E. (1938). "Fluorescence and Phosphorescence." Methuen, London.

Pringsheim, P. (1949). "Fluorescence and Phosphorescence." Wiley (Inter-science), New York.
Pringsheim, P., and Vogel, M. (1946). "Luminescence of Liquids and Solids." Wiley (Interscience), New York.
Radley, J. A., and Grant, J. (1954). "Fluorescence Analysis in Ultraviolet Light," 4th ed. Van Nostrand, Princeton, New Jersey.
Udenfriend, S. (1962). "Fluorescence Assay in Biology and Medicine." Academic Press, New York.
Venkataraman, K. (1952). "The Chemistry of Synthetic Dyes." Academic Press, New York.

INSTRUMENTATION

Chapter Three

LIGHT SOURCES

I. GENERAL COMMENTS

Light sources for fluorescence microscopy should be rich in ultraviolet and blue wavelengths, and should have high intrinsic brightness. Incandescent filament sources, such as are used for ordinary microscopy, are characterized by a spectrum relatively rich in visible and infrared wavelengths but poor in ultraviolet. Furthermore, brightness per unit area of such sources is much below levels attained in arc lamps. For these reasons filament sources in general have been ineffective in fluorescent antibody studies, although the more intense varieties may be adequate for other types of fluorescence microscopy. All present-day commercial illuminators designed specifically for fluorescent antibody work employ so-called "super high-pressure" or compact mercury vapor arcs as the light source.

Arcs are electrical discharges taking place between electrodes separated by a gas or vapor. They may be open, like carbon arcs in air, or closed, like mercury arcs in sealed quartz envelopes. The characteristics of radiation emitted by arcs are determined by the nature and pressure of the gases involved, and by the nature of the electrodes. Electrical properties of arcs are such that they are inherently unstable and require special power supplies for proper operation. Such accessories are almost always available from the specific lamp manufacturers or from the electrical supply industry in general. Mercury arcs radiate much less red and infrared than xenon and carbon arcs and are therefore relatively cool sources. Nevertheless, the absorption of any wavelength by an opaque object will raise its temperature, so that adequate heat dissipation presents a problem in housing design for all types of arcs.

II. HIGH INTENSITY LIGHT SOURCES

A. Mercury Arcs

Mercury arcs emit a line spectrum particularly rich in ultraviolet, superimposed upon a generally low-level continuous spectrum (Fig. 3). With increasing pressure the lines are broadened and intensity of the continuum increases.

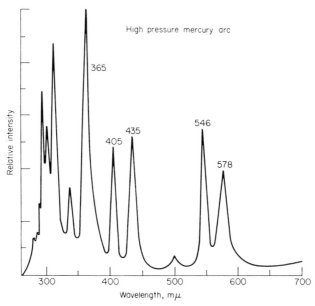

FIG. 3.   Energy distribution for high pressure mercury arc (Philips CS 100).

In the following discussion, various kinds of mercury arcs available for fluorescence work are described. Table I summarizes the technical specifications of these and other light sources.

1. HBO 200 (Osram, Germany) (Fig. 4a). This bulb may be taken as typical of this class of illuminants since it is the most widely used at the present time. Overall length is 108 mm. It is equipped with a special, side-arm, starting electrode by means of which a hot bulb may be re-ignited even though the vapor pressure of the heated mercury ordinarily would inhibit an arc from being struck between the two main electrodes. The bulb may be operated on either AC

TABLE I

HIGH INTENSITY LIGHT SOURCES FOR FLUORESCENCE MICROSCOPY

Type of arc	Lamp identification	Manufacturer	Power (watts)	Type of current	Arc size (mm)	Average brightness (candles per mm^2)	Average life (hours)	Remarks
Mercury	(a) HBO 200	Osram, Germany	200	AC or DC	2.5 × 1.3	250	200	Housings available from major microscope manufacturers
	(b) HBO 100	Osram, Germany	100	DC	0.3 × 0.3	1400	100	May be housed in the G.K. Turner "Ultra-Vis" lamp
	(c) PEK 200-3	PEK Labs, U.S.	200	AC or DC	2.5 × 1.7	250	200	May be used in some housings designed for HBO 200
	(d) PEK 107	PEK Labs, U.S.	100	DC	0.3 × 0.3	1400	100	G.K. Turner "Ultra-Vis" housing designed for this bulb
	(e) HGK 200A	Sylvania Electric Prod., U.S.	200	AC or DC	2.5 × 0.3	250	200	May be used in some housings designed for HBO 200

TABLE I (continued)

Type of arc	Lamp identification	Manufacturer	Power (watts)	Type of current	Arc size (mm)	Average brightness (candles per mm²)	Average life (hours)	Remarks
	(f) 901A	Hanovia Lamp Division, U.S.	200	DC	3.0 × 1.5	190		Housing available from Schoeffel Instrument Co.
	(g) ME/D 250	A.E.I. Lamp and Lighting Co., England	250	AC or DC	3.7 × 1.5	200	500	Housings available from W. Watson and Sons, and Cooke, Troughton and Simms
	(h) ME/D 1KW	A.E.I. Lamp and Lighting Co., England	1000	AC or DC	6.5 × 2.5	400	500	Air cooled; housing available from Schoeffel Instrument Co.
	(i) CS 150	Philips, Holland	150	AC or DC	2.0 × 1.2	250	200	Housing available from E. Leitz, Inc.
	(j) A-H6	General Electric Co., U.S.	1000	AC or DC	25.0 × 1.5	300	75	Water cooled; no commercial microscope housing currently available

		Manufacturer		AC/DC	Dimensions			Remarks
	(k) A-H4	General Electric Co., U.S.	100	AC	10.0 × ?	10	1000	Conventional screw base, glass envelope bulb
Xenon	(l) 510C1	Hanovia Lamp Division, U.S.	150	AC	3.8 × 2.0	50	200	Housing available from Schoeffel Instrument Co.
	(m) XE/D 250	A.E.I. Lamp and Lighting Co., England	250	AC	3.0 × 2.0	100	500	Housing available from Schoeffel Instrument Co.
	(n) XE/D 500	A.E.I. Lamp and Lighting Co., England	500	DC	5.0 × 3.0	80	1000	Air-cooled; housing available from Schoeffel Instrument Co.
	(o) XE/D 2KW	A.E.I. Lamp and Lighting Co., England	2000	DC	4.5 × 4.0	450	1000	Air-cooled; housing available from Schoeffel Instrument Co.
Xenon-mercury	(p) 901B	Hanovia Lamp Division, U.S.	200	DC	3.0 × 1.5	190	1000	Housing available from Schoeffel Instrument Co.
	(q) 537B	Hanovia Lamp Division, U.S.	1000	AC	5.0 × 2.5	167		Air-cooled; housing available from Schoeffel Instrument Co.
Carbon	(r)	American Optical, Bausch and Lomb, Zeiss, Reichert, others		AC or DC	Crater on horizontal carbon 3.5 mm diameter	175	About 2 hr. per set of carbons	

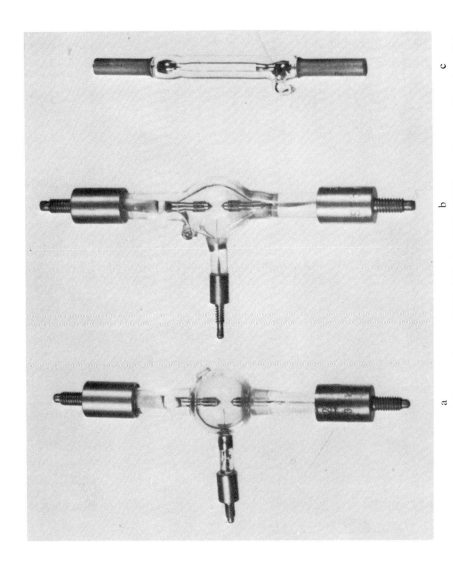

FIG. 4. Mercury arc bulbs. a. Osram HBO 200. b. PEK 200-3. c. General Electric AH-6. Note similarity in dimensions between a and b, making them virtually interchangeable in some lamp housings.

or DC; in the latter mode it shows 15–20% higher output in the blue region, the arc is much steadier, and lamp life is said to be extended.

For our purposes, the most important points about the mercury spectrum shown in Fig. 3 are the strong lines around 365, 405, and 435 mμ, all of which are important for fluorescence excitation, and the low emission in the region above 580 mμ where no activating bands are needed. The HBO 200 bulb is rated at 200 W and an average life of 200 hr. Internal pressure while burning is about

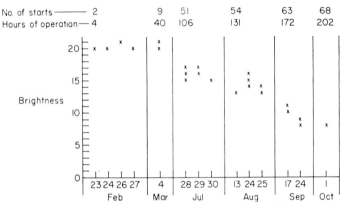

FIG. 5. Reduction in intensity of 420-mμ band of HBO 200 bulb with use. Data derived from a single bulb but are generally applicable to this class of illuminants.

40 atm, but the cold lamp has no excess pressure and may be handled without special precautions.

As is true with all such lamps, frequent starts tend to shorten the life of the bulb. Luminous output drops with use to a variable degree. The more or less characteristic history of one bulb is shown in Fig. 5. After a few hours operation on AC the arc may show a tendency to wander as the electrodes become pitted and uneven. This flickering may become progressively worse and the bulb may become unusable as a result. The quality of these lamps has varied through the years. In my laboratory, six bulbs purchased between 1957 and 1961 had an average useful lifetime of 308 hr, with 65 starts per bulb. Of five bulbs purchased between 1962 and 1963, one burned for 238 hr with 49 starts, the other four averaged only 69 hr of service with 10 starts each. Failures arose from cracks developing in the quartz envelope and, in one case, an explosion of the bulb. Early lamp failure is sometimes attributed to faulty electrical circuitry or power line fluctuations. However, the records cited above were obtained with the same power supply throughout, and repeated checks of line current failed to reveal any extraordinary fluctuations to account for the early failures.

Osram manufactures the necessary chokes and transformers for operating the HBO 200 on AC, but these items need to be mounted in suitable housings by the purchaser. All microscope manufacturers using this bulb in housings for fluorescence microscopy provide integrated power supplies which can be plugged into the house line for use. In the author's laboratory a 0–280 V Powerstat transformer (Superior Electric Co.) has been used to step up the 110-V line voltage to fit the 220-V choke for the HBO 200. This control permits feeding the bulb an increased input so that at least partial compensation can be made for reduced intensity after prolonged use. In one case it was possible to obtain as many as 435 hr at a usable level of brightness from the same bulb by this method.

2. PEK 200-3 (PEK Labs, U.S.A.) (Fig. 4B). This bulb is similar to the HBO 200 in all important respects, and will fit most housings designed for the latter bulb. However, not all power supplies provided for the HBO 200 will operate the PEK 200-3. It is about 30% cheaper on the American market. A DC power supply is available from the manufacturer. These bulbs have been used in the author's laboratory for several years and have performed very satisfactorily.

3. Sylvania HGK-200A (Sylvania Electric Prod., U.S.A.). This bulb has only recently come on the market. Physical and electrical specifications are similar to those of the first two bulbs listed above.

4. Hanovia 901 A, 510-A (Hanovia Lamp Division, U.S.A.). The former of these is a 200 W model, the latter 250 W. Both bulbs are 112 mm long and are equipped with only two electrodes. They are available for AC or DC operation. Schoeffel Instrument Company's lamp housings will accept these bulbs.

5. ME/D 250 W (A.E.I. Lamp and Lighting Co., England). The basic quartz discharge tube containing this arc is available in three different casings and bases—a rectangular metal case with glass or quartz window (130 mm long), a tubular glass envelope (141 mm), or an oval metal case with two opposing apertures (103 mm). The

lamp dissipates 250 W across an arc 3.75 mm long. It may be operated on AC or DC. The spectral distribution is similar to that shown in Fig. 3 except that when the glass envelope is used there is little or no radiation below 350 mμ. The glass envelope bulb is used as the light source in fluorescence housings put out by two British microscope firms, W. Watson and Sons, and Cooke, Troughton and Simms.

6. CS-150 (Philips, Holland). This 150 W, AC or DC source consists of a quartz discharge tube in a tubular glass envelope with a conventional bayonet base. Intrinsic brightness is the same as that of the HBO 200 and PEK 200-3 but the arc is a little smaller. The Leitz Universal housing can be fitted for this bulb as well as with the HBO 200.

7. A-H6 (General Electric, U.S.A.) (Fig. 4C). This is an extremely brilliant light source rated at 1000 W. The quartz bulb is 81 mm long, of a capillary construction, and requires water cooling during operation. (A similar, forced-air cooled unit, the B-H6, is also available.) Initial output is 65,000 lm from an arc 25.0 × 1.0 mm with a brightness of 300 candles/mm^2. Pressure within the cold bulb is less than 1 atm, building up to 110 atm within a few seconds of starting. The average rated life of a bulb is 75 hr. Suitable water jackets and auxiliary operating equipment are available from the manufacturer, but housing the lamp for use as a microscope illuminator needs to be done by the buyer.

The A-H6 served as illuminator in some of the early work with fluorescent antibody, before the lower powered, compact mercury arc lamps became generally available. There were several reasons for its displacement by the latter sources, and these are still valid. The water-cooling requirement makes for bulky and expensive auxiliary equipment. Only about one-quarter of the 25-mm-long arc can be utilized for microscope illumination, presenting a problem in shielding against the rest of the intense light flux. In the author's hands, these bulbs have been variable and unpredictable with respect to longevity and light output. Out of 50 bulbs used over a period of 4 years, 25 failed or could not be used because of excessive flicker or light loss within less than 10 starts, 22 gave fair to good service, and 3 gave exceptionally good service. Nevertheless, the superlative brilliance of a fresh bulb makes this a lamp to consider when extreme light intensities are needed. Suggestions for mounting it are given in Section III.

8. PEK Capillary High Pressure Mercury Lamps (PEK Labs, U.S.A.). This is a group of lamps of very intense energy rated at from 1000 to 2000 W. Luminous output of the various types ranges from 65,000 to 130,000 lm, with arc brightnesses of 400 to 900 candles/mm^2 for arcs 25–28 mm in length. Except for the type A-H6, which is similar to the General Electric model described above, none of these lamps has been used for microscopy. Power supplies for these bulbs are expensive (over $1,000) and unless there is special need for the extreme energies provided, they are not likely to find much use in the ordinary laboratory.

9. Miscellaneous sources. In this category are included several 100-, 500-, and 1000-W bulbs manufactured in the U.S., England, Holland, and Germany. The 100 W PEK 107 and 109 bulbs, which are similar in specifications to the Osram HBO 100 W, serve as light sources in the Turner lamp housing for fluorescence microscopy. These are small bulbs (about 80 mm long) with an extremely intense point source of 0.3 × 0.3 mm, rated at 1,400 candles/mm^2. Although this source may provide exceptionally brilliant illumination for high magnification microscopy with a bright-field condenser where only a portion of the aperture is to be filled, it is less desirable than the larger arcs for ordinary fluorescence microscopy with a dark-field condenser. The arc of the 100 W bulb needs to be enlarged 40 times as much as that of 200 W bulbs in order to fill the aperture of an ordinary microscope condenser. Since the brightness of the smaller arc is only about 5.5 times greater than that of the larger ones, a microscope field illuminated by the smaller bulb would be significantly less bright than if the larger arc were used.

The General Electric A-H4, 100 W bulb was used for fluorescent antibody work by Mellors *et al.* (724). This is a quartz discharge tube enclosed in a glass, tubular envelope with a screw base. The 10-mm arc is rated at only 10 candles/mm^2, making it a very weak source in comparison with the higher wattage, compact arc models.

Philips, PEK, Osram and A.E.I. manufacture 500- and 1000-W, convection-cooled, high intensity bulbs which may offer some advantages in terms of large arc size of great brilliance. Nevertheless, the extra size of these bulbs, problems of adequate cooling, higher power consumption, and higher initial cost have militated against their general use in microscopy. Schoeffel Instrument Company's lamp housings accept these bulbs.

B. Xenon and Xenon—Mercury Arcs

Lamps of this type are similar in construction to some of the high-pressure mercury arcs. That is, they consist of a quartz envelope which is spherical in the center and has dorsal and ventral arms through which the electrodes are led to the discharge chamber. The lamps contain xenon gas which is under pressure even when not in operation. Thus, safety goggles and shielding for other parts of the body should be worn whenever handling these bulbs.

From the standpoint of serving as sources for fluorescence excitation, this group of lamps differs in two respects from high-pressure mercury arcs. First, spectral emission consists of a strong continuum due to the xenon, from the far ultraviolet through the visible into the infrared, upon which are superimposed intense mercury lines, if the latter element is also present (Fig. 6); and second, brightness per unit area is somewhat lower in the xenon and xenon—mercury lamps for the same power input. The spectral emission and intensity of xenon lamps make them especially useful for color photomicrography, and microscope lamp housings are available for the lower powered ones.

Since most fluorescent dyes have broad absorption bands, the relatively high-level continuum in the blue and near ultraviolet of the xenon arc offers the possibility of more energy being available for excitation of fluorescence than would be the case from a line emission source (like mercury) of equal power. On the other hand, the xenon radiation continues at a high level into the region that corresponds to the fluorescence emission of the dyes with which we are concerned. This means that more restrictive primary filters may be needed to prevent the longer wavelengths from passing through the secondary filter and producing a spurious image. The net usable fluorescence obtained with these lamps, then, may well be no different from that obtained with mercury arcs, and the extra expense and hazards involved with the xenon bulbs would then make them less desirable. The fact is, however, that these lamps have not been adequately explored as sources for microfluorescence, and it is quite difficult to predict on *a priori* grounds just what results they would produce. Emmart *et al.* (285) used a 1000-W Hanovia xenon—mercury bulb for fluorescent antibody studies with apparent success. Osram, Hanovia, PEK, and A.E.I. manufacture a line of AC and DC bulbs varying in power from 40 to 2000 W, and they should be consulted for detailed specifications regarding the different types. A few examples are listed in Table I. Schoeffel Instrument Company's housings will accept convection-cooled bulbs from this group.

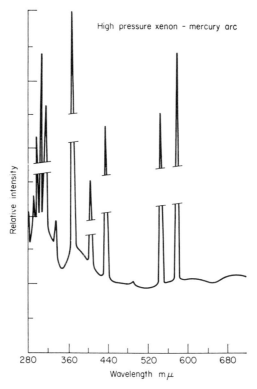

FIG. 6. Energy distribution for high pressure xenon–mercury arc (Hanovia 1000 W). The mercury lines have been reduced by a factor of ten in order to present the data more compactly [after Emmart *et al.* (285)].

C. Carbon Arcs

The carbon arc lamp consists of two pencil-like carbon electrodes between which an electric discharge occurs in air at atmospheric pressure. Unlike mercury arcs, for which the major source of light is the arc stream itself, in the ordinary, laboratory model carbon arc the incandescent electrodes provide essentially all the radiation. Spectral output is continuous and extends from about 230 mμ into the infrared. Distribution in the visible and near ultraviolet is shown in Fig. 7 for an 8-amp AC arc.

High intensity carbon arcs, operated at from 35 to over 100 amp provide extremely intense light sources of as much as 2000 candles/mm². However, they have never been adapted for microscope use and there are serious obstacles preventing such adaptation. Low intensity laboratory arcs operate at from 5 to 15 amp on either AC or DC. In the latter case, the center of the crater in the face of

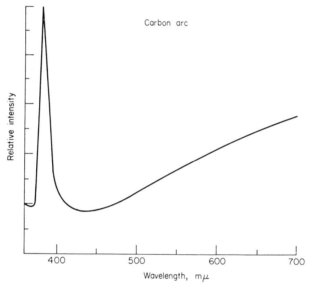

FIG. 7.   Energy distribution for carbon arc (8 amp, AC).

the positive (generally horizontal) carbon may reach the limiting brightness of 175 candles/mm² when the arc is operated at optimum current for the diameter of carbons involved. Increasing the current beyond optimum results in consumption of carbons at a faster rate without any increase in brightness. When operated on AC, the luminosity of each carbon is about half that of the positive electrode operated on DC at the same amperage.

Since the electrodes are consumed during operation at a rate of about 2 inches/hr, they must be constantly fed toward each other in order to maintain a proper spacing for the discharge. All modern carbon arc lamps accomplish this by mechanical or electrical clockwork devices. At their best, carbon arcs provide light sources of great brilliance, good daylight color, and reasonable stability at an acceptable price. But in the overall evaluation, mercury lamps must be given the edge for fluorescence work. Under ordinary laboratory conditions carbon arcs are more troublesome, produce more heat, frequently have a disturbing hum, and are less stable than the mercury lamps, which to a large extent have replaced them.

Most of the major microscope manufacturers produce carbon arc illuminators either as separate units or as integral parts of projectors or so-called "universal" microscope outfits. Each variety of lamp is rated for the specific size and type of carbon it uses, and these are generally available from the lamp manufacturer. Theater and cinema supply houses can often provide carbons and auxiliary electrical equipment to operate such lamps.

III. LAMP HOUSINGS

A. Basic Requirements

The requirements of a good housing for compact, high-pressure arcs are as follows:

1. Mechanical construction permitting adequate ventilation of the bulb, as specified by the manufacturer of the particular bulb employed; proper shielding against stray light; and adequate protection against violent failure of a high-pressure arc during operation.

2. Simple means for aligning the arc discharge in the optical axis of the collecting lens. It should be possible to do this while looking through the microscope with the lamp in operation, by means of horizontal and vertical movement controls which will not become too hot to handle.

3. A collecting lens in a sliding mount to permit focusing the light source from about 12 inches to infinity (in practice, 10–15 feet). The lens should be of such a focal length as to be capable of producing a sufficiently enlarged image of the light source in the back lens of the microscope condenser at usual working distances. For example, taking the diameter of a mercury arc as approximately 2 mm, and the diameter of a cardioid dark-field condenser as 16 mm, the light source would need to be enlarged eightfold to fill the condenser. This could be accomplished by arranging that the distance between the lamp collecting lens and the microscope condenser be 8 times as great as that between the collecting lens and the source. For a 2-inch collecting lens these distances would be about 18 and 2.25 inches, re-

spectively; for a 4-inch lamp collector the distance to the microscope would have to be on the order of 36 inches, which would be inconveniently long.

4. An iris diaphragm to permit control of the size of the illuminated field. This provides a measure of control over glare in the microscope image and is needed for centering the light source.

5. Provision for mounting at least four filters simultaneously. One mount, for a heat-absorbing glass, should be placed closest to the light in a manner that will prevent its being moved out of position accidentally. Other holders should allow for easy mounting and manipulation of standard round or square glass filters (2 inches in diameter or on a side is a good size). For greater flexibility, five holders are desirable.

6. A properly designed and adjustable reflector behind the bulb. A Leitz housing tested in this laboratory showed about 20% greater output with its mirror in proper position. It is desirable, though not essential, that the mirror be adjustable from the outside while the lamp is burning.

7. Easy accessibility to the bulb. It should be possible to replace a bulb without disrupting any of the other alignments, and without requiring more than slight readjustment of arc centration.

8. Simple mechanical adjustability. It should be possible to align illuminator and microscope on a common axis or platform to which both units can be fixed in place. If the housing is adjustable, so far as tilting, raising, etc., are concerned, movements should be easy to perform with positive locking in any position.

B. Miscellaneous Comments

If it is intended that the fluorescence microscope be used also for conventional microscopy, then dual lamp housings incorporating a tungsten filament source are handy, since filament bulbs are easier and cheaper to use for ordinary work than mercury arcs. However, if the only purpose of the tungsten source is to visualize the fluorescent field with non-fluorescent light, then that purpose can be perfectly well served by the mercury lamp itself at a considerable savings in cost as compared to the dual lamp housings. With dark-field illumination it is only necessary to replace the fluorescence excitation filter with a clear red filter to render all light-scattering objects in the field completely visible. With bright-field illumination an opal glass diffusion screen can be substituted in the light path. Red is preferable to the white or yellow light of a tungsten filament since red will not affect adaptation of the eye to the yellow–green of fluorescein fluorescence as much as the other colors will. In addition, it will not cause any fading of fluorescence. Recommended filters for this purpose are described in Chapter 4.

Carbon arc housings need to be designed quite differently from closed arc housings because of the special nature of the electrodes and arc discharge. In addition to general requirements applicable to all lamps, such as a good collector lens, etc., two special needs of the carbon arc are an effective carbon feeding mechanism so that spacing between the electrodes remains optimal at all times, and a carrier for a water cell. Carbon arcs radiate much more red and infrared than mercury arcs, and a water filter is necessary to protect glass color filters against overheating and cracking.

Commercial housings currently available meet the above requirements to a greater or lesser degree. Although most are made by microscope manufacturers, generally with the parent microscope in mind, the housings can sometimes be used with other microscopes with little or no adaptation. Thus, one can pick a lamp and microscope independently on their own merits, at least on the first go-round. Final decisions will, naturally, depend on the extent to which difficulties in adaptation may outweigh the merits of a particular housing or microscope.

In the following list of lamp housings (Table II), the Osram HBO 200 bulb is ordinarily provided except where noted otherwise. No attempt has been made to quote individual prices because these vary from place to place and time to time. It is sufficient to say that housings of comparable elaborateness are of comparable price, about $700–$800 for the more complete units, including necessary electrical auxiliaries.

Carbon arc lamps for use in metallurgical microscopes, microprojectors or as general microscope lamps are made by American Optical Co., Bausch and Lomb, Cooke, Troughton and Simms, Leitz, Zeiss, and probably others. Since they are not a first choice for purposes of this book, the various models are not evaluated here, but descriptive literature is readily available from the manufacturers.

A specially designed housing for putting the water-cooled A-H6 mercury bulb into use as a microscope illuminator was described by

TABLE II

LAMP HOUSINGS FOR HIGH PRESSURE MERCURY ARCS

Housing manufacturer	Requirements[a]								Power supply	Remarks
	1	2	3	4	5	6	7	8		
(a) American Optical Co.	+	+	+	+	+	+	+	+	AC	Water cell or glass heat-absorbing filter; lamp slides on track to permit use of built-in, filament light source; enclosed light-path; fan for cooling bulb
(b) Bausch & Lomb	⊕	+	+	+	⊕	0	+	+	AC	Power supply does not provide for high-voltage starting pulse to third electrode of the HBO-200 bulb used
(c) Cooke, Troughton and Simms	+	+	+	+	⊕	NI	⊕	⊕	AC or DC	Uses ME/D 250-W bulb
(d) Galileo	+	+	+	+	+	0	+	+	AC or DC	Enclosed light-path; swing-out mirror to allow use of filament light source; fan for cooling bulb
(e) Leitz, Inc.	⊕	+	+	0	+	+	+	+	AC	Can be used also for Osram XBO 150 (xenon) and Philips CS 150 bulbs; built-in filament light source; enclosed light-path
(f) Nikon	+	+	+	+	+	+	+	+	AC	Built-in filament source; enclosed light-path
(g) Reichert	+	+	+	+	+	+	+	+	AC or DC	Built-in filament light source; enclosed light-path

TABLE II (continued)

Housing manufacturer	Requirements[a]								Power supply	Remarks
	1	2	3	4	5	6	7	8		
(h) Schoeffel Instrument Co.	+	⊕	+	0	⊕	+	+	⊕	AC or DC	Will accept very wide range of high-pressure arcs (up to 5000 W) and spectral discharge lamps; has blower fan for cooling bulb; attachable quartz monochromator
(i) G. K. Turner Assoc.	+	0	0	0	0	NI	+	+	DC	Uses PEK 107 bulb; enclosed light-path
(j) Vickers Ltd.	+	+	+	+	+	NI	+	+	AC	Built-in filament source; enclosed light-path
(k) W. Watson & Son Universal Lamp	⊕	0	+	+	⊕	NI	⊕	⊕	AC	Uses ME/D 250 W bulb; can be used also for ribbon filament and Pointolite tungsten sources
(l) Wild Heerbrugg	+	⊕	+	+	+	+	⊕	⊕	AC	Can be used also for Osram XBO 162 (xenon), ribbon filament, tungsten sources and electronic flash equipment
(m) Zeiss (West Germany)	+	⊕	+	+	+	+	⊕	+	AC	Can be used also for tungsten filament, electronic flash and sodium spectral bulbs

[a] 1, Mechanical construction; 2, alignment; 3, collecting lens; 4, iris diaphragm; 5, filter mounts; 6, reflector; 7, bulb accessibility; 8, adjustability. +, fulfills requirement; 0, does not fulfill requirement; ⊕, requirement partially fulfilled; NI, no information.

Tobie (1056). This is an elegant but unnecessarily complicated and expensive design. The major problem encountered in using this bulb is overheating of elements exposed to its extremely high light flux. This is most readily prevented by fitting a machined aluminum or brass sleeve *inside* the water jacket. A 0.25-inch hole can be drilled opposite the center of the arc discharge, and the water jacket can be fitted into a partially dismantled Bausch and Lomb research lamp housing or similar box equipped with a collector lens. A Pyrex water cell, such as is available with the Bausch and Lomb housing, can be filled with copper sulfate solution and the primary filters immersed in the cell. No additional cooling with running water beyond that provided for the bulb itself is needed for any part of this system, and the lamp housing will remain cool at all times.

BIBLIOGRAPHY

Koller, L. R. (1952). "Ultraviolet Radiation." Wiley, New York.

Chapter Four

FILTER SYSTEMS

I. GENERAL COMMENTS

Filter systems are used in fluorescence microscopy to prevent the fluorescence image from being swamped by non-fluorescent light from the illuminator. It is hardly necessary to add that filters always *remove* radiation; unless fluorescent themselves, they do not contribute any wavelengths not already present in the first place. Filter systems (Fig. 8) typically involve *excitation* or *primary* filters placed between the light source and the object that pass essentially only those wavelengths necessary to stimulate fluorescence; and *barrier* or *secondary* filters that, placed between the object and the observer, remove excitation radiation not absorbed by the object, but pass fluorescent light that is emitted. Properly matched primary and secondary filters should appear opaque when held in tandem against the light source with which they are intended to be used. This is sometimes called a "crossed" filter system, by analogy to polarizing screens which appear opaque when crossed at right angles to each other.

Filters are of two general types: absorption, in which organic or inorganic substances with suitable absorption spectra are dispersed in media like water, gelatin, or glass; and interference, in which thin metallic layers sandwiched between protective glass sheets serve to reflect some wavelengths and to pass others, depending upon the spacing between the layers and the angle of the incident beam. Interference filters are more efficient than absorption types in isolating narrow spectral lines, but since fluorescence excitation is frequently best accomplished with broad bands, absorption filters are more commonly used in fluorescence microscopy.

Water filters are awkward because of their bulk, tendency to form air bubbles as they warm up, and general inconvenience if one wishes to maintain a set of filters with different absorption properties. On the other hand, a single cuvette of 20–30 mm thickness, containing

41

dilute copper sulfate solution, makes an admirable heat-absorbing filter if the lamp housing can accommodate it conveniently. Gelatin filters are sensitive to heat and therefore should be avoided in the primary position with high intensity light sources. However, they make excellent secondary filters, although their transmittance may change in time. For permanent use they should be mounted in glass, since the gelatin surface itself is easily scratched or marred in handling. Glass filters are most convenient in the primary position provided that, if the filter itself is not heat-resistant, suitable heat-absorbing

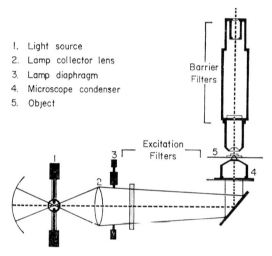

1. Light source
2. Lamp collector lens
3. Lamp diaphragm
4. Microscope condenser
5. Object

Barrier Filters

Excitation Filters

FIG. 8.   General arrangement of excitation and barrier filters for fluorescence microscopy.

glasses or water filters are interposed between the source and the color filter. A variety of absorption glasses are available in various thicknesses, providing in all a large range of systems that can be assembled.

Primary filters can be mounted anywhere between the light source and the microscope, but generally they are found on the lamp housing itself. Heat-absorbing filters or cuvettes should, naturally, be closest to the lamp collector lens and preferably in a fixed mount that is not readily movable. Secondary filters are often dropped onto the field diaphragm of the microscope oculars or are mounted as caps above the oculars. The preferred position is in the body tube where the filter is out of focus and slight surface imperfections or filter fluorescence will be invisible. This location also permits a single filter to control the light going to binocular and trinocular heads, eliminating the problem of matching two or three separate filters for visual and photographic work. It is especially convenient for the secondary to be mounted on a slide or wheel in the body tube, so that filters can be changed easily to match the particular primary being used.

Choice of filters is influenced by absorption and emission spectra of fluorescent materials under study, and by the spectral character of the illuminating source. Ideal systems based upon these considerations are rarely attainable because of practical limitations. The problem of fluorescence observations with fluorescein will serve to demonstrate these limitations. Fluorescein shows absorption maxima around 280, 320, and 490 mμ, and an emission maximum at about 517 mμ. In the ordinary microscope, glass (rather than quartz) is used for lamp collector lens, substage condenser, and microscope slide. As a consequence, the absorption peaks at 280 and 320 mμ are unavailable for purposes of excitation because optical glass is relatively opaque to wavelengths shorter than 350 mμ. Similarly, the main absorption peak around 490 mμ cannot be taken advantage of because, first, it is so close to the emission band at 517 mμ that ordinary color filters cannot efficiently segregate the two bands; and second, the mercury arc emits only low-level radiation at 490 mμ. Thus, filter systems actually used for fluorescein can only represent compromises between what one would like to have and what is practically available.

A further consideration influencing choice of filters is arrangement of the light path through the microscope. Bright-field condensers are designed to put a maximum of light into the microscope objective. As a result, dense primary and secondary filters are necessary to block unwanted wavelengths so that the fluorescence image will be visible. On the other hand, dark-field condensers are designed so that no light enters the objective except by reflection and scatter, and therefore more transparent filters can be used.

It is evident, then, that different combinations of dyes, light sources, and microscope condensers demand different filter systems for optimum results, and the possible permutations are considerable. However, in practical fluorescent antibody work, the almost universal use of fluorescein for labeling and mercury arcs for illumination narrows the choice of filters greatly. In particular, the line spectrum of the mercury arc provides only three feasible excitation systems for fluorescein, each based upon a major cluster of lines, namely, ultraviolet irradiation with the 350–390 mμ region, blue–violet irradiation with the 405–450 mμ region, and combined ultraviolet–blue irradiation with the entire range from 350 through 450 mμ. For orange- and red-fluorescing dyes, like the rhodamines and Evans blue, the mercury bands at 546 and 577 mμ could be made available. However, inasmuch as the latter dyes are used primarily as counterstains for fluorescein preparations, the longer wavelengths cannot be tolerated in the excitation system since they fall within the fluorescence band of fluorescein.

Lists of specific filters provided later in this chapter include appropriate representatives from the major American, British, and German manufacturers. For each type of illumination examples have been given which provide a range of densities to meet most requirements. The accompanying transmission curves have been drawn for the filter thicknesses actually recommended; thus all curves of a particular type are directly comparable, allowing easy determination of relative densities.

It is well to recognize that, in commercial lamps, filters with the same color specification may be provided in different thicknesses from time to time. Since such variations can introduce significant differences in transmission, it is good practice to measure the thickness of each filter and to record this information (and the filter number) along the periphery of each glass where there will be no interference with the light beam. Since each air–glass surface involves a transmission loss from reflection of about 4%, it is preferable to work with single, thick filters rather than with multiple, thinner ones, if overheating is not a problem.

The effectiveness of a filter system is influenced by the efficiency of the microscope and lamp optics, the intensity and type of light source, and the innate variability of filters bearing the same color specification number. Thus, a combination acceptable under one set of circumstances may appear too dark or too light under other conditions. Good results are generally attainable by following specifications found in the literature or provided by manufacturers; *best* results may come only by individual juggling of various combinations to fit the particular equipment and problem under consideration.

A word needs to be added here concerning health hazards of exposure to ultraviolet radiation. Radiation capable of reddening or "tanning" human skin, inducing conjunctivitis, and showing bactericidal effects, falls in the short wavelength end of the ultraviolet spectrum, below about 310 mμ. As stated earlier, transmission of optical glass fall off sharply below 350 mμ and is negligible at 310 mμ. Thus, light from an ultraviolet source that has passed through several thicknesses of glass in the form of lenses and filters is entirely deficient in short wavelengths of possible hazard. Nevertheless, such light is still capable of exciting fluorescence in the lens of the human eye and needs to be removed by the secondary filter before fluorescence observations can be made. Unfiltered radiation scattered through ventilating baffles on the light housing, however, contains the full ultraviolet spectrum and should be screened by some type of shield. Persons who have suffered surgical removal of an eye lens are much more sensitive than normal to even long-wave ultraviolet, and are probably best advised to avoid the fluorescence microscope.

II. FILTERS FOR DIFFERENT PURPOSES

A. Heat-Protective Filters*

Heat may be produced in primary filters from absorption of both red and infrared radiation from the mercury arc, and of the strong green and yellow lines at 546 and 577 mμ. Ultraviolet-passing filters are also heated by absorption of the violet and blue lines at 405 and 435 mμ. The most transparent, usable filters passing both blue and ultraviolet radiation transmit on the order of less than 20% of the energy radiated by the mercury lamp. Ultraviolet-passing filters transmit less than 10%. The remaining 80–90% of the energy must therefore be absorbed either by the primary filters themselves or by some other component of the light-transmitting system. A glass lamp collector lens will absorb the far ultraviolet, accounting for about 15–20% of the total. Protective filters are necessary in order to prevent the primary filters from overheating and possibly cracking as a result of absorbing the remaining 60–75% of the lamp emission.

* Filters are identified as follows: C-P., Chance-Pilkington Optical Works; C, Corning Glass Works; I, Ilford Ltd.; S, Schott & Gen.; W, Eastman Kodak Wratten Filters. For addresses see Appendix A.

The amount of this radiation which can be absorbed by any filter without cracking is determined in part by the efficiency with which heat is dissipated from the glass by conduction and convection, and by the degree of concentration or diffusion of the light beam at the point where it passes through the filters. Because of these considerations, heat-absorbing filters that are adequate for one type of housing may offer insufficient protection in a different housing. Occasionally, the use of a new bulb with an especially high light flux may result

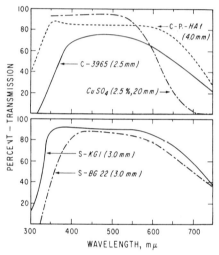

FIG. 9.   Transmission spectra for heat-absorbing filters. S-KG 2 and KG 3 are similar to the KG 1 shown.

in the cracking of a primary filter in the presence of heat-absorbing filters that were adequate previously. Such events are not readily predictable and one can only begin with a tried system and add further protective filters as needed.

It is useful to consider protective filters in two separate groups: heat-absorbing and red-absorbing. Heat-absorbing filters (Fig. 9) are more or less colorless, heat-resistant glasses which absorb strongly beyond 700 mμ, in the region accounting for about 30% of the lamp energy. These filters may generally be left in the light path indefinitely without fear of breakage. Red-absorbing filters (Fig. 10) consist of blue–green glasses with high transmission at shorter wavelengths and reduced transmission above 500 mμ. They absorb strongly in a region

accounting for an additional 15% of the lamp energy. Such filters
are useful for reducing the intensity of the 546 and 577 mμ lines of
the mercury arc, and for eliminating visible red radiation passed by
heat-absorbing filters. Unfortunately, red-absorbing glasses are not
notably heat-resistant and may themselves crack if left continuously
in the light path of a particularly intense source. Aqueous $CuSO_4$
solutions are very effective filters that possess both heat- and red-
absorbing qualities. Concentrations of from 1 to 25% have been
used in cuvettes ranging from 10 to 32 mm thick, but a common
combination is 5–10% in a 20-mm cuvette. The solution is generally
acidified by addition of a few drops of H_2SO_4.

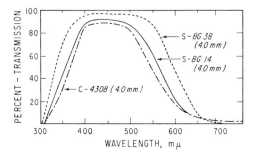

FIG. 10.   Transmission spectra for red-absorbing filters.

As a practical matter, if the lamp housing does not permit use of
$CuSO_4$, one may start with a heat-absorbing filter from the list given
below in Table IV, mounted in a more or less permanent position
in the housing. For observations with a dark-field condenser there is
generally no need for red-absorbing filters from a visual standpoint.
That is, adequate primary filters do not in general transmit enough
red to confuse or degrade the contrast in the fluorescence image stimulated by dark-field illumination. However, with bright-field illumination a red-absorbing filter is a necessary supplement to practically all
ultraviolet-passing and some blue-passing primary filters. Regardless
of the condenser system, the red-absorbing filter may be needed to
protect the primary filter from overheating, particularly when a very
bright bulb is used. For these purposes, a red-absorbing filter from
the list in Table IV may be mounted in a swing-out position between
the heat-absorbing and primary filter. The red-absorbing and primary
filters may then be swung in and out of the light path as needed for

fluorescence observations with a new bulb. As the bulb decreases in intensity it may be possible to dispense with the red-absorbing glass, or to leave all the filters in the light path continuously.

B. Ultraviolet Excitation Systems

The low absorption that fluorescein and its protein conjugates possess for the near ultraviolet make that portion of the spectrum an inefficient source of fluorescence excitation for such solutions. Nevertheless, the near ultraviolet is widely used for this purpose because of other important considerations. Since radiation in this region is largely invisible, secondary filters can be used that are practically colorless, excluding only the invisible ultraviolet and visible violet but passing all other visible wavelengths. Thus, an ultraviolet filter system permits observation of fluorescence of any color. Furthermore, the strong mercury line at 365 mμ corresponds to the peak transmission of several ultraviolet-passing filters. The relatively high energy thus available compensates in part for the low absorption of fluorescein in this region.

Primary filters for ultraviolet excitation are black-appearing filters that, upon being held up to a strong light, show blue, violet, or reddish images, depending upon the specific type. Peak useful transmission occurs at about 360 mμ in all cases and some pass considerable red light, although absolute transmissions for given filters vary. Characteristic curves are shown in Fig. 11. Photometric data on intensity of fluorescence stimulated by radiation transmitted by some of these filters are presented in Table III. The data were obtained by measuring through the microscope the fluorescence of a dilute solution of fluorescein (5 × 10⁻⁵ M) in a special cuvette, 4 μ deep. Irradiation was accomplished with a cardioid dark-field condenser, and measurements were made through a 16-mm objective. A BG 22 (2 mm) heat-absorbing filter was in the lamp housing, and the light source was a PEK 200-3 mercury arc. A Wratten 2A secondary filter was in the body tube, and a 0.9 density neutral filter was used to reduce the light intensity so that fading of fluorescence was negligible. The photometric data were supplemented by visual examination with a binocular microscope of microorganisms stained with fluorescein-labeled antibody. The dark-field image described in the last column refers to the appearance of strongly light-scattering particles occurring on some of the smears.

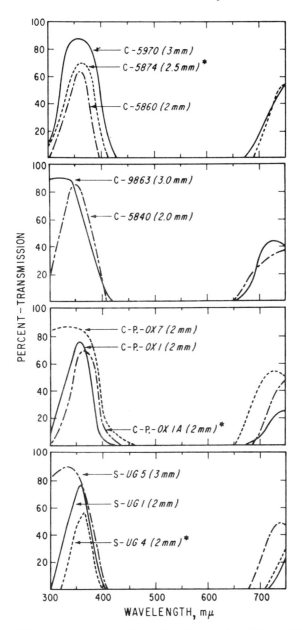

Fig. 11. Transmission spectra for ultraviolet-passing filters. S-UG 2 is similar to the UG 1 shown. Asterisk denotes heat-resistant glass.

The table shows clearly that the presence of a 4-mm red-absorbing filter in the light path involves a decrease of about 35% in the brightness of the fluorescence image. For this reason it is an advantage to dispense with such a filter if possible, by using heat-resistant ultra-

TABLE III

FLUORESCENCE INTENSITY EXCITED BY ULTRAVIOLET RADIATION

Filter	Thick-ness (mm)	Brightness of fluorescence (arbitrary units)		Appearance of light-scattering particles with dark-field condenser
		With red-absorbing filter, BG 14	Without red-absorbing filter	
S-UG1	2	30	47	Not visible
S-UG1	4	21	33	Not visible
C-5840	2	40	61	Very dim red–violet without red-absorbing filter
C-5840	4	28	44	Not visible
C-5874	2	72	—	Fairly bright yellow–white with or without red-absorbing filter
C-5874	3	42	62	Yellow–white of low intensity
C-5874	4	38	—	Essentially invisible
C-5970	2	98	—	Fairly bright yellow–violet with or without red-absorbing filter
C-5970	4	58	86	Very dim reddish–violet without red-absorbing filter
C-9863	3	57	86	Red–violet without red-absorbing filter; dark blue–violet with latter

violet-passing filters in the primary position. These are identified by an asterisk in Table IV. In working with "clean" smears of bacteria, fungi, or similar materials with little tendency to scatter light in dark-field illumination, brighter fluorescence images are possible with the thinner filters shown in Table IV, wherever a range of thickness is indicated. However, where many brightly reflecting particles occur

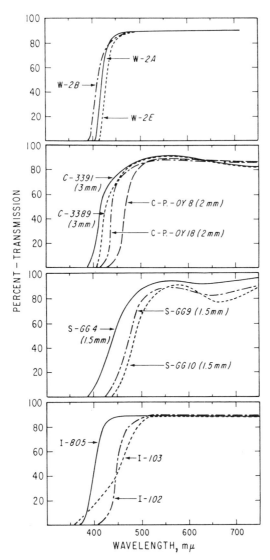

Fig. 12. Transmission spectra for secondary filters in ultraviolet excitation systems. Leitz "Euphos" is similar to S-GG 10.

TABLE IV

FILTER SYSTEMS FOR ULTRAVIOLET EXCITATION

Heat-absorbing	Red-absorbing	Primary	Secondary
Dark-field illumination			
$CuSO_4$, 2–10%	None needed	C-5840	W-2B
(20–30 mm)	for certain	(2 mm)	(gelatin)
S-BG22	types of	C-5874	W-2A
(2–4 mm)	preparations	(2–4 mm)[a]	(gelatin)
S-KG1, 2, or 3	(see text) or	C-5970	W-2E
(2–4 mm)	if $CuSO_4$ is	(2–4 mm)	(gelatin)
C-3965	used	C-9863	C-3391
(2–4 mm)	S-BG14 (4 mm)	(3 mm)	(3 mm)
C-P.-HA1	S-BG38 (4 mm)	C-5860	C-3389
(2–4 mm)	C-4308 (4 mm)	(2 mm)	(3 mm)
		S-UG1	C-P.-OY18
		(2 mm)	(2 mm)
		S-UG2	C-P.-OY8
		(2 mm)	(2 mm)
		S-UG4	S-GG4
		(2 mm)[a]	(1–2 mm)
		S-UG5	S-GG9
		(2–4 mm)	(1–2 mm)
		C-P.-OX1	S-GG10
		(2 mm)	(1–2 mm)
		C-P.-OX1A	I-805
		(2 mm)[a]	(gelatin)
		C-P.-OX7	I-102
		(2–4 mm)	(gelatin)
			I-103
			(gelatin)
			L-Euphos
			(2–3 mm)
Bright-field illumination			
As for dark-field	Always neces-	C-5840	As for dark-
illumination	sary; same as	(4 mm)	field but fa-
	for dark-field	C-5860	voring the
	illumination	(4 mm)	denser fil-
		S-UG1	ters
		(2–4 mm)	
		S-UG2	
		(2–4 mm)	
		C-P.-OX1	
		(4 mm)	

[a] Heat resistant.

on the slides, it is necessary to increase filter thickness for proper observations.

Suitable gelatin and glass secondary filters to match the ultraviolet-passing primary glasses are colorless or pale greenish-yellow filters with high absorption in the ultraviolet and high transmission in the blue and longer wavelengths (Fig. 12). Some secondary filters are in themselves fluorescent in ultraviolet light. If they are used in a position in which this interferes with the observed or photographed fluorescence image, a colorless UV-absorbing filter, e.g., W-2B, may be placed beneath them to absorb the exciting radiation.

Table IV lists ultraviolet excitation filter systems suitable for both dark- and bright-field illumination. Filters in any one column are more or less interchangeable, but the accompanying transmission curves can serve as guides to preparing specific systems of greater or lesser light passage. In our laboratory, dark-field illumination with a cardioid-type condenser has invariably given brighter fluorescence images of better contrast than bright-field illumination with achromatic high-aperture condensers oiled to the slide.

C. Blue and Ultraviolet–Blue Excitation Systems

Excitation by combined ultraviolet and blue radiation provides the brightest fluorescence with fluorescein-stained material, for two reasons: (1) such a system draws energy from the spectral region accounting for about 25% of the lamp emission, compared to about 10% for an ultraviolet system; and (2) the absorption spectrum of fluorescein begins to rise at about 410 mμ toward its maximum at 485–495 μ. Thus, photons of blue light at 450 mμ, for example, have about a threefold greater probability of being absorbed and exciting fluorescence than photons of ultraviolet light at 360 mμ. The main disadvantage of this system is that it requires yellow secondary filters to block the visible blue light of the primaries. As a consequence, fluorescence colors which can be observed range from green through red; blue fluorescence cannot be recognized as such. These remarks apply equally well to excitation with purely blue wavelengths, with the exception that the blue spectral region accounts for only about 15% of radiated energy from the lamp. However, since this energy occurs in a more favorable region of the spectrum for fluorescein excitation than ultraviolet radiation, fluorescence tends to be brighter with this system than with the latter, even though the energies involved are similar.

Primary filters in this category all appear almost the same shade of blue to the eye, but they differ significantly in the amount of near ultraviolet and red wavelengths transmitted (Fig. 13). Except for the C-5850, no red-absorbing filters are needed from the visual standpoint in either dark- or bright-field illumination. Where a red-absorb-

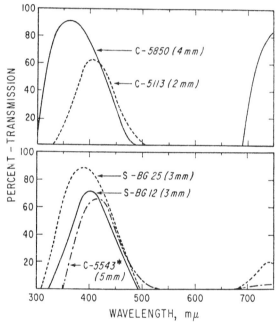

FIG. 13. Transmission spectra for blue and ultraviolet–blue passing filters. Klett 420 is similar to C-5113. Asterisk denotes heat-resistant glass.

ing filter like the S-BG 14 (4 mm) is employed for heat protection, one may expect a reduction in fluorescence of 15–20%. Table V presents photometric data on the brightness of fluorescence stimulated by light transmitted through some filters of this group. The data were obtained in the manner described above for ultraviolet filters, with the exception that the secondary filter used was a yellow Wratten 12 instead of a colorless Wratten 2A. A representative ultraviolet system, C-5840 plus Wratten 2A, is included for comparison purposes. (Absolute values are not comparable between Tables III and V).

Secondary filters to match this group of primaries are yellow glass or gelatin filters which characteristically possess sharp cutoffs at about 500 mμ (Fig. 14). Wavelengths longer than this are transmitted with high efficiency. There is an unfortunate tendency in the literature to use deeper colored yellow or orange filters than is necessary, resulting in fluorescence images that are 30–50% less bright than they might be. Perhaps more unfortunate than the light loss is the fact that the denser filters alter color values to the extent that the characteristic emission of fluorescein is seen as yellow rather than green.

TABLE V
FLUORESCENCE INTENSITY EXCITED BY BLUE AND ULTRAVIOLET-BLUE
RADIATION

Filter	Thick-ness (mm)	Nature of radiation	Brightness of fluorescence (arbitrary units)
S-BG12	3	UV + blue	46
C-5850	3.8	UV + blue	44
C-5113	2.0	Blue	40
C-5113	4.0	Blue	18
C-5840[a]	2	UV	5

[a] With a colorless Wratten 2A secondary filter instead of the yellow Wratten 12 employed in the rest of the determinations.

In Table VI, which presents filters for blue and ultraviolet–blue excitation, the secondary filters are listed with the less dense filters first. Whenever possible, preference should be given to filters in the upper part of the column. Since it may not always be possible to try different filters, the W-12 is recommended as a good compromise between high transmission of fluorescence and complete blocking of exciting light.

D. Miscellaneous Filters and Accessories

It is frequently desirable or necessary to visualize all the elements in the microscope field, including those not fluorescent. This can be accomplished on some lamp housings by switching from the filtered mercury arc illuminator to an incandescent source which bypasses the primary filters. In cases where this mechanical arrangement is not

available, a simple and practical alternative is to swing out the primary filter and replace it with a red-transmitting glass. With a dark-
field condenser this will produce a bright red, dark-field image which
can be studied at length. Since fluorescein does not absorb in the red,
there is no danger of fading any fluorescence even during prolonged

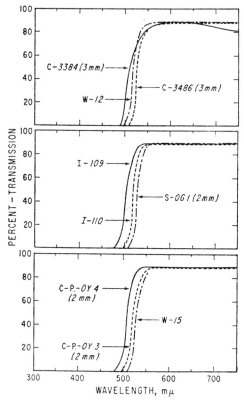

Fig. 14.   Transmission spectra for secondary filters in blue and ultraviolet–
blue excitation systems. S-OG 4 is similar to C-P.-OY 3.

examinations. Furthermore, dark-adaptation of the eye to green light
will not be lost during examination of a red-illuminated object. Depending upon the type of housing, it may be possible to arrange the
filters so that a single movement will place either the red or the ex-
citer filter in the light path while at the same time removing the other.
    Heat-resistant red glass should be employed if the filter is to be

TABLE VI

BLUE AND ULTRAVIOLET-BLUE EXCITATION SYSTEMS

Heat-absorbing	Red-absorbing	Primary	Nature of radiation	Secondary
	Dark-field illumination			
$CuSO_4$, 2-10% (20-30 mm cuvette)	None needed for visual purposes	S-BG25 (3 mm)	UV + blue	I-109 (gelatin)
		S-BG12 (3-4 mm)	UV + blue	C-3384 (3 mm)
S-BG 22 (2-4 mm)	For additional heat protection when $CuSO_4$ solution is not used			
S-KG1, 2, or 3 (2-4 mm)		C-5850 (4 mm)	UV + blue	C-P.-OY4 (2 mm)
	S-BG14 (4 mm)	C-5133 (2 mm)	Blue	S-OG4 (3 mm)
C-3965 (2-4 mm)	S-BG38 (4 mm)	C-5543 (5 mm)[a]	Blue	W-12 (gelatin)
C-P.-HA1 (2-4 mm)	C-4308 (4 mm)			C-P.-OY3 (2 mm)
				I-110 (gelatin)
				W-15 (gelatin)
				C-3486 (2 mm)
				S-OG1 (2 mm)
	Bright-field illumination			
As for dark-field illumination	Necessary for visual purposes only with primary filter C-5850. Otherwise not needed except for additional heat protection; as for dark-field	S-BG12 (6 mm)	UV + blue	As for dark-field, but favoring the denser filters
		S-BG25 (8 mm)	UV + blue	
		C-5850 (8 mm)	UV + blue	
		C-5113 (4 mm)	Blue	

[a] Heat resistant.

mounted on the lamp housing; otherwise gelatin filters may be used, but with the realization that a few minutes of continuous exposure can harm the gelatin film even at a distance from the housing. There is nothing critical about the transmission requirements for these red filters. However, only the Corning glasses are specifically designated as heat-resistant; four of the eight Corning glasses from orange to red are 2434, 2418, 2408, and 2403, all in 3-mm thickness. Number 2434 has been most useful in my laboratory. Other possibilities are Wratten 24, 25, and 26; Ilford 203, 204, 205; Schott RG series, 3 mm.; and Chance-Pilkington OR 1 and OR 2, 2 mm.

If the red filter is employed with a bright-field condenser, it is necessary to reduce the light intensity before examining the field. An opal glass diffusion screen is best for this purpose because not only will the intensity be reduced to about 0.1%, but the field will be more evenly illuminated. Opal glasses are available from photographic supply houses and as standard equipment with some light housings. Non-diffusing, neutral density filters are useful adjuncts to any serious microscopy. Sets consisting of a range of densities are available from microscope manufacturers or general laboratory supply catalogs. Another useful accessory is a block of fluorescent glass or plastic which can be placed over the microscope condenser to visualize the path of the light rays. Corning's fluorescent glass No. 3750 may be used for this purpose.

Carbon arc and xenon light sources emit a high proportion of their radiation in the red and infrared regions. Should such light sources be used, copper sulfate solutions should be resorted to for proper heat protection, particularly with carbon arcs.

If the background of the fluorescence image excited by bright-field illumination shows a high luminosity, it may arise from inadequate blocking of the source by the filter combination, or from fluorescence of an optical component in the light path. Price and Schwartz (866) list steps that can be taken to determine the cause. (1) Reverse positions of the primary and secondary filters. Complete darkening of the field means that leakage of source light is not the trouble, and that the background light was due to fluorescence. (2) Return the filters to their proper positions and remove the object slide. If light is still seen, (3) place the primary filter on the stage. Darkening of the field shows that the fluorescence was coming from the substage condenser. If the field is still luminous, then either the filters, objective, or ocular are at fault. (4) The filters can be checked by direct observation in ultraviolet light, and the objective and ocular by comparison with other similar components.

BIBLIOGRAPHY

Price, G. R., and Schwartz, S. (1956). Fluorescence microscopy. *In* "Physical Techniques in Biological Research" (G. Oster and A. W. Pollister, eds.), Vol. 3, pp. 91-148. Academic Press, New York.

Richards, O. W. (1955). Fluorescence microscopy. *In* "Analytical Cytology" (R. C. Mellors, ed.), 1st ed., pp. 5/1-5/37. McGraw-Hill, New York.

Young, M. R. (1961). Principles and technique of fluorescence microscopy. *Quart. J. Microscop. Sci.* **102**: 419-449.

Chapter Five

MICROSCOPY

I. GENERAL COMMENTS

The main purposes of this chapter are first, to provide background information on microscope components so that a rational choice can be made from the overwhelming variety available; and second, to describe rather simple methods for aligning and using the fluorescence microscope.

Since the microscope sits at the very heart of fluorescent antibody work, no effort should be spared to ensure its employment at peak efficiency. Poor microscope practices, which only hinder or handicap conventional studies, can utterly ruin a project in fluorescence since the latitude in visibility is much more limited.

The fluorescence microscope is optically and mechanically identical to the conventional microscope. Too frequently it is incorrectly called an "ultraviolet microscope." The latter term is properly restricted to instruments with quartz elements above and below the object, capable of transmitting ultraviolet radiation as far down as, say, 250 mμ. In marked contrast, the ordinary fluorescence microscope possesses no quartz elements at all; if specially fitted with a quartz substage condenser, it will still have ordinary glass elements above the object, since the fluorescence image consists entirely of visible, rather than ultraviolet, radiation.

II. MICROSCOPE ELEMENTS

A. Mirrors

In some of the literature on fluorescence microscopy front-surfaced, aluminized mirrors are strongly recommended because of the higher reflectivity of such surfaces for ultraviolet radiation below 350 mμ

61

(1039). Since this portion of the spectrum plays no part in fluorescent antibody work there is no advantage, even theoretically, in such reflectors over conventional, back-surfaced, silvered mirrors. This is borne out in practical experience. On the other hand, if the fluorescence microscope is to be used also for ordinary bright-field microscopy, and if the mirror is mounted so that it is protected from dust and handling, the front-surfaced mirror is preferred. This is because it presents a single, rather than multiple, image of the light source to the condenser. A plane-surfaced mirror, mounted so that it can be adjusted and then locked into position, is most desirable. Unfortunately, this modest design feature is lacking on some of the most expensive microscope stands, where mirrors are either fixed in position at the factory, or, if movable, lack devices for securing the alignment.

B. Condensers

1. BRIGHT-FIELD CONDENSERS

In ordinary microscopy, the image of the light source formed in the plane of the object by the substage condenser introduces a complex interrelationship between condenser and objective which affects resolving power and effective aperture. In fluorescence microscopy, on the other hand, the object is self-luminous, and the only function of the condenser is to bring the greatest concentration of exciting radiation to bear on the object under observation. Thus, some of the more sophisticated refinements of condenser construction are superfluous for fluorescence microscopy.

Bright-field condensers are of three general types: (1) The Abbe condenser of two or three lenses with little or no correction; (2) the aplanatic condenser of three lens elements corrected for spherical aberration; and (3) the achromatic condenser of four lens elements corrected for chromatic and sometimes for spherical aberration. The aplanatic type of 1.3 or 1.4 numerical aperture is probably best suited for bright-field fluorescence microscopy. It provides a better focused cone of light than the Abbe condenser, and its construction with fewer elements involves less loss of light by internal reflection than the achromatic condenser. If the field of view of the 16 mm (10X) objective is not filled by the complete condenser, the top element can generally be unscrewed or swung out of line to provide a condenser of longer focal length and bigger field. The increase in illuminated area, however, is obtained at the expense of reduction in overall intensity of illumination.

Regardless of the type of condenser, oiling it to the bottom of the slide increases the amount of light transmitted and thus provides brighter fluorescence (Fig. 15). Indeed, without immersion, the maximum aperture attainable is 1.0 regardless of the rating of the condenser. (The significance of numerical aperture in defining the light-gathering or transmitting capacity of a lens is explained in Section II. D.) It is essential that the condenser be capable of precise centration in the optical path and that it possess an iris diaphragm. The

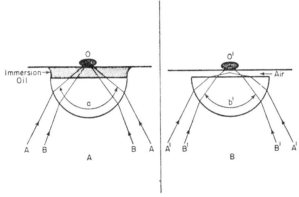

FIG. 15. The effect of immersion oil contact between condenser and slide on the light-transmitting power of the condenser. In the presence of oil (*A*), light cone *AOA* can be brought to focus on the object; in the absence of immersion contact (*B*), the maximum angle transmissable to the object is *B'O'B'*.

latter is normally left wide open in fluorescence work in order to accommodate the greatest possible cone of light, but improved contrast is sometimes attainable by cutting the iris down some. In addition, the diaphragm is necessary during the process of aligning the microscope and adjusting the light source.

2. DARK-FIELD CONDENSERS

Dark-field condensers focus a hollow cone of light onto the object in such a manner that no direct radiation enters the objective (Fig. 16B). Only those rays reflected or scattered by particles in the object plane are seen by the observer, and the microscope image thus consists of brightly outlined objects set against a dark background.

The great advantage of this type of illumination is that it provides reasonably strong radiation for exciting fluorescence, without at the same time swamping the fluorescence image with a strong beam of direct light.

Dark-field condensers fall into two main categories: refracting and reflecting types. Refracting dark-field condensers are readily made in the laboratory by the simple device of placing a central stop in the

Objective   Objective

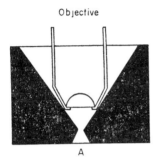 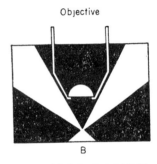

A   B

FIG. 16. Comparison of the solid light cone provided by bright-field condensers (A), with the hollow cone provided by dark-field condensers (B). No direct light enters the objective in B.

light path of any of the ordinary bright-field condensers (Fig. 17A). Such an obstruction results in an annular beam that is refracted through the peripheral portion of the condenser lens system, and is brought to a focus at the same point to which the solid, unobstructed beam would have been brought. The diameter of the stop to be used varies with the type of objective and other factors, but is approximately 9 mm for the 10× objective, 15 mm for the 20×, and 18 mm for the 45×. This system is not practical for higher magnifications because of the poor efficiency of such dark fields in comparison to the special high-power condensers described below. Microscope manufacturers frequently provide different-sized stops which can be slipped into a holder beneath the bottom lens of the substage condenser. The simple Abbe condenser with a suitable stop provides good images for the 10× and 20× objectives, but aplanatic or achromatic condensers are better suited for high-dry objectives of 40–50×. Such condensers may be used dry but immersing them to the slide increases the amount of light transmitted.

For observations with objectives of greater than 50× magnification, reflecting condensers should be used. There are two major types of reflecting condensers: those with a single reflecting surface (paraboloids), (Fig. 17B), and those with two reflecting surfaces (cardioids, bicentrics, bispherics) (Fig. 17C).

The paraboloid condenser consists of a solid glass block ground to the shape of a truncated paraboloid. Central light rays are ob-

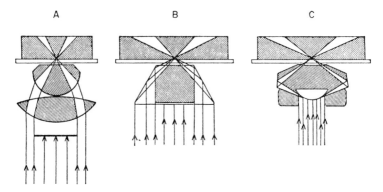

FIG. 17. Types of dark-field condensers. A. Abbe-type condenser provided with a central stop; light is refracted around the stop. B. Paraboloid condenser; single reflecting surface. C. Cardioid condenser; two reflecting surfaces.

structed by a stop, but peripheral rays are reflected from the silvered sides of the lens to a focus in the plane of the object. The focus of paraboloid condensers is not as sharp as that obtained with the double reflecting surface types, and the illuminated spot is not as intense. Paraboloids are very good for medium and lower magnifications for which they provide a bigger illuminated field than the other reflecting condensers. The lower limiting aperture of paraboloids is generally about 0.85. A useful feature of paraboloids is that closing the iris diaphragm eliminates light rays of lesser obliquity, thus providing darker background and improved contrast.

Condensers of the cardioid type possess a central, silvered hemisphere that reflects incident light to a second reflecting surface which, in turn, focuses the beam in the object plane. The hollow cone thus formed has the greatest apical angle of any of the dark-field condensers, and permits use of high magnification objectives of high aperture. The illuminated spot provided by these condensers does not fill the field of low power objectives, although there is generally adequate illumination for scanning purposes. Lower limiting apertures are of the order of 1.15, although with certain special models the full 1.30 aperture of 2-mm oil immersion objectives may be used. High-powered, bireflecting condensers are very sensitive to errors of alignment or focusing and if not adjusted properly will give inferior images. Properly used, they provide beautiful, intense images suitable for examination with the highest-powered objectives. Most of the published work with fluorescent antibody has been done with cardioid-type condensers.

TABLE VII

LIGHT TRANSMISSION OF BIREFLECTING, DARK-FIELD CONDENSERS

Manufacturer	Image brightness (arbitrary figures)
1. American Optical	42
2. Bausch and Lomb	41
3. Leitz (from Labolux microscope)[a]	7
4. Leitz (from Ortholux microscope)[a]	13
5. Reichert (standard, old type)	24
6. Zeiss-Jena (East Germany)	46

[a] Both Leitz condensers carried the same markings and appeared similar grossly.

Both types of reflecting condensers are more efficient in light-concentrating power than the refracting types, but by the same token they are more demanding in their requirements. Proper centration to the objective is of critical importance in all cases. The condensers must always be immersed to the slide, since otherwise the very oblique light rays, whose angle exceeds the critical angle of glass to air, will not emerge. Slide thickness must conform closely to the requirements generally indicated on the condenser mount. If the slide is too thick, the object plane cannot be reached by the light cone; if too thin, difficulty is experienced in maintaining oil contact through the large gap between condenser and slide. Numerical apertures (N.A.) of objectives must be matched to lower limiting apertures of condensers. For example, an oil immersion objective of N.A. 1.30 cannot be used with a condenser of 1.2 lower limit unless the objective aperture is reduced by a built-in iris, or by a reducing cone dropped into the back of the objective. Otherwise, the field will appear flooded with light in the manner of ordinary bright-field illumination.

In a series of measurements made by the author, considerable variation was encountered in the light-transmitting capacity of bireflectors made by different manufacturers. Results are shown in Table VII.

When objectives of high magnification and aperture are employed, the Bausch and Lomb cardioid condenser is very useful. The simple construction of this unit as a small cylinder with a Royal Microscopical Society objective thread facilitates its adaptation to substage mounts of different microscopes.

3. Special Purpose Condensers

The following condensers possess special qualities which may render them useful in special circumstances. There have been few or no reports of their use in fluorescence microscopy but they are presented here for the sake of completeness.

1. Long-focus, dry, dark-field condensers are made by Leitz and Reichert for low and medium magnifications. The illuminated spot fills the field of a $10\times$ objective and slide thickness is not critical. When the highest light intensities are not required they are convenient and simple to use.

2. High-aperture, reflecting dark-field condensers. Watson and Son's Cassegrain, Zeiss' luminous spot ring, and Leitz's bicentric reflecting condenser D 1.40 are all examples of reflecting condensers whose lower limiting aperture is high enough to allow use of the full aperture of a 1.30-N.A. oil immersion objective. The object to be studied must be mounted in medium of refractive index greater than 1.45. (Glycerine, the usual mountant for fluorescent antibody preparations, has an index of 1.460.) The top lens of these condensers has an exceptionally large diameter, all of which must be kept in oil contact with the object slide.

3. Quick changeover condensers. Leitz at one time manufactured a unit designed to give either bright- or dark-field illumination, depending upon the position of a substage stop and iris diaphragm. This condenser provides rather good dark field of the bireflecting type, but poor bright-field illumination. It may be useful when the major purpose is dark-field fluorescence and when the bright field is to be used primarily for scanning and locating purposes. Baker makes a condenser (Trilux) that provides bright-field, dark-field, and phase contrast illumination, all with the same unit. Each type of illumination

is said to be designed for full efficiency, with the dark-field comparable to the usual cardioid condenser. Changing illumination is accomplished by rotating a wheel beneath the condenser to the desired position.

4. Phase contrast—fluorescence condenser. Reichert manufactures a unit intended for use with their "Binolux" combined mercury arc–tungsten illuminator. It consists of the usual type of phase condenser with a series of annular diaphragms for different objectives. The diaphragms are designed to transmit visible light through the annular rings in the usual manner, but the rest of the diaphragm plate, instead of being opaque, transmits ultraviolet light. With phase objectives and suitable filter combinations, a mixture of light from both the mercury and tungsten sources will produce simultaneous phase and fluorescence images in different colors in the same field. Alternatively, pure phase or pure fluorescence images are possible. This is an expensive system which may, however, be worthwhile in special circumstances. Directions for constructing such a unit are given by Price and Christenson (867).

4. Relative Advantages of Bright- and Dark-Field Condensers

Both categories of condensers include a variety of specific types to match different-powered objectives—thus, choice of one or the other category can be made directly on the basis of over-all usefulness and versatility. Two major advantages of bright-field illumination are the more intense beam of light brought to bear on the object [about threefold greater than with a cardioid condenser according to Young (1147)], and the ability to work dry, i.e., without immersion oil. The first of these advantages loses considerable force when filter systems needed for the two types of illumination are compared. Primary filters for bright-field excitation are in general twice as dense as those required for dark-field illumination. Thus, the filtered light actually presented to the condenser is about 30–50% less intense for bright-field than for dark-field condensers. The difference is even greater for microscopic preparations that do not contain much scattering material, because then even thinner filters can be used with a dark-field condenser, whereas no corresponding reduction in thickness is tolerable with the bright field. As for the second point, the dry condenser is likely to be practical only at low magnifications with rather brightly fluorescent preparations. At the higher magnifications frequently necessary in fluorescent antibody work, oiling the condenser to the slide is almost as necessary for the bright field as for the dark field, in order to obtain maximum illumination and fluorescence.

The two major disadvantages of bright-field illumination are, first, the solid cone of light directed through the condenser and into the objective excites autofluorescence and makes for light scatter throughout the optical system of the microscope. This tends to produce a relatively high background luminosity that degrades the contrast upon which the fluorescence image depends for its effectiveness. Second, it is frequently necessary or desirable to examine a field with non-fluorescent illumination. It is difficult or impossible to visualize transparent, unstained, non-fluorescent particles or structures in wet mounts with the bright-field condenser. The first of these disadvantages can be partially overcome by careful selection of optical components for minimal autofluorescence. Or special objectives with ultraviolet—excluding cover slips cemented over the front lens may be used to reduce autofluorescence of the objectives. Neither solution is as simple or convenient as using a dark-field condenser in the first place. The direction of the dark-field beam away from the objective reduces autofluorescence of lenses to a minimum, and provides for dark backgrounds of high contrast for the fluorescence image. The second disadvantage of the bright field can be overcome by reducing the light intensity and manipulating diaphragms and condenser position until a bright-field image of sufficient visibility (generally of low resolution and poor contrast) is produced. However, it is much easier to produce an image of high resolution and excellent contrast with the dark-field condenser, by simply switching a filter or mirror to change the illumination from fluorescence excitation to white or red light.

The three major disadvantages of dark-field condensers (particularly the high-powered, reflecting types) are: (1) the reduced tolerance for variations in focusing, alignment, and slide thickness compared to bright-field condensers; (2) the need for matching the numerical aperture of the objective to the limiting aperture of the condenser; and (3) the necessity of immersing the condenser to the slide. There is no bypassing the first two difficulties. Operation of high-powered dark-field condensers presupposes a higher level of experience in microscopy than is the case for bright-field condensers, but it is not difficult to acquire a reasonable facility with these optical elements. Some of the messiness and inconvenience of working continuously with an immersed condenser can be alleviated by using a microscope stage that allows the object slide to be carried about 1.0 mm above the stage platform. This is discussed in the next section.

Overall, in the experience of many workers, dark-field illumination is superior to bright-field for fluorescence work. Images appear brighter and of greater contrast in the former instance. A possible exception occurs in the case of low-magnification studies (less than 100×) when differences between the two systems may be minimal.

C. The Stage

Unless there is a known need for a circular, revolving stage, the ordinary square stage is generally suitable in fluorescence work. It

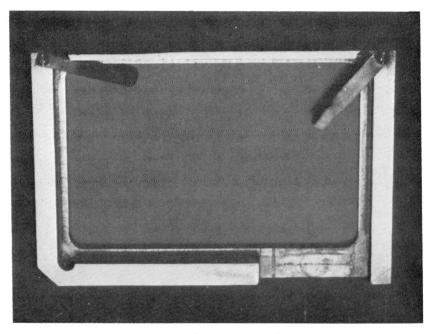

FIG. 18. Slide-carrying frame for raising the slide above the microscope stage when working with an immersed condenser. The frame accepts 1 × 3 or 2 × 3 inch slides. The cut-out in the lower right corner allows easy finger access to a 2 × 3 inch slide.

is essential that it be provided with mechanical controls for lateral and fore-and-aft motions, with vernier scales reading to 0.1 mm on both movements. Ideally, the excursion of the stage should allow complete coverage of a 50 × 75 mm slide, although this is seldom the case. Stage movements should, obviously, be smooth and easy, and the slide should be held firmly in the same plane while in traverse.

Since, in most instances, the slide will be oiled to the condenser, it is desirable that the slide clips be fashioned with narrow ledges to carry the slide a short distance above the stage surface. Otherwise, the stage is soon soiled with immersion oil and, worse, movements of the slide may become jerky and uneven. If the microscope is not equipped with this type of clip, a frame similar to that shown in Fig. 18 may be fabricated in the shop to fit the particular microscope in use. The task is simplified if the distance between the stage clips can be increased by about half an inch, to accommodate the additional width of the frame, and more importantly, if the condenser can be raised sufficiently to reach the slide, now 1.0 mm higher than before. Unfortunately, many of the newer microscope models do not possess the necessary flexibility in both regards.

D. Objectives

1. NUMERICAL APERTURE

Any discussion of objectives must inevitably include reference to an important lens constant—numerical aperture. Numerical aperture enters into many equations dealing with lenses but its greatest significance for fluorescence microscopy is that it defines the light-gathering power of an objective. The light-gathering power of a lens varies according to the refractive index of the medium in which it is immersed, being greater the higher the index. This is taken into consideration by defining N.A. as equal to the refractive index (n) of the medium times the sine of half the angular aperture of the lens (Fig. 19), or

$$N.A. = n \sin \theta$$

Since the value of n for air is taken as 1.0, and since the maximum sine of an angle is also 1.0, it is obvious that the greatest theoretical N.A. of a dry objective cannot exceed 1.0. The practical limit is about 0.95. For objectives immersed in oil of refractive index 1.52, the highest N.A. commonly encountered is 1.30 or 1.40.

Light-gathering power varies directly as the square of the N.A.*
If this were the only consideration, objectives of choice for fluorescence work would be simply those with the highest aperture for a
given magnification. Indeed, this recommendation is sometimes made.
However, as will be seen below, other factors should also be considered in choosing optical units.

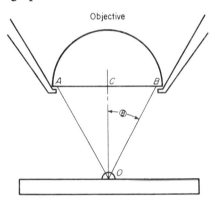

FIG. 19.   Angular aperture (*AOB*), and angle used in computing the numerical aperture of an objective (*BOC*).

2. TYPES OF OBJECTIVES

There are three major classes of objectives, grouped according to
their correction for chromatic and spherical aberrations. Achromats
are corrected chromatically for two colors and spherically for the
yellow-green region. They form the bulk of objectives in routine use
since they are very adequate for visual work and their cost is mod-
erate. For a given magnification, the N.A. of an achromat is practically always lower than that of a comparable lens from the other
two groups.

Fluorite objectives are corrected for two colors spherically as well
as chromatically. Their cost is intermediate between achromats and
the highest priced group, the apochromats. For a given magnification, the N.A. of a fluorite objective is likely to be the same or very

* The relative brightness of a microscopic field is defined by the relationship: $B = \text{N.A.}^2/\text{magnification}^2$; thus, although higher powered objectives generally have higher numerical apertures than low power objectives, brightness
to the eye may actually be less at high magnifications because of the magnification factor.

close to that of an apochromat. Fluorites often represent very good choices of fine lenses at reasonable cost.

Apochromat objectives are corrected for three colors chromatically and for two colors spherically. For the advanced worker who knows how to arrange his illumination and alignment, apochromats possess the highest potential for visual and photographic work. These objectives are expensive and, in general, should not be purchased unless there is a known specific need for them. For general work the cheaper lenses can be expected to perform as well or even better because of the more demanding requirements of the apochromats. The N.A. of lenses in this group are the highest available for a given magnification.

In addition to these general types, special-purpose objectives are available for extra-long microscope tube lengths, metallography, flat-field photography, low-power magnification, etc. These provide a sometimes confusing array of choices to the buyer but, unless there is a known special need involved, one can safely restrict his attention to the standard, biological microscope objectives.

3. Recommended Objective Combinations

For low-power, long focal length objectives of less than $10\times$ magnification, essentially only achromats are available. Such lenses are not commonly employed in fluorescent antibody work. For most purposes, the 16 mm $10\times$ achromat, of N.A. 0.25 provides a perfectly satisfactory lens for scanning slides preparatory to more careful study at higher magnification. The comparable apochromat of N.A. 0.30 furnishes a brighter image, but unless there is to be considerable detail work or photography at this magnification, the extra cost of the apochromat cannot be justified.

For medium powers of $200–400\times$, the 8 mm, $20\times$ apochromat of N.A. 0.65, in conjunction with $10\times$ and $20\times$ oculars, has much to recommend it. The aperture is as high as that of a 4 mm, $40–50\times$ achromat but the working distance is about 0.2 mm longer and there is greater depth of focus. The quality of the image formed by the highly corrected apochromat is such that it readily takes $20\times$ magnification by the ocular without breaking down. A further advantage is that the N.A. of the 8-mm objective allows it to be employed without modification with low-power, dark-field condensers whose lower limiting N.A. equals 0.85. The 4-mm, $50\times$ dry apochromat, N.A. 0.95, in conjunction with $5\times$ and $10\times$ oculars might appear to offer an even better choice in this magnification range because of the higher N.A. provided. There are, however, two serious inconveniences that mitigate against routine use of this system. First, the working distance of the 4-mm apochromat is only about 0.2 mm compared to 0.7 mm for the 8-mm apochromat. Second, the combination of high aperture and dry usage makes the 4-mm objective extremely sensitive to cover-glass thickness. This is provided for by a correction collar on the objective which must be adjusted for each preparation. Aside from the nuisance value of this adjustment in the routine examination of a series of mounts, there is the further fact that a poor adjustment yields a very inferior image. On the other hand, for detailed study of a particular mount, or for photography, the 4-mm apochromat may be the objective of choice, especially for low-intensity fluorescence.

For the magnification range of 500–1000×, the 4-mm, 40–50× oil immersion fluorite of N.A. 0.95–1.0, in conjunction with 10× and 20× oculars, has been the writer's choice for many years. The necessity for immersing these objectives is a disadvantage, but the alternatives are even less attractive, in the writer's experience. Thus, the 50×, dry achromat of N.A. 0.65 collects less than half the light of the immersion objectives, 0.65^2 (0.4225) vs. 0.95^2 (0.9025); and the 4-mm dry apochromat of N.A. 0.95 requires adjustment for cover-glass thickness. Another means of achieving this magnification range is with a 2-mm, 90–100×, oil-immersion achromat or apochromat of N.A. 1.25–1.30, in conjunction with 5× and 10× oculars. The higher N.A. of the 2 mm objective loses its significance when dark-field illumination is used, as is almost universally the case. The lower limiting aperture of dark-field condensers demands that the N.A. of the objective be reduced to about 1.05 or less by means of a built-in iris or by a special dark-field funnel stop dropped in behind the back lens of the objective. In contrast, the 4-mm fluorite objective needs no adjustment or modification for use with high-power dark-field condensers. A further disadvantage of the 2-mm objective is the shorter working distance, about 0.1 mm compared to 0.2 mm for the 4-mm objective. With a thick mount, this may spell the difference between reaching or not reaching the desired object plane.

For magnifications greater than 1000×, a 2-mm, 90–100×, oil-immersion achromat of N.A. 1.25, with a built-in iris, may be used with greater than 10× oculars. If the objective is to be used for fluorescence work exclusively, there is little justification for going to the more expensive fluorite or apochromat lenses of N.A. 1.30. With dark-field illumination the N.A. will need to be reduced anyhow, and with bright-field illumination the extra elements in the more highly corrected lenses may vitiate the slight increase in light-gathering power resulting from the higher aperture. A continuously variable iris diaphragm built into the objective is a convenience, but an ordinary objective with the proper aperture-reducing stop added is also effective for dark-field work. It is only fair to mention, however, that fluorescence microscopy at these magnifications is a challenge to the most experienced, and is effective only under the most favorable conditions of illumination and fluorescence.

E. Oculars

Most microscope manufacturers make either simple or improved Huygenian-type oculars that are perfectly satisfactory, particularly for lower magnification objectives. For objectives of 40× or higher, compensating eyepieces are more desirable. Oculars of from 8 to 20× are most useful for visual work. Since the image formed by the objective is bowl-shaped rather than flat, low-magnification oculars of 4 and 5× present highly curved fields of which only small portions can be brought into focus at a time. At the other end of the scale, oculars of greater than 20× are likely to present somewhat fuzzy images in all but the most exceptional instances. In determining the ocular magnification desired, the enlargement of the image resulting from auxiliary lenses built into the body tubes of some microscopes should be taken into consideration.

F. Body Tubes and Observation Heads

Although ordinary body tubes are acceptable, models containing slides or discs for inserting barrier filters are more convenient. Such models are sometimes available on research-type microscopes, or body tubes from polarizing microscopes may be interchangeable or adaptable to medical stands. As mentioned in the previous chapter, the best location for the secondary filter is in the body tube, away from the focal plane of the eyepiece.

Binocular observation heads provide the most comfortable viewing, but at the expense of considerable loss in light transmission. Measurements by the author on representative models of Leitz, Spencer, Wild, and Zeiss microscopes show the image to each eye through the binocular head to be only 0.33–0.20 as bright as that through the straight monocular tube. In spite of this light loss, many workers prefer binocular viewing in fluorescent antibody studies because of the greater comfort, particularly for prolonged examinations.

It is a definite convenience for photographic purposes to use a head equipped with a straight photographic tube as well as an inclined monocular or binocular visual tube. In such cases it is important to be able to direct *all* the light either to the camera or the eye. Tubes with permanently mounted prisms which split the light beam to both directions simultaneously are unsatisfactory when working at the low light levels characteristic of fluorescence.

III. ALIGNMENT AND CENTRATION OF THE MICROSCOPE

A. Rationale

To the beginner, the manipulations of the more advanced microscopist as he aligns his equipment may appear a cabalistic ceremony. Actually, the principles that govern these manipulations meet the tests of common sense as well as of theoretical optics, and no one seriously interested in microscopy can afford to ignore them. This is particularly true in fluorescence microscopy, where poor alignment of the microscope can easily nullify the most expensive equipment and render a program difficult, if not impossible, to carry out.

The principles of proper alignment are simply these: (1) The entire light train from source to eye must be put onto a single optical axis, so that the light beam is not deviated from its course to produce an unevenly illuminated field; and (2) an image of the light source or its surrogates, the collector lens or a diffusion screen, must be projected into the plane of the object. The Kohler method of illumination provides for these requirements and is the basis of the following step-by-step procedure for aligning microscope and lamp. It is recognized that it may not always be possible to follow each step as given, because of the varying designs of microscopes and lamp housings. For example, some microscopes have fixed mirrors, or the lamp may lack an iris diaphragm. Generally, such features are the result of factory "pre-setting," and one should proceed as if the settings were accurate. If it becomes obvious that they are not, compromise adjustments may be made with components that are adjustable, or the unit should be returned to the dealer for appropriate corrections.

B. Steps in Aligning the Microscope and Illuminator

It is most convenient to make basic adjustments with a bright-field condenser, and then to switch to dark field, if that is how the work is to be done. Separate directions to be followed when only a dark-field condenser is available are given further below.

1. Turn on the microscope light, direct the beam grossly at the microscope mirror, and adjust the latter to illuminate a test slide through a bright-field condenser. A stained tissue section serves well for this purpose. *Important caution:* Unfiltered light from the mercury arc is literally blinding. Be sure to reduce the intensity by means of dense color or neutral density filters. A ground glass diffusion screen may be used but it will have to be removed at step 6.

2. Focus on the test section with a $10\times$ objective and $10\times$ ocular. The slide may then be moved to a clear area.

3. Close down the diaphragm on the substage condenser, and rack the condenser up or down until an image of the diaphragm comes into focus.

4. Center the diaphragm image in the field by manipulating the condenser centering screws.

5. Open the condenser diaphragm and close down the diaphragm on the lamp housing.

6. Again, rack the condenser up or down until an image of the lamp diaphragm is in focus in the plane of the test section. Leave the condenser in this position.

7. Center the image of the lamp diaphragm by adjusting the microscope mirror.

8. Open the lamp diaphragm enough to see the field properly, and focus the lamp collector lens until an image of the light source (for the mercury arc, two pencil-shaped electrodes) becomes visible.

9. Close down the lamp diaphragm slightly and center the image of the light source in the resultant circle by adjusting the bulb-centering controls. If the lamp design permits adjusting the lamp mirror

from the outside, the reflected image of the electrodes can also be brought into centration at this point. If the mirror adjustment cannot be made from the outside, ignore the reflected image for the time being and consider only the original. Adjustment of the mirror can be done later after the lamp has been turned off (step 17).

10. Switch to the objective and oculars actually to be used and, if necessary, recenter the image of the light source by adjusting the substage condenser.

11. Focus the lamp collector lens until the field is just filled with an image of the electrodes.

For work with a bright-field condenser the alignment is now complete. By replacing the ocular with a Bertrand lens, such as is provided for aligning the phase microscope, and observing the various diaphragm images at the back lens of the objective, all of the above adjustments can be made directly with the objective one plans to use, even a 2-mm objective.

To switch to dark-field illumination, proceed as follows:

12. Replace the bright-field with the dark-field condenser. Switch back to a low-powered objective. If the dark-field condenser has a centering circle engraved on its upper surface, illuminate the surface with a table lamp, focus the objective on it, and bring the circle to the center of the field by means of the condenser centering screws.

13. If there is no centering circle on the condenser, add a drop of immersion oil and raise the condenser into contact with the test slide. Bring the tissue section into focus and lower the condenser very slowly until the illuminated circle is brightest and has clean, sharp margins. Drop the condenser a little more until a dark spot appears within the illuminated circle.

14. By manipulating very slightly the condenser centering screws and the microscope mirror, bring both the illuminated circle and the dark spot to the center of the field.

15. Switch to the objective to be used and if necessary, bring the centration into line by slight adjustments of the condenser.

16. Focus the lamp collector lens until the field appears brightest, and leave in that position.

17. After the light has been turned off, remove the lamp housing or tilt it so that it is possible to look directly into the lamp collector lens. Focus the collector until the original and reflected images of the

electrodes can be seen and adjust the mirror so that the reflected image is superimposed on the original. *Do not* change the position of the bulb in this operation. The lamp can then be returned to the microscope, and the microscope mirror and lamp tilt adjusted as described in steps 5–7 above.

If the microscope lacks a bright-field condenser, precise alignment is more difficult since the lamp diaphragm and source cannot be seen as such with a dark-field condenser. The following steps, however, may be followed with reasonably good results.

1. Remove the lamp from the microscope and point at a distant wall. Place dense filters in the path of the light source.
2. Turn on the light.
3. Close down the lamp diaphragm a little and place a ground glass close to it.
4. Focus the lamp collector lens on the ground glass until an image of the electrodes can be seen in the circle formed by the lamp diaphragm.
5. Center the electrodes in the diaphragm circle by adjusting the bulb centering controls. Adjust the mirror image as described above.
6. Turn off the light and return lamp to the microscope.
7. With a test-slide in the field of a 10× objective and ocular, turn on the lamp, point the beam as carefully as possible onto the center of the microscope mirror, and adjust the mirror to illuminate the condenser.
8. Proceed from step 12 above.

IV. PHOTOMICROGRAPHY

Contrary to general opinion, photomicrography of fluorescence is fundamentally a more simple procedure than general photography with the microscope. Two of the major difficulties in conventional photomicrography, obtaining adequate contrast and high resolution, are self-resolving in fluorescence work because of the nature of the image—self-luminous objects set on a dark background. The main difficulties in fluorescence photomicrography relate to the relatively low image brightness, and to the tendency of fluorescence to fade or change color during continuous irradiation.

Modern film emulsions for black and white photography are fast enough to provide good fluorescence photographs with exposures of from about 15 sec to 5 min, even at magnifications of 1000×. Special film developers may allow these exposure times to be reduced considerably and with Polaroid film, ASA 3000 speed, exposures of

TABLE VIII

FILMS SUITABLE FOR FLUORESCENCE PHOTOMICROGRAPHY

Manufacturer	Film	ASA exposure index
Black and white		
Agfa	Isopan ISS	200
	Isopan Ultra	500
	Isopan Record	1250
Ansco	Super Hypan	500
Dupont	Superior 4	625
Gevaert	Gevapan 33	250
	Gevapan 36	500
Ilford	HP3	400
	HPS	800
Kodak	Tri-X Pan	400
Color		
Agfa	Agfachrome CT-18	50
Ansco	Anscochrome Daylight	32
	Super Anscochrome Daylight	100
Ilford	Ilfochrome Daylight Type 32	32
Kodak	Kodachrome II	25
	Kodachrome-X	64
	Ektachrome-X	64
	High Speed Ektachrome Daylight	160

1–2 sec are feasible. Ordinary color film is considerably slower than this, but extra-fast films are available whose speed approaches that of ordinary black and white types. Table VIII presents a list of fast films available in 35 mm, the size commonly used in photomicrography.

Generally, "daylight" color film is preferred, but it must be recognized that absolutely true color values may not always be attained.

Variations in fading rates of different objects in the field, and inherent variability in films and processing contribute to the difficulty of true color rendition. For many purposes black and white prints are perfectly suitable, and the range of film types available is considerably broader than in the color series.

Because of the low brightness of fluorescence images, the only generally practical type of camera is one having a side-arm telescope through which the image may be focused. Ground glass focusing is out of the question in any but the most exceptional cases. The 35 mm photomicrographic cameras made by all the major microscope manufacturers are very convenient, but larger sizes using Polaroid film are also practical. It is preferable to choose a model in which the camera tube directs all of the light either to the viewer or the camera by means of a swing-out reflector. Such an arrangement allows for easier focusing and shorter exposures than is possible with fixed beam-splitting designs.

Determining proper exposure is generally less of a problem in fluorescence than in ordinary bright-field photography. Assuming a good crossed-filter system, it is almost impossible to overexpose a fluorescence image. I have obtained good photographs of organisms from the same slide using exposures of 15 sec to 2 min. Under such circumstances, there is little justification for purchasing expensive, sensitive photomultiplier photometers in order to get instrumental readings for exposure determinations. In my laboratory, where such an instrument has been available, I have found it more convenient and as reliable to work from the written record of relevant data maintained for each roll of film used. A simple record of the material being photographed, film, optics, filters, exposure times, and whether the exposure was good or bad, provides in a short time enough information to determine exposures for most any new photographs that need to be made.

If the filters being used for visual examination are leaking near-UV or blue light, the film will be fogged and contrast degraded. In that case a colorless or pale yellow secondary filter chosen from Table IV may be added to the system to block those wavelengths.

Microfluorimetric data collected in my laboratory show that brightly fluorescent organisms irradiated continuously with a high light flux can lose more than 60% of their fluorescence during the first 15 sec, and more than 80% by the end of 1 min. Less bright organisms exposed to reduced irradiation have shown a 40% reduction during the first quarter minute, and a 65% reduction at 1 min. The reduction in fluorescence is correspondingly less with material of lower initial fluorescence irradiated with less efficient filter and condenser systems. The obvious moral for the photographer is to minimize exposure of his field to the excitation irradiation before he is ready to snap the shutter. This can be achieved by using red light to perform all the preliminary operations of locating a proper field, centering it in the camera frame, and focusing it. Final focusing must be done with fluorescent light but a neutral filter of suitable density can be employed to reduce fading to a minimum during this step. The photograph can then be taken with the full excitation beam with the fluorescence at its highest point.

V. QUANTITATION OF MICROFLUORESCENCE

Subjective estimates of fluorescence intensity, generally expressed in the form of plus marks, are necessary, valuable, and certainly the simplest kind of "quantitation." With experience, such evaluations provide a good, rough guide for the individual worker. However, the ability of human vision to adapt itself readily to variations in illumination makes this method unreliable in judging brightness values that differ by less than about twofold. Variation in the brightness distribution of individual cells or particles also contributes to the difficulty of accurate, subjective evaluations. Finally, plus marks do not lend themselves to statistical or mathematical manipulation.

Conceptually, obtaining instrumental measurements of microfluorescence is a simple problem. All that is needed is a sensitive detector in the image plane of the microscope which will respond in direct proportion to the intensity of fluorescence. Modern photomultipliers connected to amplifiers, recorders, and cathode ray tubes can readily respond accurately to incredibly low light fluxes, so that the low intensity of the fluorescence image is not a particularly serious difficulty. In spite of this fact, objective quantitation of microfluorescence is rarely encountered in the literature, and this entire area remains relatively unexplored except for the few instances cited below. The main reason for this seems to be that there is as yet no commercial instrument of an appropriate level of sophistication designed specifically for microfluorimetry. The effort necessary to assemble such an instrument individually appears to have inhibited consideration of problems for which quantitation of fluorescent antibody reactions could be helpful.

Mellors *et al.* (724) photographed fluorescent fields on conventional films which, after processing, were analyzed with a microdensitometer. Numerical values for relative brightness of structures within each field where then compared. The photographic approach has the virtue that no special microfluorimetric gear needs to be attached to the microscope. However, the necessity of photographing, processing and analyzing on an expensive microdensitometer every single field to be measured adds up to a very bulky operation. Furthermore, differences in the rate of fading of different objects could introduce serious errors during exposures of several minutes.

A hand-held, photographic exposure meter (S.E.I. photometer, made by Salford Instruments) was used by Curtain (214) to obtain estimates of microfluorescence intensity. This photometer provides a small, self-illuminated comparison spot in the center of the visual field that is matched by eye to the brightness of the field being measured. Since Curtain provided no information on his use of the instrument, which is designed for conventional, large-scale photography, it is hard to judge its value for measurements through the microscope.

Completely instrumental evaluation of the brightness of microscopic fields containing fluorescent bacteria was accomplished by Ehrlich and Ehrmantrant (278). They mounted the ocular of a microscope into the housing of a photomultiplier tube whose output could be read on the meter of the attached amplifier, a Photovolt Model 520-M. This system was also used by de Repentigny *et al.* (249) for unstained bacteria, and by Pittman *et al.* (852) for stained tissue culture cells. A basically similar mechanical arrangement was used by Holter and Marshall (464) to measure the fluorescence of solutions in capillary microcuvettes. The Evans Electroselenium Ltd. microphotometer is specifically constructed for this type of application. In all of these cases the total field was measured, and different ancillary techniques of counting cells, standardizing suspensions, etc., were used to relate observed readings to a given number or volume of fluorescent cells. Obviously, in order for this method to be useful, background fluorescence must be low and relatively uniform throughout the slide, and the measured fields should be highly if not entirely homogeneous.

Where these two conditions cannot be met, it becomes necessary to include a diaphragm in the light path above the ocular, so that portions of the field can be isolated and measured independently of the rest of the field. Unfortunately, this seemingly simple requirement introduces an extraordinary mechanical complexity into the system. The photometer head now needs to be provided with a viewer to allow centering and focusing the object in the plane of the diaphragm, and with a sliding platform, rotating mirror, or other device to allow the phototube to be brought to the light beam or the latter to be directed into the phototube. Such a device needs to be machined with a precision comparable to that of the microscope itself if readings are to be dependable enough to compensate for the problems of constructing the instrument in the first place.

A number of designs have been described for use in microspectrophotometry by Pollister and others (619, 857, 858, 1024). In the author's laboratory an instrument of this type was assembled from commercial components and adapted for microfluorimetry. It was easily sensitive enough to measure fluorescence emitted from single bacterial cells or smaller particles (367, 375). A similar, but more advanced, instrument that takes advantage of the extra stability afforded by double-beam ratio recording was described more recently by Goldman (372). By and large, assembly and operation of such microfluorimeters are within the budget and technical competence of a medium-sized biological research laboratory.

Microfluorimeters whose construction and operation require considerably greater mechanical and electronic sophistication have been assembled for automatic scanning and selection of cells showing predetermined levels of fluorescence (682, 725); comparing autofluorescence of small areas with the same cell (129); and determination of fluorescence spectra of tissues and suspensions (801, 816, 930, 954). None of the above instruments is available commercially as an integrated system. However, Kunz (598) has used a Reichert microphotometer for microfluorimetry with apparently satisfactory results, and the Leitz microspectrophotometer may also be adaptable for this purpose. For the system described by Goldman (372), which represents a practical compromise between capabilities and expense, components such as photomultipliers, amplifiers, and recorders can be used as obtained from ordinary commercial sources. Photometer heads may be constructed from photomicrographic tubes that already possess the basic design features needed (69).

It should be obvious from the above that prototype microfluorimeters have by now been described for the simplest to the most complicated applications. The ready measurement of as little as 10^{-7} μg of labeled antibody on individual cells (375), and the extremely refined antigenic studies possible (373, 377–379) would seem to offer opportunities in immunohistochemical research that have hardly been touched as yet.

VI. MISCELLANEOUS OBSERVATIONS

A. Incident Illumination

Illumination from above the object has an appeal for fluorescence microscopy, because the excitation beam is directed away from the objective and only fluorescent and scattered excitation light is seen by the viewer. Zeiss, Leitz, Reichert, and Wild make special objectives that, with the help of other accessories, provide incident illumination by means of reflecting and condensing elements surrounding each objective. In general, such accessories are attached to the larger research stands or to expensive, "universal," microscopes. In spite of the seeming attractiveness of these designs, they have been used to only a limited degree in fluorescent antibody studies. Various practical difficulties operate to reduce the efficiency of such units [in Danielsson's hands (230) staining titers were sixteenfold lower than with conventional units], and their expense plus the general unfamiliarity of biologists with such equipment has limited their use.

The Russian ML-2 fluorescence microscope possesses a built-in vertical illuminator in addition to the usual substage gear. Illumination can be readily switched from substage to vertical by sliding appropriate levers. The same objectives are utilized in both cases. In the author's laboratory, results with this system have been comparable in brightness to those obtained with conventional dark-field, substage illumination. Advantages of the vertical illuminator are that high magnification objectives can be used at full aperture, and various combinations of incident and substage lighting may be utilized for special effects.

B. "Universal" Microscopes

In recent years, some of the larger manufacturers have put out "universal" microscopes of frequently radically different appearance from conventional or classic microscopes. Such stands, or consoles, have accessories either built in or available at extra cost for conventional, phase, fluorescence, polarization, and other kinds of microscopy. Photography is facilitated by convenient arrangements for plates, 35-mm rolls, and sometimes by automatic exposure meters. Various filament or arc light sources are provided for and, often, the impression is given that such stands make the more sophisticated types of microscopy easy even for the tyro.

Before investing in such expensive instruments, it should be realized that alignment and proper use of the various accessories available often require more than passing experience with the particular type of microscopy involved. Furthermore, it is unlikely that one stand will be used for all the specialized purposes of which it is capable, if for no other reason than that very few workers are competent in all phases of microscopy, and multiple usage of a microscope for critical purposes hardly ever works out. Finally, the true usefulness of a microscope is determined more by its optical and mechanical quality and the knowledgeability of the worker, rather than by gadgetry which may sometimes actually frustrate good practice. For these reasons, the beginner in fluorescence microscopy is well-advised to stick to a simple instrument with which he can become thoroughly familiar. There is no need to buy a yacht when a rowboat will do.

BIBLIOGRAPHY

Gage, S. H. (1947). "The Microscope," 17th ed. Cornell Univ. Press (Comstock), Ithaca, New York.
Needham, G. H. (1958). "The Practical Use of the Microscope." Thomas, Springfield, Illinois.
Shillaber, C. P. (1944). "Photomicrography in Theory and Practice." Wiley, New York.

TECHNIQUES

Chapter Six

PREPARATION AND FRACTIONATION
OF ANTISERUM

I. GENERAL COMMENTS

Antiserum for labeling purposes differs in no way from that used in general immunological work. The two general procedures for developing antibodies are: active infections of suitable hosts with living agents, or repeated inoculations of suspensions or solutions of antigen into laboratory animals. The rabbit is most commonly used for the latter purpose, but the chicken, horse, goat, and other species are also employed. Antigen may be introduced by practically any route other than orally, although the intravenous method is probably most common. There is no evidence that the titer of antibody produced is particularly influenced by small variations in immunization schedules; the main requirement appears to be gradual introduction of a rather large total dosage of antigen over a period of several weeks or longer.

Many antisera are now available commercially in the labeled or unlabeled condition (see Appendix A for a listing of suppliers). Anti-agent serum for direct staining, and anti-species serum for the indirect method can frequently be provided out of stock for many microbial agents and species used in antibody production. A few suppliers will prepare antiserum against antigens provided by the buyer or will label antisera prepared by the buyer. The main caution in using purchased antiserum is to subject the reagent to the same critical evaluation for specificity and titer as would be applied to one made in the laboratory. Claimed standards of purity and activity cannot be taken for granted in subtle reagents like antisera.

II. PRODUCTION OF ANTISERUM

A. Bacteria and Fungi

Antibacterial and antifungal serum is commonly prepared by intravenous inoculation of rabbits with living material or with non-viable intact cells treated with formalin, heat, phenol, alcohol, or thiomersal. Adjuvants, non-specific substances whose presence in the immunizing inoculation enhances antibody production, are useful when preparing antisera against soluble antigens such as culture washings or organism extracts. Different types of adjuvants are described in Section II, D, which deals with soluble antigens. Most immunization schedules involve 2–3 inoculations a week for 3–5 weeks, with blood being drawn 7–10 days later. Individual injections are often in the range of 10^9– 10^{10} organisms, with a total mass of 10 mg or more for the complete series. Frequently the course of antibody production is followed by

TABLE IX

REFERENCES TO PRODUCTION OF ANTIBODIES DIRECTED AGAINST
BACTERIA AND FUNGI

Organism	Reference
Actinomyces	990
Aspergillus	956
Bacillus	140
Candida	388
Clodosporium	7
Chrysosporium	538
Clostridium	76
Escherichia	929, 1049, 1121
Haemophilus	248
Histoplasma	389, 538, 870
Leptospira	155, 219, 759
Malleomyces	747
Mycoplasma	30, 115, 144, 639
Pasteurella	532, 1100, 1136, 1144
Proteus	856
Pseudomonas	1144
Salmonella	1051
Sepedonium	538
Sporotrichium	525
Staphylococcus	159
Streptococcus	284, 409, 527
Treponema	236

agglutination, precipitin, or complement-fixation reactions, although these do not necessarily exactly parallel fluorescent staining titers (527). Agglutination titers of 1:1000 or more are aimed at for preparing the labeled antibody, but sera with lower titers have also been used successfully.

Table IX presents selected references in which details of antibody production against specific bacterial and fungal agents may be found. In this table, as in those following, only references dealing with antisera subsequently labeled for fluorescent staining are given, since more general bibliographies are widely available in reviews and texts.

B. Protozoa and Helminths

In this field most antisera have been obtained from humans or laboratory animals carrying active infections, so that few generalizations can be made about dosages or schedules. When immunization

TABLE X

REFERENCES TO PRODUCTION OF ANTIBODIES DIRECTED AGAINST
PROTOZOANS AND HELMINTHS

Organism	Reference
Amoeba	1140
Ascaris	204, 1029
Entamoeba	363, 364, 377
Nippostrongylus	489
Paramecium	39
Plasmodium	482, 587, 1000, 1058, 1091
Schistosoma	18
Toxoplasma	222, 365
Trichinella	488
Trichomonas	707

has been achieved without infection, the usual procedure of repeated inoculations has been followed. Table X presents a list of references dealing with specific agents in this group.

C. Viruses and Rickettsia

Antiserum production against viruses may be complicated by "contaminant" antigens derived from infected tissues or cultures with which the virus is associated. This problem is not peculiar to fluorescent staining and the usual immunological and methodological solutions apply, e.g., absorption of antisera or purification of virus preparations. Convalescent sera of high titer in conventional tests are frequently taken for labeling purposes. Immunization schedules follow the usual pattern except that they may extend over a longer period

TABLE XI

REFERENCES TO PRODUCTION OF ANTIBODIES DIRECTED AGAINST
VIRUSES AND RICKETTSIAE

Agent	Reference
Anaplasma	914
Canine distemper	644
Colorado tick fever	102
Egypt 101	803
Fowl plague	87
Hog cholera	1014
Influenza	74, 328, 636
Mumps	139
Murine leukemia	311
Myxoviruses	444
Newcastle disease	869
Poliomyelitis	443
Polyoma	932
Reovirus	901
Rickettsiae	103, 387
Rous sarcoma	719
Shope papilloma	805
Swine influenza	783
Tobacco mosaic	772
Trachoma	792
Vaccinia	584, 806
Wound tumor	774
Venezuelan equine encephalomyelitis	728

of time than those used for bacteria, periods of several months being not uncommon. Table XI presents selected references concerned with antibody production against some viruses and rickettsiae.

D. Soluble Antigens and Tissue Homogenates

Antibody production methods in this category differ from those mentioned previously in the almost universal use of adjuvants to improve the antibody response, and in the generally greater mass of antigen inoculated. As much as 1–2 gm of protein may be inoculated into a rabbit over a 2-month period, although a more common figure is 100–200 mg. Where antibody production has been followed during the immunization period, good titers have been detected after as little as 11 mg of inoculated protein (291). Nevertheless, titers increase with increasing dosage, and repeating an immunization schedule after a rest period of 3–4 weeks is sometimes necessary. Spacing of injections may vary from three times a week to once in 2 weeks, and a series is continued, sometimes for as long as 3 months, until antiserum of good titer is developed. Qualitative and quantitative estimations of antibody potency may be checked by test-tube and gel diffusion precipitin reactions. As a result of the widespread use of adjuvants, inoculation is more often by the subcutaneous, intramuscular, or intraperitoneal routes, and only occasionally intravenous.

Freund's adjuvant, a mixture of nine parts light mineral oil, one part emulsifier (Arlacel A, Atlas Powder Co.), and killed *Mycobacterium butyricum* cells (2 mg/ml) is the most commonly used potentiating agent. The prepared mixture is available from Difco Laboratories. It is mixed with an equal volume of aqueous antigen solution in a blender (very brief mixing suffices), or by other means, to form a smooth water-in-oil emulsion. Subcutaneous inoculation of such mixtures produces sterile abscesses but the antibody response is greatly enhanced. Alternatively, antigen solutions may be precipitated with sterile potassium alum [$Al_2(SO_4)_3 \cdot K_2SO_4 \cdot 24H_2O$], or mixed with aluminum hydroxide gel to provide immunizing suspensions that are more effective than saline solutions alone.

The problem of contaminant antigens is perhaps most acute when dealing with tissue extracts. Preparation of enzymes, hormones, or serum fractions in pure condition for immunization purposes is frequently difficult or impossible. Resultant antisera may have titers to different antigen components out of all proportion to the concentration of these components in the inoculated material, and staining results may be correspondingly misleading. For example, antiserum with a high *in vitro* inhibition titer against an enzyme may also possess a high undetected activity against contaminant components of the enzyme preparation. Tissue sections stained with such a labeled antiserum may show brightly stained structures unrelated to the enzyme under investigation. The resolution of such problems is often difficult and depends upon the individual case. Table XII presents references

TABLE XII

References to Production of Antibodies Directed Against
Soluble Antigens

Antigen	Reference
Serum components	55, 94, 134, 153, 299, 360, 444, 461, 716, 795, 887, 929, 1085
Hormones	23, 210, 290, 691
Enzymes	288, 289, 291, 751, 777
Organ and tissue extracts	287, 309, 361, 440, 521, 547, 548, 745, 778, 850, 891, 921, 946, 1016, 1036
Tumor extracts	314, 450, 452, 454, 456

dealing with preparation of antibodies to different categories of soluble or tissue antigens.

E. Antiglobulins

Antibodies directed against human or animal globulins are so frequently used in the indirect staining method that their preparation deserves to be described in some detail. Injection schedules differ in the various laboratories. The two methods presented below may be considered representative of two extremes. Method A is lengthy and intended to yield very high precipitin and staining titers. Method B is simpler but is also effective. It is noteworthy that high-titered antisera may cross-react with serum components of species other than the one used for immunization (431). In both methods, antibody development should be followed by trial bleedings during immunization and the schedule terminated when satisfactory titers have been reached.

Serum globulins for immunization may be isolated by the usual physical methods (see Section III), or immunological techniques may be employed to prepare highly purified antibody globulins (55, 461, 724). There is no critical experimental evidence to indicate that staining results are necessarily superior following immunization with specially purified antibody globulins, but on general principles the more precise the activity of the labeled serum the better.

1.   Method A [Adapted from Niel and Fribourg-Blanc (795)]

To 10 ml of globulin containing 16.5 mg of protein/ml in 0.05M phosphate buffer, pH 7.2, are slowly added 10 ml of 2% potassium alum [$Al_2(SO_4)_3 \cdot K_2SO_4 \cdot 24H_2O$]. The pH is controlled constantly by adding a few drops of alcoholic bromthymol blue and maintaining a jade green color by the addition of $0.2N$ NaOH. The suspension keeps well at 5°C when penicillin (20,000 units) and streptomycin (20 mg) are added as preservative. Rabbits are injected intravenously twice a week for 5 weeks with doses increasing from 0.3 to 1.0 ml. The spacing may be spread out somewhat if the animals evidence too strong a shock following the injections. After a rest period of 15 days three more injections are given. Thirty days later a final inoculation is given and the animal is bled 8 days after that. The complete course involves about 80 mg of protein. Mellors *et al.* (716) administered a small intravenous dose 6–12 hr before the scheduled immunizing dose, in order to reduce the anaphylactic shock. Better protection may be afforded by introducing the first dose of each series of injections by the subcutaneous or intraperitoneal route.

2. METHOD B [ADAPTED FROM FAHEY AND HORBETT (299)]

Rabbits are inoculated subcutaneously or intramuscularly with 5 mg of globulin plus an equal volume of Freund's adjuvant at 2-week intervals for the first three inoculations. Subsequent inoculations are performed weekly until a satisfactory titer is obtained.

Anticomplement, necessary in the complement-staining technique (386), is prepared by essentially the same procedures as antiglobulin, using fresh guinea pig globulin as the antigen (444).

III. SEPARATION OF GLOBULIN FOR LABELING

Labeled whole serum has been used for staining in a sufficient number of instances to be certain that this is a feasible procedure. Nevertheless, most investigators have preferred to work with more-or-less purified globulin fractions according to the lead of Coons and his original group. Less labeling compound is required, since none is wasted on the non-antibody-containing albumins, and more importantly, greater staining specificity may result (337). At the other extreme, there appears to be no staining advantage to labeling only highly refined globulin fractions in place of the more conveniently obtained crude fractions (381).

By far the commonest methods used for separation of globulins are precipitation with ammonium sulfate or cold ethanol. These methods are described below in detail. Diethylaminoethyl (DEAE)-cellulose column chromatography is useful for purification of labeled globulins, but has been little employed in fluorescent antibody work for isolating globulins before labeling. However, both column and batch methods using DEAE-Sephadex, and scaled to handle 50 ml or more of serum at a time, have been described (37, 244). Riggs *et al.* (907) proposed the labeling of whole serum and the separation of globulin by chromatography on DEAE, while simultaneously removing unreacted dye. Both Riggs and Frommhagen and Martins (336), however, have shown that elution characteristics of serum proteins are changed after reaction with fluorescein isothiocyanate. Thus the slight savings in time which the Riggs procedure offers may be more than offset by the variability of elution pattern and waste of labeling compound. Precipitation of non-globulin serum proteins by 2-ethoxy-6,9-diaminoacridine lactate (Ethodin, Winthrop Laboratories), with subsequent separation and labeling of the globulins remaining in solution, has been described (392). This procedure is presented here, together with the ammonium sulfate and ethanol methods, because of its simplicity.

O'Berry (808) and Lewis *et al.* (628) compared staining results obtained with antibacterial serum fractionated by ammonium sulfate, ethanol, and ethodin. In both laboratories the best staining occurred with the ammonium sulfate fractions. However, until unequivocal evidence from several different laboratories points to a particular technique as superior, it is probably wisest at the beginning to become proficient in the one particular method for which the laboratory is best equipped, rather than to cast about with a variety of techniques.

A. Ammonium Sulfate Method [Adapted from Kendall (546)]

To one volume of stirred serum in a water–ice bath add slowly 1.0 volume of saturated $(NH_4)_2SO_4$ solution. After allowing the precipitated globulin to aggregate for a few hours, the suspension is centrifuged in the cold and the precipitate redissolved in a measured volume of water about equal to the original volume of serum. Saturated ammonium sulfate solution is again added equal in volume to that of the water used, and the precipitated globulin is again centrifuged. If the serum was strongly colored from hemolysis, or if a purer globulin fraction is desired, this step may be repeated several times. Otherwise, the precipitate is redissolved, dialyzed against running water till frèe from sulfate, and then against 0.85% saline. The precipitate which may form is discarded and the supernatant globulin solution is recovered for use.

Variations in the above procedure include precipitation of globulin from diluted serum by addition of solid $(NH_4)_2SO_4$ to the extent of 0.5 saturation (about 2.1 moles or 271 gm/liter); and the washing of the precipitate with 0.5 saturated $(NH_4)_2SO_4$ solution instead of by repeated dissolving and precipitation. Kaufman and Cherry (540) have shown that contamination of globulin with $0.08M$ or greater concentration of ammonium sulfate interferes with conjugation to fluorescein isothiocyanate. However, precipitated globulins dialyzed in 27/32-inch dialysis tubing against 200 volumes of saline lose over 99% of their ammonium sulfate within 6 hr (428). Thus, small volumes of globulin can be cleared of interfering levels of ammonium sulfate relatively simply and quickly.

B. Cold Ethanol Method [Adapted from Nichol and Deutsch (791)]

Fractionation with ethanol depends upon precise control of temperature, pH, alcohol concentration, and ionic strength. The method is thus inherently more demanding than precipitation with ammonium sulfate, and it is strongly recommended that anyone attempting this technique familiarize himself with the rationale behind the various steps. The review by Deutsch (253) is useful for this purpose.

One volume of serum is diluted to four volumes with distilled water and the pH at 25°C is adjusted (if necessary) to 7.7 with $0.05M$ Na_2HPO_4 or $0.05M$ acetic acid. The diluted serum is cooled until a small amount of ice forms. Fifty percent ethanol, pre-cooled to $-10°$ to $-20°C$, is added slowly to the stirred serum to yield a final concentration of 20% (2.67 volumes). The temperature of the serum is lowered to $-6°C$ during this step by keeping the beaker immersed in an ice–salt mixture or in a cold alcohol bath containing small pieces of solid CO_2. The precipitate, which consists of a crude globulin fraction of the serum, is separated by centrifugation at $-5°$ to $-7°C$.

Additional purification is effected by suspending the precipitate in cold, distilled water, and further manipulating pH and alcohol concentration to yield essentially pure γ-globulin. For ordinary labeling purposes, the first fraction obtained is adequate. When highly purified fractions are desired for immunization or other special purposes, it is best to consult the original references since details vary with the animal species involved.

The crude globulin sediment may be dissolved directly in water or buffer and then dialyzed in the cold against buffered saline to remove the alcohol in the precipitate.

C. Ethodin Method [Adapted from Gordon et al. (392), and Horejsi and Smetana (467)]

Ethodin is the generic name for 2-ethoxy-6, 9-diaminoacridine lactate (Winthrop Laboratories). To one volume of serum at room temperature are added 2.8 volumes of 0.5% ethodin in $0.15M$ NaCl solution buffered at pH 7.4 with $0.035M$ phosphate. The precipitate, which contains the non-globulin serum components, is removed by centrifugation and discarded. Globulin is then precipitated from the supernatant with an equal volume of cold acetone (392) or with ammonium sulfate (336).

The globulin sediment is cleared of ethodin by repeated washings with cold 50% acetone or by solution in saline and reprecipitation with acetone. Residual ethodin after a single acetone precipitation does not interfere with the fluorescein labeling process, and is removed after labeling by procedures used for removing unreacted dye.

BIBLIOGRAPHY

Campbell, D. H., Garvey, J. S., Cremer, N. E., and Sussdorf, D. H. (1963). "Methods in Immunology." Benjamin, New York.

Carpenter, P. L. (1965). "Immunology and Serology," 2nd ed. Saunders, Philadelphia, Pennsylvania.

Cohn, M. (1952). Production of antibodies in experimental animals. *Methods Med. Res.* **5**: 271–283.

Kabat, E. A. (1961). "Experimental Immunochemistry," 2nd ed. Thomas, Springfield, Illinois.

Raffel, S. (1961). "Immunity," 2nd ed. Appelton, New York.

Chapter Seven

LABELING AGENTS AND PROCEDURES
FOR CONJUGATION

I. FLUORESCEIN DERIVATIVES

The factors that determined the choice of fluorescein as a protein label by Coons and his associates in 1942 carry equal weight at the present time, and derivatives of fluorescein are by far the most popular labels in fluorescent antibody work. Free fluorescein in alkaline solution emits a high percentage of the light it absorbs (80–95%, depending upon the author) as green fluorescence, the region of maximum sensitivity for the human retina. This high efficiency is reduced to considerably less than half upon conjugation of fluorescein to proteins through the thiocarbamide linkage (337, 375, 706), but the color of emitted light remains unchanged. Autofluorescence of this color is uncommon in vertebrate tissue or in microorganisms, so that structures stained with fluorescein are easily traced with the fluorescence microscope.

In a comparison of staining titers obtained with samples of the same antiserum labeled with fluorescein isothiocyanate, tetramethyl-rhodamine isothiocyanate, lissamine rhodamine B 200, and 1-dimethylaminonaphthalene-5-sulfonic acid, Lewis and Brooks (627) found the brightest fluorescence to occur with the fluorescein isothiocyanate conjugate. Titers were from two- to sixteen-fold greater than the next best dye, lissamine rhodamine B 200. Similar results were obtained by Hiramoto *et al.* (446).

A. Fluorescein Isocyanate and Isothiocyanate

1. SYNTHESIS AND GENERAL CHARACTERISTICS

Fluorescein isocyanate (FIC) (187) and fluorescein isothiocyanate (FITC) (908) (Fig. 20) are the only derivatives of fluorescein that

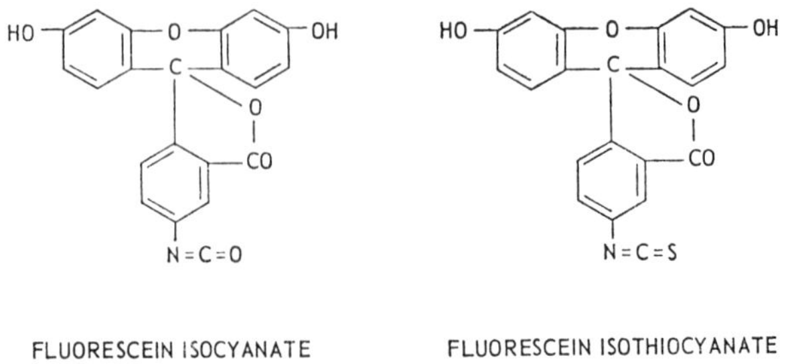

FLUORESCEIN ISOCYANATE   FLUORESCEIN ISOTHIOCYANATE

FIG. 20.   Structural formulas for the isocyanate and isothiocyanate derivatives of fluorescein.

have been successfully employed as protein labels. Others derivatives,
such as diazotized aminofluorescein (179), acid chlorides of fluorescein (125), and sulfofluorescein (1075) do not produce useful conjugates.

FIC may be synthesized by reacting 4-nitrophthalic acid with resorcinol to produce 4-nitrofluorescein, reducing this to aminofluorescein by catalytic hydrogenation, and finally converting the
amine to isocyanate with gaseous phosgene (188) (Fig. 21). The

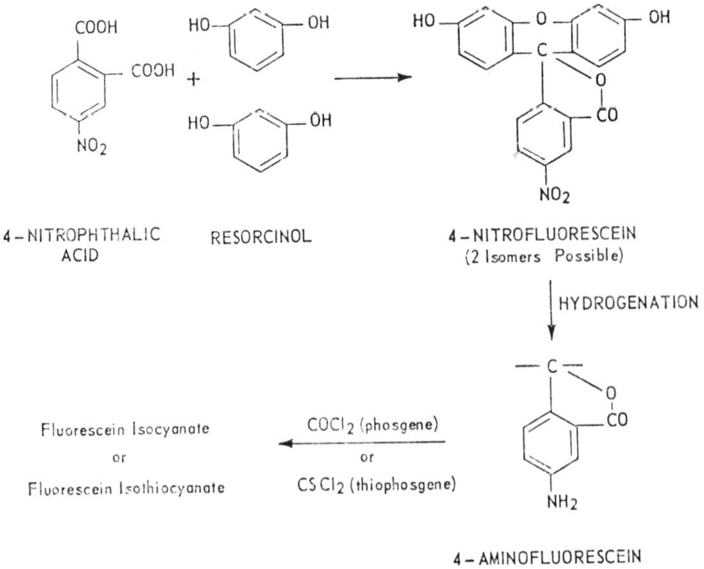

FIG. 21.   Synthesis of fluorescein isocyanate and isothiocyanate starting with
nitrophthalic acid and resorcinol.

isocyanate is unstable in the presence of moisture and, in the original description, conjugation to protein was carried out immediately following phosgenation. However, Marshall (691) found that acetone solutions of FIC could be stored for at least a year protected from moisture, light, and heat; and Goldman and Carver (374) preserved FIC by drying it on filter paper and storing the pads at $-20°C$. About the time that experiments with preserved FIC were being attempted, the much more stable isothiocyanate was synthesized by Riggs *et al.* (908). This rapidly replaced FIC in fluorescent antibody work, and methods involving the isocyanate are more of academic than practical interest now.

Synthesis of FITC is analogous to that of FIC (Fig. 21), except that the more easily handled liquid thiophosgene is used in the final step instead of gaseous phosgene (689, 908). Aminofluorescein, which may be obtained commercially, is dissolved in dry acetone and added dropwise over a period of hours to an acetone solution of thiophosgene. After removing the thiophosgene by evaporation, an acetone suspension of the reaction product is washed with a large excess of petroleum ether and the yellow or orange isothiocyanate collected by filtration. Although synthesis of FITC is relatively simple, it may be cheaper to buy quantities of less than 1–2 gm from commercial sources. The dry powder shows no deterioration upon storage in a desiccator for at least 1 year, as determined by infrared analysis (712). In the author's laboratory a single batch of FITC, stored in an evacuated desiccator jar at $5°C$, has continued to give excellent results over a 5-year period.

Fluorescein isothiocyanate synthesized by the methods mentioned above is a yellow to red mixture of two isomers plus impurities, and contains only 20–60% FITC. Purified fractions can be prepared by chromatography (192, 303, 337). Labeling efficiency of the purified compound, which is available commercially from Baltimore Biological Laboratory, appears to be about twice that of the ordinary crude material (381). With regard to other characteristics, however, for example, staining titers or non-specific staining qualities of resulting conjugates, the refined product appears to offer no advantages over the crude dye (381, 706).

Freshly prepared alkaline solutions of crude FITC are only one-half or one-third as fluorescent as comparable solutions of sodium fluorescein (375). Aqueous solutions of unconjugated dye stored in the cold show stable absorbance over long periods of time (several years in the author's laboratory), but fluorescence emission decreases in an irregular pattern at a rate that appears to be related to concentration (375, 540). This is probably the result primarily of development of aminofluorescein by hydrolysis, since the amine is much less fluorescent than FITC. Polymerization of isothiocyanate with amine residues may also contribute to the phenomenon.

Labeling with FIC or FITC is accomplished by exposing the alkaline-buffered protein solution to the dye over a period of hours. By analogy with the chemistry of other isocyanates, it appears that ε-amino groups of lysine residues and terminal amino groups of protein chains are the major sites of reaction with both FIC and FITC, although accessible sulfhydryl groups may also be involved (1017) (Fig. 22). Within the framework of the simple reaction conditions cited above, a variety of labeling methods were followed for many years, differing from the original technique of Coons and Kaplan (188) in apparently unimportant details. For example, protein concentration was varied from 10 to 50 mg/ml; dye was added in acetone suspension or as the dry powder; carbonate or barbital buffers were used in the range of pH 8.5–9.0.*

More recently, critical studies have delineated some of the para-

---

* The original method of coupling with FIC was based on earlier chemical studies that employed purified 1,4-dioxane and acetone in the reaction mixture (208, 466). Goldman and Carver (374), acting upon a recommendation by Goldwasser, found that organic solvents were unnecessary when labeling with FIC dried on filter paper. Since no protein denaturation occurred in the latter method, in contrast to the considerable denaturation when the Coons procedure was followed, the erroneous notion is sometimes expressed that organic solvents per se are responsible for protein precipitation during labeling. It is readily demonstrated that chilled globulin solutions are quite insensitive to the small volumes of acetone and dioxane employed in the original technique. Protein precipitation occurs only when the organic solvents which are added contain FIC in solution. The basis for this appears to be rapid local reaction, over-labeling, and immediate denaturation of some of the protein. Slow release of dried FIC from filter paper avoided this undesirable effect, even in the presence of organic solvents. There is a similar lack of precipitation at the time of labeling when FITC is used, presumably because of its lower reactivity and generally slower release into the medium when added as the dry powder or as a slurry in acetone. Regardless of whether organic solvents are used or not, precipitation of protein may occur after the reaction period, when the pH is lowered to a little above neutrality, as a result of the reduced solubility of globulins carrying a heavy fluorescein load.

meters affecting labeling with FITC. At room temperature the reaction proceeds at a much faster rate than at 5°C, so that equivalent levels of binding are reached in about 3 and 18 hr, respectively (568, 711, 1003). No loss in antibody activity or staining titer occurs as a result of labeling at the higher temperature, but overlabeling may occur if the reaction is allowed to continue overnight.

Labeling efficiency is significantly improved with increasing alkalinity of the reaction mix in the pH range 6.0–10.0, reaching a maximum around pH 9.5. Varying the protein concentration in the range 5–50 mg/ml has little effect on the final degree of labeling achieved. Albumins bind FITC much more rapidly and to a greater degree than

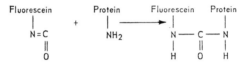

FIG. 22. Conjugation of fluorescein to protein by means of the isocyanate–amine linkage. Reaction of the isothiocyanate is comparable.

globulins (628, 711), emphasizing the importance of removing such non-antibody-containing proteins before labeling.

2. LABELING WITH FLUORESCEIN ISOTHIOCYANATE

Two methods of labeling with FITC are presented, each representing a somewhat different approach. Method (a) yields conjugates with higher ratios of fluorescein to protein but with appreciable non-specific staining under certain conditions; it is perhaps best suited for antibacterial or antifungal conjugates where non-specific staining is not a serious problem. Method (b) tends to minimize non-specific staining and may be most useful when staining antigens in association with tissue cells. Both methods can be carried out at either refrigerator or room temperatures, without any detectable difference in results.

a. Adapted from Cherry et al. (134)

1. Determine the concentration of protein in the solution to be labeled and adjust to 10–30 mg/ml with saline.

2. To the chilled protein in an ice bath add $0.5M$ carbonate buffer in saline, pH 9.5, to the extent of 10% by volume.

3. Add FITC powder to the buffered protein in the proportion of 25–50 μg of dye per milligram of protein for crude FITC, or half that for the purified compound. The higher proportions of dye to protein

result in more highly labeled conjugates, but non-specific staining may also be increased.

4.   Stir gently overnight in the cold. (To perform the reaction at room temperature, dissolve the required amount of FITC in the volume of $0.5M$ buffer determined in step 2, add to the protein solution adjusted as in step 1, and allow the reaction to proceed for 2–3 hr at 20°–25°C. The FITC must be in solution when added to the protein, otherwise it will not dissolve rapidly enough in the diluted buffer to react properly in this short period of time.)

5.   Remove for further processing. (See Section I, 3.)

b.   *Adapted from Clark and Shepard* (143)

Steps 1 and 2 as in *a*.

3.   Place the buffered protein solution into dialysis tubing.

4.   Prepare $0.05M$ carbonate buffer in saline, pH 9.5, in a volume ten times that of the protein solution.

5.   Add FITC (purified or crude) to the buffer in the proportion of 0.1 mg/ml of buffer.

6.   Fold or suspend the dialysis tubing in the FITC solution so that it is completely submerged. Cover the container with aluminum foil or equivalent to retard evaporation.

7.   Stir overnight in the cold. (Alternatively, the reaction may be carried out at room temperature for 4–6 hr. Dissolve the necessary amount of FITC in $0.5\,M$ carbonate buffer before diluting the latter to $0.05M$ concentration. For example, to label 10 ml of protein solution, dissolve 10 mg of FITC in 10 ml of $0.5M$ buffer, and make up to 100 ml with saline.)

8.   Remove dialysis tubing for further processing of the contained conjugate.

Note: In method *b* the amount of FITC used is based upon volume of buffer solution, rather than upon mass of protein being labeled. It is thus feasible to estimate rather than to determine the amount of protein to be labeled, since a wide range in the ratio of dye offered to protein appears acceptable under these conditions.

An ultrarapid method of labeling has been described in which FITC adsorbed onto finely dispersed Celite powder is added to the appropriately buffered globulin solution as in method *a* (909, 910). Labeling is said to occur within less than an hour because of the high availability of the dye under these conditions. That labeling does indeed take place has been confirmed, but there are insufficient data concerning the efficiency of the method in terms of yield of suitably labeled protein to recommend this technique for routine purposes at present.

3. REMOVAL OF UNREACTED DYE FROM FLUORESCEIN CONJUGATES

a. Dialysis. Unreacted FITC and small molecule derivatives of FITC are most simply removed by dialyzing the reaction mixture against repeated changes, first of water and finally of cold $0.01M$ phosphate-buffered saline, pH 7.0–7.5. Under ordinary conditions, it may be a week before the dialyzate appears free of fluorescence when examined with a long-wavelength ultraviolet lamp following overnight dialysis. Dialysis time may be reduced significantly by adding to the dialysis vessel about 10 gm of Dowex 2-X4, 20–50 mesh (Dow Chemical Co.) per 25 ml of conjugate. Dowex absorbs FITC as it passes into the dialyzate, resulting in a more efficient gradient at all times. The final dialysis should be against buffered saline alone. Critical studies of conjugates treated in this manner reveal that a small amount of unreacted dye remains even after prolonged dialysis (125, 701), but for many routine applications such conjugates are quite adequate. Precipitate that appears during dialysis may be centrifuged or filtered out. The cleared supernatant should be stored at 5°C or lower after addition of thiomersal (Merthiolate, Lilly), 1:10,000, or other bacteriostatic agents.

b. Gel Filtration. Molecules may be separated on the basis of size by means of so-called "molecular sieves" (861). Sephadex (Pharmacia Ltd.), a cross-linked dextran, and Bio-Gel P (Bio-Rad Lab.), a polyacrylamide gel, are examples of chromatographic materials by which proteins may be separated from smaller molecules such as FITC. The filtration method given here is based upon Sephadex (322, 354, 381, 392, 551, 635, 1155).

About 10 gm of Sephadex G-25 or G-50 (100–250 mesh) are suspended in water and washed free of "fines" by repeated sedimentation and decanting. The slurry is poured into a column, allowed to pack by gravity, and equilibrated with phosphate buffered saline, pH 7.0–7.5. The fluorescein–protein reaction mixture is delivered to the column by pipet and, when the last portion has soaked into the Sephadex, elution is begun using the equilibration buffer. A front of conjugated protein is seen to separate quickly from unreacted dye and may be collected in its entirety. A column of 20×110 mm will handle 10–15 ml of crude conjugate, delivering 90–100% of the separated protein in the first 10–20 ml of eluate after the bed volume. Further elution with large volumes of buffer removes the slower band of unreacted dye (not always completely), allowing the column to be used again. This method of removing unreacted dye from crude conjugates is the method of choice since the technical simplicity, thoroughness of clearing, and high yield of undenatured conjugates are unequaled by any other procedure.

c. *Extraction with Charcoal.* This method cannot be recommended for routine use because of the great loss of protein involved, about 40% (322). However, since it is said to reduce non-specific staining, which gel filtration and dialysis do not accomplish, the method is presented here. Powdered activated charcoal (British Drug Houses, Ltd.) at the rate of 2.5 mg/mg of protein, is washed thoroughly in buffered saline to remove soluble substances that may affect the pH of the solution. The conjugate is shaken for 1 hr with charcoal and then centrifuged. Free fluorescein derivatives, as well as those adsorbed onto labeled protein, are removed with a resultant decrease in staining titer but with improvement in specificity.

4. FRACTIONATION ON DEAE-CELLULOSE

Conjugates labeled by the methods given above and freed of unreacted fluorescein, generally stain certain types of tissues and cells in a non-specific manner. This subject is dealt with in greater detail in Chapter 11. However, in connection with processing conjugates, it is pertinent to indicate here that chromatography on the anion exchanger, DEAE-cellulose (Schleicher and Schnell Co.), yields fractions with high specific activity and minimum non-specificity (214, 381, 706, 907). The rationale for this procedure appears to be that globulin molecules carrying a low load of fluorescein retain the charge characteristics of native globulin, and may be eluted from DEAE-cellulose with low salt concentrations at a pH of 6.3 (625). Such molecules also show the highest staining specificity. On the other hand, overlabeled globulins, which are associated with non-specificity, are retained on the column at low salt concentrations. This difference in behavior provides a simple method for separating the more specific components of the conjugate from other undesirable portions. The method presented here is based on Riggs *et al.* (907).

1. Dry DEAE-cellulose (40–100 mesh, 0.96 meq/gm), about

1 gm/20–30 mg of protein to be fractionated, is sedimented for 0.5 hr in distilled water. Non-settling "fines" are decanted with the supernatant and the remainder is washed successively with 1.0N NaOH, 1.0N HCl, 1.0N NaOH, and then to neutrality with large volumes of water. In preparing large batches, filtration through several thicknesses of cheesecloth on a Büchner funnel facilitates the washing process. The slurry is finally made up and stored in phosphate buffer, 0.0175M, pH 6.3 after several suspensions and decantations in this "starting buffer."

2.   The slurry is packed into columns with the aid of gentle air pressure not exceeding 5 psi. A column of about 20 $\times$ 110 mm will handle 10–15 ml of conjugate.

3.   Conjugated globulin is equilibrated against phosphate buffer, 0.0175M and pH 6.3, either by eluting from a Sephadex G-25 column with this buffer, or by overnight dialysis. Precipitate forming during this process may be discarded.

4.   The conjugate is loaded onto the column and elution carried out in three steps, as follows:

Fraction I—elution with 0.0175M, pH 6.3, phosphate in distilled water.

Fraction II—elution with 0.0175M, pH 6.3, phosphate in 0.125M NaCl.

Fraction III—elution with 0.0175M, pH 6.3, phosphate in 0.250M NaCl.

5.   At each step a colored (and fluorescent) fraction may be seen to emerge. When the major portion of distinctly colored effluent has been collected for a particular fraction, the eluting solution containing the next higher salt concentration is added. Intermediate, dilute effluents should not be discarded because they may possess considerable staining activity if the original conjugate had a high antibody titer.

6.   The volume of conjugated protein collected at each elution step depends upon the labeling procedure. For example, with either heavily labeled or very lightly labeled proteins little or no conjugate may be eluted in Fraction I: in the former instance because of the strong binding of heavily labeled proteins to the DEAE, and in the latter instance because a proportion of the protein may be too lightly labeled to be recognized by color, and may pass through the column undetected. Molarities of NaCl higher than that used for Fraction III elute highly colored fractions which, however, possess considerable non-specific staining activity.

7.   The collected fractions should be dialyzed against phosphate-buffered saline, pH 7.0–7.5 and 0.01M, and should be evaluated for staining properties. The fraction showing the best combination of titer and specificity, generally I or II, can then be used. Twenty-five to 50% of the applied protein may be recovered in the good fractions.

5.   CONCENTRATING DILUTE PROTEIN SOLUTIONS

Conjugates that have been chromatographed on columns or otherwise diluted may need to be concentrated before they can be used for staining or be analyzed for protein and fluorescein content. Older methods for accomplishing this are lyophilization, with subsequent redissolving to the desired volume; or pervaporation, by suspending the solution in a dialysis sac in front of a fan and evaporating excess water. Aside from the awkwardness of these methods which, in the case of lyophilization, also requires special equipment, a fundamental objection is that salt concentration increases while water is being removed to the point at which irreversible changes may be induced in the proteins. In both methods, the concentrated solutions need to be dialyzed against appropriate buffered saline solutions to restore the conjugates to a useful condition.

The availability of water-soluble, high molecular weight polymers such as dextran (Commercial Solvents Corp.), polyethylene glycol (Carbowax, Union Carbide Chemical Co.), polyvinylpyrrolidine (Plasdone, General Aniline and Film Corp.), and carboxymethyl cellulose salts (Aquacide, Calbiochem) makes possible much simpler concentration techniques, with the additional virtue that the ionic concentration of solutions being concentrated remains essentially the same throughout the procedure (400, 574, 635). An appropriate amount of dry dextran, Carbowax 4000 (or higher molecular weight), Plasdone C 788–50, or Aquacide is poured into a dialysis tube that is then suspended in the solution to be concentrated. A graduated cylinder or a conical centrifuge tube of suitable size makes an efficient container for this purpose. The tube containing the polymer must be left open at the top to allow for expansion of contents as water is absorbed from the protein solution and held by the polymer. Since electrolytes pass freely through the dialysis membrane, the proteins are not subjected to changes in salt concentration as water is removed. Rate of concentration is dependent upon the initial water content of the protein solution, but eluted conjugate fractions from a chromatographic column may be reduced to one-third or one-fourth of the original volume within several hours and to smaller volumes overnight. A variation of this method is to add the protein solution to the *inside* of the dialysis tubing and to suspend this in a 20–30% solution of polyvinylpyrrolidine until it has been concentrated to a suitable level.

Rapid concentration within definite volume limitations may be achieved by adding molecular sieve materials like Sephadex or Bio-Gel P directly to the protein solution until a thick suspension is formed. The water regain rate per gram of dry gel can be determined from charts furnished by the manufacturers. The slurry may then be filtered or centrifuged to recover the concentrated protein that, again, has not suffered any essential change in ionic condition during removal of water.

Pressure dialysis, whereby protein solution inside a dialysis sac enclosed in a supporting cloth web is subjected to high internal pressure against a suitable dialyzing solution may also be used to concentrate conjugates (381). This method requires a source of nitrogen or other gas under pressure and lacks the convenience of the dialysis methods described above.

II. RHODAMINE DERIVATIVES

The desirability of having available protein labels fluorescing in different colors was recognized from the very beginning. Such reagents could facilitate simultaneous studies of more than one antigen in the same smear or section, and provide flexibility in the study of antigen–antibody reactions in general. The only feasible direction in which to move to provide a contrast color to fluorescein and to blue autofluorescence of tissues was toward the longer wavelength end of the spectrum, and thus red-fluorescing compounds were investigated. Only two of the many such compounds tested have proven useful. Both are derivatives of rhodamine, which is closely related chemically to fluorescein.

A. Rhodamine Isocyanate and Isothiocyanate

1. SYNTHESIS AND GENERAL CHARACTERISTICS

Silverstein (985) and Chadwick *et al.* (124) labeled proteins with tetraethylrhodamine isocyanate, but found the conjugates either difficult to reproduce or of an unsatisfactory level of fluorescence. Hiramoto *et al.* (447) synthesized tetramethylrhodamine isocyanate and obtained successful conjugations. However, the introduction about the same time of the more stable isothiocyanate derivative of tetraethylrhodamine (908) quickly suppressed interest in the previous unstable isocyanates. At the present time, tetramethylrhodamine iso-thiocyanate (MRITC) (Fig. 23) is available commercially from Baltimore Biological Laboratory (996). There are no data compar-ing the relative merits of the ethyl and methyl derivatives as protein labels.

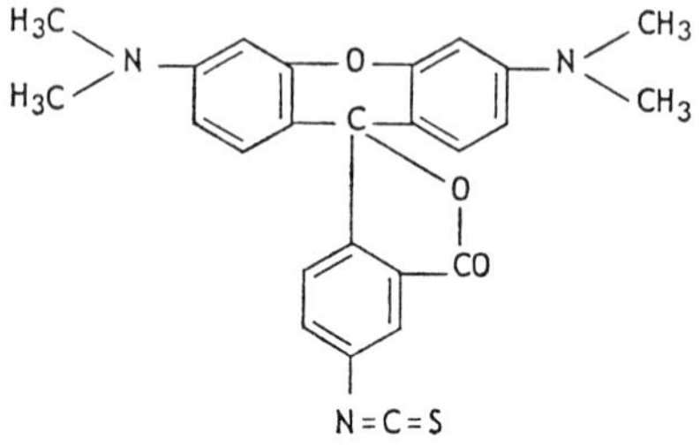

TETRAMETHYLRHODAMINE
ISOTHIOCYANATE

FIG. 23.   Structural formula for tetramethylrhodamine isothiocyanate.

MRITC is synthesized by converting 4-nitrophthalic acid to the anhydride, reacting this with *m*-dimethylaminophenol to produce nitrorhodamine, reducing this by catalytic hydrogenation to amino-rhodamine, and finally converting the amine to the isothiocyanate with thiophosgene (447, 908). The final product is a magenta mixture of two isomers whose solutions show bright orange–red fluorescence. Stability of the powder upon dry storage appears to be comparable to that of FITC.

2.   LABELING WITH TETRAMETHYLRHODAMINE ISOTHIOCYANATE

Since the isothiocyanate radical for coupling to protein is the same as in FITC, it is assumed that the same protein sites are involved. Both the crude dye or its chromatographically separated isomers have been used. Reaction conditions are the same as for fluorescein and method (a) above may be followed. Conjugation through a dialysis sac, method (b), has not yet been reported for MRITC but would seem to be feasible. Unreacted dye is removed as for fluorescein.

B. Lissamine Rhodamine B 200 Sulfonyl Chloride (RB 200SC)

1. SYNTHESIS AND GENERAL CHARACTERISTICS

The parent substance for this compound is lissamine rhodamine B 200 (Fig. 24), a commercial dye (C.I. 748) that is stable upon shelf storage without special precautions. Reaction with PCl_5 produces the sulfonyl chloride derivative that Chadwick *et al.* (124)

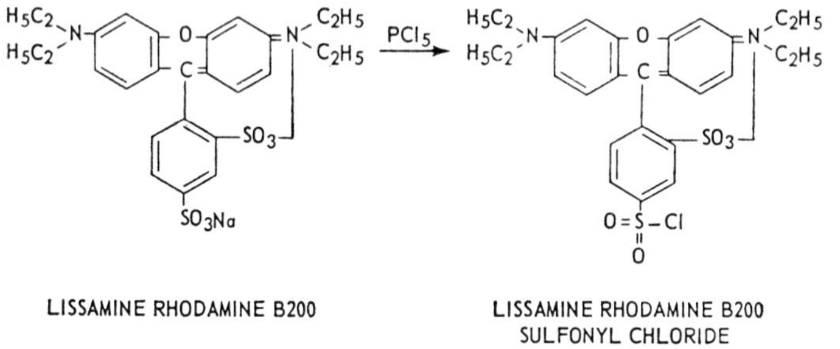

FIG. 24. Preparation of the sulfonyl chloride derivative of lissamine rhodamine B 200.

were able to introduce into proteins to produce orange–red fluorescing conjugates of adequate intensity for microscopic work.

RB 200SC is unstable in the presence of moisture but remains reactive for at least 1 year when stored as an acetone solution in sealed ampules at $-15°C$. (9). In common with the compounds discussed previously, the commercial dye is impure and shows different fluorescence spectra with different excitation wavelengths (321, 419). Nevertheless, it consists predominantly of an orange-fluorescing compound with a peak absorption in the yellow region. Indirect evidence based on other compounds bearing the sulfonyl chloride radical again points to the ε- and α-amino groups of protein chains as the major sites of reaction, with accessible sulfhydryl groups also taking part (1017) (Fig. 25). Labeling conditions are essentially the same as for the isothiocyanates, with a special requirement for strong alkaline buffering capacity in the reaction mixture to compensate for the acidity of PCl_5 used in preparing the sulfonyl chloride, and for the chloride released by the dye during conjugation. The dye is available in the sulfonyl chloride form adsorbed on Celite for ultra-rapid labeling (909, 910).

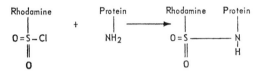

FIG. 25. Conjugation of rhodamine to protein by means of the sulfonyl chloride–amine linkage.

2. LABELING WITH RB 200SC [ADAPTED FROM CHADWICK AND FOTHERGILL (122)]

1.   RB 200 (0.5 gm) is ground thoroughly in a mortar with fresh PCl₅ (1.0 gm), under a fume hood for about 5 min.

2.   Dry acetone (5.0 ml) is added and the slurry mixed for an additional 5 min.

3.   The mixture is filtered through paper to recover the sulfonyl chloride–acetone solution. Sediment containing inert filler and un-reacted dye is discarded. The solution may be stored for as long as 48 hr in a stoppered container at room temperature.

4.   Protein solution containing 20–60 mg/ml is diluted with two volumes of 0.5M carbonate buffer, pH 9.5, and the solution is chilled in an ice bath.

5.   RB 200SC in acetone solution is added slowly over a period of 15 min., in proportions of 0.1 ml/60 mg of protein. Alkalinity of the reaction mixture should be spot-checked with litmus paper and more buffer added if necessary. The mixture is stirred gently for an additional 30 min.

6.   Removal of unreacted dye and further processing is carried out as described for fluorescein.

III. 1-DIMETHYLAMINONAPHTHALENE-5-SULFONYL CHLORIDE (DANSC)

1.   SYNTHESIS AND GENERAL CHARACTERISTICS

Prior to introduction of the stable isothiocyanate derivative of fluorescein there was considerable interest in developing other fluorescent labels, not necessarily differing in color, but which would be more stable than FIC and easier to prepare. Weber (1109) had prepared fluorescent protein conjugates with the sulfonyl chloride derivate of 1-dimethylaminonaphthalene-5-sulfonic acid for his studies of fluorescence polarization, and Clayton (146) had reported briefly on use of such a conjugate as an immunohistological stain. Thus, although this dye, with its yellow fluorescence, was of little use as a contrast stain to fluorescein, it was studied as a general substitute or replacement for FIC. With the advent of FITC, the use of DANSC had to be justified on grounds other than stability. One of these was the claimed reduction in non-specific staining as compared to fluores-

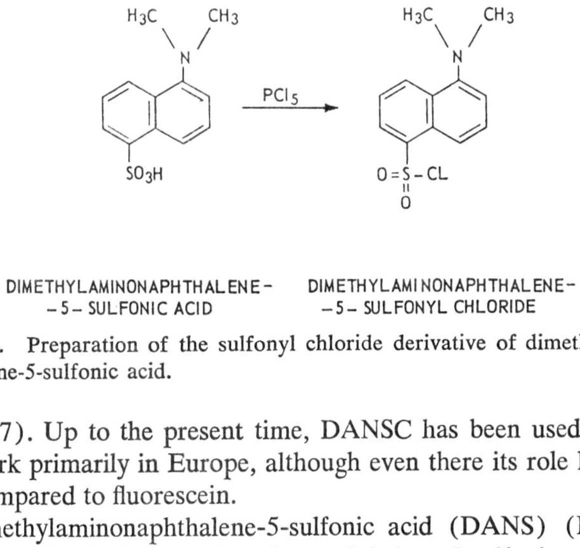

DIMETHYLAMINONAPHTHALENE-
—5— SULFONIC ACID

DIMETHYLAMINONAPHTHALENE-
—5— SULFONYL CHLORIDE

FIG. 26.   Preparation of the sulfonyl chloride derivative of dimethylamino-naphthalene-5-sulfonic acid.

cein (697). Up to the present time, DANSC has been used in antibody work primarily in Europe, although even there its role has been small compared to fluorescein.

1-Dimethylaminonaphthalene-5-sulfonic acid (DANS) (Fig. 26) may be synthesized from 1-aminonaphthalene-5-sulfonic acid and methyl iodide reacting under pressure in a bomb tube (Fussgänger's procedure), or by methylation of the aminonaphthalene sulfonic acid with dimethyl sulfate at atmospheric pressure (608, 697). The stable sulfonic acid thus formed is converted to DANSC by grinding DANS with PCl_5 in a mortar, washing the resulting melt exhaustively with cold water, extracting with acetone, and finally precipitating DANSC by dilution of the acetone solution with water (608, 697, 1109).

The yellow or orange crystals of DANSC are almost insoluble in water and can be kept over $CaCl_2$ for months without apparent deterioration. They are readily soluble in organic solvents such as acetone, ethanol, and dioxane, and react readily with ammonia and aliphatic amines (1109). DANSC is available commercially from Calbiochem.

By reacting DANSC with a series of amino acids under conditions comparable to those used for labeling proteins, Hartley and Massey (423) demonstrated that strong binding took place with ε- and α-amino groups, with the thiol group of cysteine, and with the phenolic group of tyrosine. Interestingly, the fluorescence color produced by these small-molecule conjugates was blue–green for the cysteine conjugate although yellow for all the others. Reaction conditions are similar to those used for fluorescein and rhodamine compounds with the special requirement of keeping the concentration of DANSC below a certain maximum level. DANSC in water–acetone solutions occurs as finely dispersed particles which may agglomerate into crystals if limiting concentrations are exceeded. Since reaction with protein occurs most efficiently with the dispersed particles, it is advantageous to adjust the reaction mixture to minimize crystal formation. Volume relationships in the conjugation procedure below are adjusted to keep the concentration of DANSC below 0.5 mg/ml of reaction mixture.

2.   LABELING WITH DANSC [ADAPTED FROM MAYERSBACH (697) AND ALBRECHT AND SOKOL (6)]

1.   Determine the concentration of protein in the solution to be labeled and adjust to 10–20 mg/ml with saline.

2.   To the chilled protein add $0.5M$ carbonate buffer, pH 9.5, to twice the volume of protein used.

3.   Prepare a solution of DANSC in dry acetone according to the following specifications: Amount of DANSC computed on the basis of 50 μg of dye/mg of protein; volume of acetone computed as 5% of the volume of protein–buffer solution, but not to exceed 1.0 ml.

4.   Drip the DANSC–acetone solution into the protein slowly over a 15-min period with gentle shaking.

5.   Allow reaction to proceed in the cold overnight or until the milkiness clears; no stirring.

6.   Centrifuge to remove undissolved sulfonyl chloride and remove supernatant for further processing as described for fluorescein.

TABLE XIII

UNCOMMON FLUORESCENT DYES FORMING USEFUL CONJUGATES WITH PROTEINS

Name	Fluorescence color	Reactive group[a]	Source	Reference	Remarks
Aminorosamine B (2,6-tetraethyldiamino-9-phenylxanthene amine)	Orange, changes to yellow after 5 min no fading	IC, ITC, N≡N	Laboratory synthesis	78	Fluorescent at pH 3, which is too low for most work
Anthracene	Blue	IC	Laboratory synthesis	186	Color poor for tissue work
Calcein	Yellow–green	Sulfonyl chloride	Laboratory synthesis	125	Less intense than fluorescein
Fluolite C	Blue	Sulfonyl chloride	Imperial Chemical Industries	124	Color poor for tissue work
Lissamine flavine FFS	Blue–green	Sulfonyl chloride	Imperial Chemical Industries	124	Color poor for tissue work
Lissamine rhodamine GS	Orange–yellow	Sulfonyl chloride	Imperial Chemical Industries	124	Fluorescence less than that of RB 200
Triazine chloride dyes	Various possible	Chloride	Imperial Chemical Industries	438	Chadwick and Nairn (125) could not obtain useful conjugates with two members of this group

TABLE XIII (continued)

Name	Fluorescence color	Reactive group[a]	Source	Reference	Remarks
2,2',4-Trihydroxy-4'-aminoazobenzene	Yellow	ITC	Laboratory synthesis	266	Requires chelation for fluorescence
3-Hydroxypyrene-5,8,10-trisulfonic acid	Yellow–green	Sulfonyl chloride	Laboratory synthesis	125, 1074	Good possibilities because of absorption curve at pH 7

[a] IC, isocyanate; ITC, isothiocyanate; N $\equiv$ N, diazonium.

IV. MISCELLANEOUS DYES

A number of fluorescent dyes other than those described above have been tested for possible use as protein labels. Table XIII lists dyes from which fluorescent conjugates have been prepared, but which have not enjoyed widespread acceptance because of not being commercially available, showing poor color, or for other reasons indicated in the column headed Remarks.

Other dyes whose conjugates have been tested and shown to be quite useless for staining purposes are: alizarin S, brilliant-sulfoflavin, geranin, thioflavin S, thiazinrot, and sulfoacridin-orange (1074); aminoeosin, aminorhodamine B, 3-phenyl-7-isocyanatocumarin, 5-carboxyethyl aminoacridine, and R 4388 (124); and glycine or taurine derivatives of fluorescein, and a dichlorocyclopropyl derivative of a stilbenesulfonic acid (125).

V. DOUBLE LABELING

Preparation of conjugated proteins carrying more than one type of label has been reported, but the technique appears still to be in its infancy. Vazquez and Dixon (1085) introduced ^{131}I into fluorescein-tagged globulin in an effort to obtain quantitative data on the antigen–antibody reaction that was being visualized by fluorescence. Jackson (488) labeled antisera with diiodofluorescein isocyanate into which ^{131}I had been introduced, also for purposes of quantitation. Distribution by electron micrography and light microscopy of the same antibody is possible by double labeling with fluorescein and mercury (840, 841), or with ferritin (471).

None of these procedures is well enough characterized to warrant detailed description at this point, and the original papers should be consulted for further information.

VI. FLUORESCENT COUNTERSTAINS

Counterstaining fluorescein-stained sections or organisms is often desirable in order to quench non-specific green fluorescence and heighten contrast between specific staining and background. Serum albumin (993) or the enzyme papain (9), labeled with one of the rhodamine derivatives described above, have been used for this purpose. They may be prepared by the same methods used for labeling globulin [Smith *et al.* (993) add 0.5% phenol to the protein before labeling]. The fluorescence color of those conjugates is orange and similar to that of globulin conjugates.

Hall and Hansen (412) screened a series of 2,2'-dihydroxyazo dyes that form fluorescent chelates with aluminum, for possible use as

TABLE XIV

DYES FORMING FLUORESCENT CHELATES USEFUL AS COUNTERSTAINS

Dye	Color index (first edition numbers)	Fluorescence color	Source[a]
1. Acid Alizarin Garnet R	168	Yellow	Du Pont
2. Pontachrome Violet SW	169	Yellow	Du Pont
3. Superchrome Blue B Extra	202	Cherry red	National Aniline
4. Eriochrome Black A	204	Orange	Geigy
5. Diamond Red ECB	652	Orange–yellow	General Aniline
6. Flazo Orange	—	Orange–red	Du Pont

[a] Nutritional Biochemicals, Inc. markets the entire series of dyes.

counterstains. Table XIV lists six suitable dyes, as well as their sources and fluorescence colors. Staining for 1–3 min is performed with dilutions of stock solutions of chelated dyes that are prepared as follows: 1.7×10^{-5} mole of dye is dissolved in 1 ml of N,N-dimethylformamide, and 5 ml of chelating reagent is added slowly with shaking. The composition of the chelating agent is N,N-dimethylformamide, 50 ml; distilled water, 20 ml; $0.1M$ aluminum chloride 10 ml; and $1M$ acetic acid; 10 ml. The reagent is adjusted to pH 5.2 with $1M$ sodium hydroxide and made up to 100 ml with distilled water.

Simple counterstains that provide deep red fluorescence are Congo red (C.I. 22120) and Evans blue (C.I. 23860) (792). These commercially available dyes are employed in aqueous solutions of about 0.01% to 0.005% concentration, depending upon the material being stained. Because of its color and simplicity of use, Evans blue is my own choice of counterstain under ordinary conditions.

BIBLIOGRAPHY

Cebra, J. J., and Goldstein, G. (1965). Chromatographic purification of tetramethylrhodamine-immune globulin conjugates and their use in the cellular localization of rabbit γ-globulin polypeptide chains. *J. Immunol.* **95**: 230-245.

Dedmon, R. E., Holmes, A. W., and Deinhardt, F. (1965). Preparation of fluorescein isothiocyanate-labeled γ-globulin by dialysis, gel filtration, and ion-exchange chromatography in combination. *J. Bacteriol.* **89**: 734-739.

Nairn, R. C. (1962). "Fluorescent Protein Tracing." Williams & Wilkins, Baltimore, Maryland.

Wood, B. T., Thompson, S. H., and Goldstein, G. (1965). Fluorescent antibody staining. III. Preparation of fluorescein-isothiocyanate-labeled antibodies. *J Immunol.* **95**: 225-229.

Chapter Eight

PROPERTIES OF CONJUGATED SERA

I. DEGREE OF CONJUGATION

A. General Comments

The most significant parameter of a labeled serum compared to the parent substance is the number of dye moieties attached per protein molecule, all other characteristics being influenced by this underlying physical fact. Relative data concerning degree of conjugation are readily obtained by relating absorption or fluorescence of conjugates, in arbitrary terms, to protein concentration. Such information can be very useful to individual laboratories in comparing staining capacities and other characteristics of conjugates prepared under similar or different conditions. However, absolute data concerning degree of labeling are more difficult to ascertain because of the uncertainty concerning absorption and fluorescence characteristics of dyes attached to large protein molecules. Absorption maxima tend to shift toward longer wavelengths when free dyes are bound to protein, and extinction coefficients change. A thorough discussion of these problems as they relate to fluorescein conjugates is given by Jobbagy and Kiraly (500).

Goldman and Carver (375) demonstrated that free FITC (not purified) passed quantitatively through a dialysis sac over a period of 16 days, and that the amount in the dialyzate could be determined by absorption measurements, with FITC solutions as reference standards. They then determined the amount of FITC bound to protein in a labeling experiment by calculating the difference between dye passing out in dialysis and the original amount of FITC added to the protein. This value was about 25% higher than the value determined by direct absorptiometry on the conjugate itself, using FITC as a standard. This suggests that the extinction of bound FITC was lower than that of free dye. In contrast, the greater absorbance of aminofluorescein and of purified fluorescein, both sometimes used as standards for establishing the fluorescein content of labeled protein, rendered them entirely inadequate as direct reference standards for FITC conjugates.

These results, based on impure FITC samples, were confirmed in principle by McKinney *et al.* (711) who determined extinction coefficients for purified aminofluorescein in alkaline solution, and for purified FITC bound to protein. The latter values were determined by passing an FITC–protein reaction mixture through Sephadex and subtracting the amount of free dye eluted from the column from the amount added to the protein. The optical density of the labeled protein was then divided by the calculated concentration of bound dye. The extinction coefficient of aminofluorescein in $0.1N$ NaOH (expressed as optical density of 1 µg/ml in a 1-cm cell) was found to be 0.250, and that of FITC bound to protein 0.176–0.190. It followed from these results that fluorescein/protein (F/P) ratios based on McKinney's fluorescein or aminofluorescein reference standards were also about 25% lower than true values.

Similar studies by Wells *et al.* (1115) and Jobbagy and Kiraly (500) have confirmed that the extinction maximum of FITC bound to protein is about 24–30% lower than that of the free dye or of fluorescein.

McKinney *et al.* recommended that purified FITC be taken as an absolute reference standard for FITC conjugates, but it is not clear that the pure dye is really suitable for conjugates prepared from impure commercial samples. Frommhagen and Spendlove (337) showed that "degradation products" of FITC, which possessed an orange hue, coupled with serum proteins in the same manner as undegraded FITC. Pure FITC, lacking this component, may thus yield erroneous absolute F/P values. In addition, three out of four crude commercial samples of FITC tested by McKinney *et al.* possessed extinction coefficients which were closer to that of protein-bound pure FITC than the purified reference compounds. Jobbagy and Kiraly recommended purified fluorescein as a reference standard, with appropriate corrections for differences in molecular weight and extinction maxima compared to FITC.

Although the foregoing has been concerned only with the fluorescein label, similar considerations must undoubtedly affect proteins tagged with rhodamine or DANS. In the latter instance, for exam-

ple, Weber (1109) ascribed a molar extinction coefficient of 4.3 ×
$10^6 cm^2$/mole to protein-bound DANS, based upon extinction of the
sulfonamide formed by reacting DANSC with ammonia. However,
Hartley and Massey (423) determined the extinction of bound DANS
to be 3.3 × $10^6 cm^2$/mole, or about 25% lower than Weber's figure,
based upon the difference between the amount of DANSC offered
to proteins and the amount dialyzing freely from the reaction mixture.

Fluorimetric determinations on conjugates are useful as a guide to
staining potential of labeled proteins which, after all, are detected by
fluorescence and not by absorption. However, determination of absolute dye content by fluorimetry is beset by even more uncertainties
than absorptiometry. Differences in fluorescence efficiency with varying loads of dye per protein, instability of fluorescence in reference
standards, and possible changes in fluorescence spectra upon binding
to proteins are added complications to the intrinsically more demanding techniques of quantitative fluorimetry.

B. Determination of Relative and Absolute Dye Concentrations of Conjugates

Relative dye concentrations of conjugates are readily determined
by reading optical density of suitable dilutions of conjugate at the
absorption maximum of the free dye, and relating this to the density
of known, standard concentrations of free dye by means of the equation:

$$\text{Conc. of dye in conjugate} = \frac{\text{Conc. standard} \times \text{OD conjugate}}{\text{OD standard}}$$

In the case of RB 200 and DANS, if the sulfonic acids are taken as
standards, concentrations so determined in micrograms per milliliter
need to be multiplied by the factor 0.93 to compensate for the lower
molecular weights of the attached dyes. This results from the split-
ting off of an oxygen molecule during formation of the sulfonyl chloride from the sulfonic acid. Table XV presents absorption maxima
that have been found by various authors for the four main protein
labels, but this information should be taken only as a general guide.
In any individual laboratory precise maxima may vary depending
upon the batch of dye and instrumentation. Molecular weights are

indicated for those wishing to prepare reference standards in terms of molarity. Because of the fact that pH and the nature of the ionic environment may affect absorption measurements, conjugate dilutions and standards should be made up in the same medium. Phosphate-buffered saline, pH 7.5, 0.01M, is a convenient diluent since in many cases the conjugate will have already been equilibrated against this buffer. Solutions of FITC in phosphate-buffered saline have shown stable absorbance for 3 years in our laboratory when stored at 5°C, providing reliable standards for conjugates prepared from the same batch of dye over a long period of time.

TABLE XV

ABSORPTION MAXIMA AND MOLECULAR WEIGHTS
OF THE MOST WIDELY USED FLUORESCENT LABELS FOR PROTEINS

Dye	Molecular weight	Absorption maximum	Concentration for absorption measurements (μg/ml)
FITC	389	490-495	2–5
MRITC	444	536-550	2–5
RB 200 (Na salt)	580 (541 for the attached dye)	564-575	2–5
DANS	251 (235 for the attached dye)	300-360	10

To determine *absolute* dye content of a conjugated protein it is necessary to take into consideration the different absorption maxima of free and bound dyes, and the change in extinction coefficients. Absorption maxima can be determined readily in the individual laboratory, and although extinction coefficients are more difficult to obtain, it is only necessary to know the ratio of the coefficients for free and bound dye in order to determine bound dye concentration. In the case of FITC, maximum absorbance is at about 490 mμ for unbound dye in pH 7.5 buffer, and at about 496 mμ for the dye bound to protein, in the same buffer; the extinction of bound FITC in a concentration of 1 μg/ml at pH 7.2 is about 0.15 (1115) and is approximately 75% of the extinction of free dye in the same concentration (500, 1115). Thus, absolute FITC content can be solved for by the following equation:

Conc. bound FITC (μg/ml) =

$$\frac{\text{Conc. free FITC standard (μg/ml)} \times \text{OD}_{496} \text{ conjugate}}{\text{OD}_{490} \text{ FITC standard} \times 0.75}$$

The above computation applies when purified FITC is used both for labeling and as a standard. If crude FITC is used, the computed concentration cannot be regarded as absolute because of the unknown and probably varying relationships between the absorbances of the free and bound dyes.

C. Determination of Protein Concentration of Conjugates

Any of the general methods for protein determination may be used for labeled proteins provided that, in the colorimetric techniques, due attention is paid to absorption characteristics of the label involved. The biuret method (393) may be used for fluorescein conjugates, in which case absorption is read at 540–565 mμ (386, 444, 500) instead of the usual 520 mμ. Reading at the longer wavelengths avoids the contribution from fluorescein to the optical density of the reaction mixture. The method is also suitable for DANS conjugates since DANS does not absorb in that region, but it cannot be applied to rhodamine conjugates, which absorb most strongly between 500 and 600 mμ. For proteins labeled with rhodamine the nesslerization method has been recommended (321).

A colorimetric technique which is suitable for all conjugates is the Folin–copper method of Lowry *et al.* (656). Maximum absorbance of the colored reaction product is at about 750 mμ, but the broad nature of the absorption band allows sensitive readings to be made starting at about 600 mμ. This technique has the additional advantage of being applicable to protein concentrations as low as 50 μg/ml, compared to about 1500 μg/ml for the biuret. The extra sensitivity is valuable in determining fluorescein/protein ratios on small volumes of dilute fractions eluted from columns such as DEAE-cellulose.

Absorption at 280 mμ may be used for protein determinations of fluorescein and rhodamine conjugates, after correcting for absorption of the dyes at that wavelength. For example, since the ratio of the absorbance of conjugated FITC at 280 and 496 mμ has been reported as 0.35–0.38 (500, 1141), and since the absorbance of globulin at 280 mμ is 1.4 for 1 mg/ml in a 1-cm cuvette, protein concentration of FITC conjugates can be determined by ultraviolet absorption as follows:

$$\text{Conc. of FITC–protein (mg/ml)} = \frac{OD_{280} - (0.36 \times OD_{496})}{1.4}$$

In spite of the high extinction of DANS in the ultraviolet, Sokol *et al.* (1002) have described an absorption method for DANS conjugates involving readings at 278 and 315 mμ maxima for protein and DANS, respectively.

The Kjeldahl method for nitrogen determination, or one of the micromodifications, represents the most standard technique for proteins in general and is applicable as well to labeled proteins. However, it is not a convenient procedure to set up for intermittent use on just a few samples.

D. Dye/Protein Ratios

The ratio of dye to protein in a conjugate may be calculated from the values determined for each separately by any of the methods described above. Wells *et al.* (1115) have published a nomograph from which FITC and protein concentrations and F/P ratios can be derived solely on the basis of absorbance of conjugates at 276 and 493 mμ (Fig. 27). Approximate conversions of dye/protein ratios from a weight to molar basis or the reverse can be made with the

TABLE XVI

CONVERSION OF DYE/PROTEIN RATIOS FROM A MOLAR
TO WEIGHT BASIS OR THE REVERSE

1[a]	2	3
FITC	2.4	0.41
MRITC	2.8	0.36
RB 200	3.4	0.29
DANS	1.5	0.67

[a] To convert molar dye/globulin ratios to micrograms of dye per milligram of globulin, multiply by figures in column 2; for the reverse, multiply by figures in column 3.

factors given in Table XVI. The factors are based on a molecular weight for globulin of 160,000 and the weights indicated for the respective dyes on Table XV.

Fluorescein/protein ratios on whole conjugates reflect the *average*

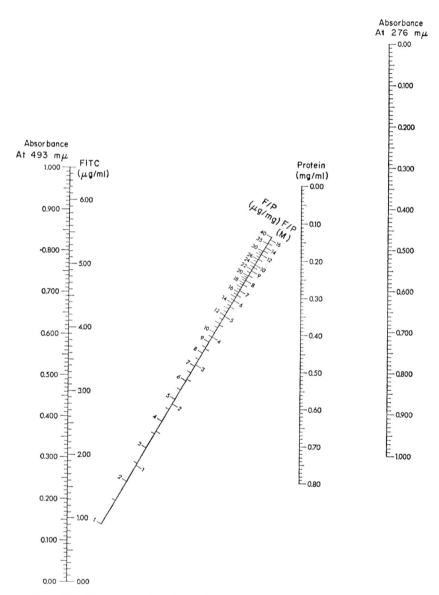

Fig. 27. Nomograph for determination of FITC and protein in FITC-globulin conjugates [after Wells *et al.* (115)].

load of fluorescein per protein molecule, but do not reveal the heterogeneity of the molecular population. The different mobility patterns of labeled globulins in electric fields, and their elution characteristics from DEAE columns show that globulins labeled by methods now available invariably consist of a spectrum of molecular species, so far as the FITC load is concerned (212, 214, 337, 381, 706, 907). Table XVII shows the range of F/P ratios obtained in fractions eluted from DEAE columns following various labeling procedures.

TABLE XVII

HETEROGENEITY OF GLOBULINS LABELED WITH FITC
AS REVEALED BY DEAE-CELLULOSE CHROMATOGRAPHY

Labeling method[a]	FITC Offered (μg/mg protein)	Molar F/P ratio of conjugated globulin[b]				Reference
		Orig-inal	Fract. I	Fract. II	Fract. III	
(1) (a)	8	2.1	1.4	2.7	3.4	381
(2) (a)	10	0.98	0.25	—	1.4	382
(3) (a)	20	7.0	2.1	4.1	5.3	381
(4) (a)	25-50	4.0	1.0	2.0	6.1	706
(5) (b)	—	2.6	0.46	2.2	4.6	Goldman, unpublished
(6) (b)	—	3.1	1.4	3.2	8.2	Goldman, unpublished

[a] (a) = FITC added directly to the protein solution; (b) — protein labeled through dialysis sac.

[b] In all cases fractions were eluted from DEAE-cellulose columns with increasing salt concentrations; precise details differed in each laboratory.

The average number of fluorescein moieties introduced per globulin molecule may vary from less than 1.0 to as many as 22, depending upon reaction conditions. There appears to be general agreement that an average molar ratio of about 1.5–4 is optimal for fluorescein in situations where non-specific staining may pose a problem. Below this level staining intensity may be too low, and above it (say at ratios above 10) antibody inactivation and high non-specific staining may vitiate the usefulness of the conjugate. However, I have found that if antibody activity of the conjugate is high enough, DEAE fractions with molar ratios as low as 0.4 may stain brilliantly and with great specificity when used in dilutions containing about 1 mg of protein/ml. Conversely, fractions or whole conjugates with high molar ratios may still be usable if taken in high dilutions, say, about 0.1 mg of protein/ml or less.

Information concerning degree of conjugation with serum proteins when dyes other than fluorescein are used is considerably more limited. For DANS, molar ratios of 1–9 have been reported (6, 895, 1109); for RB 200 the figure is about 3 (124). Binding rates of albumin with DANS are about twice as high as for γ-globulin (895).

E. Kinetics of Labeling

The degree to which proteins become labeled with FITC increases with reaction time. This is true for temperatures between 5° and 35°C, and for dye to protein offerings ranging from 6 to 100 μg/mg. Table XVIII presents data covering the more common labeling conditions and based upon purified FITC. Aside from the lower rate reported by McKinney *et al.* (711), it appears that under common labeling conditions (FITC: protein offering, 25 μg/mg; reaction temperature, 5°C) some 60–80% of maximum binding takes place within the first 6 hr. The proportion of offered FITC (purified) that reacts with globulin after overnight exposure at 5°C has been variously reported as from 20 to 86% (381, 397, 706, 711). A value of 50–60% is probably most common. The proportion combining after 1–2 hr at 25°C is approximately the same (568, 711). Lower or higher ratios of dye to protein can be attained by decreasing or increasing the amount of dye offered, and by shortening or extending reaction times.

Critical information for reactions in which crude FITC is used are scarce, but indications are that such samples are about half as reactive, *in toto*, as the crystalline product. The reported range for the proportion of FITC offered which reacts with globulin is 12–54% (94, 321, 337, 375, 381, 444, 628, 1003, 1062). With the usual methods of conjugation, 20–30% may be taken as the expected value.

McKinney *et al.* (711) found that rabbit and bovine α-globulins reacted with FITC at a faster rate than horse α-globulins. In all three species, albumin fractions reacted much more rapidly than γ-globulin. The reaction rate of rabbit γ-globulin was higher at protein concentrations of 25 mg/ml than at 5 mg/ml, although final levels reached after 4 hr at 25°C were about the same.

Conjugation with RB 200 increases linearly with increased dye

TABLE XVIII

EFFECT OF REACTION TIME AND TEMPERATURE ON DEGREE OF CONJUGATION WITH FITC

Reaction Temperature (°C)	µg FITC offered/ mg protein	Reaction period in hours										Reference
		0.5		1		2–3		6		18–24		
		a[a]	b[b]	a	b	a	b	a	b	a	b	
5	12.5	75%	2.7	108%	3.9	—	—	95%	3.4	100%	3.6	397
5	20–25	65	4.1	65	4.1	—	—	84	5.3	100	6.3	397
5	20–25	—	—	17	0.39	23%	0.55	—	—	100	2.3	711
5	20–25	—	—	—	—	61	4.3	—	—	100	7.1	381
5	40–50	55	5.9	58	6.2	32	3.2	69	7.4	100	10.3	397
5	40–50	—	—	—	—	52	3.3	60	6.0	100	10.0	568
25	25	—	—	36	2.3	—	—	—	—	100	6.3	711
25	40	—	—	—	9.2	—	—	—	—	—	—	568

[a] a = Percentage of maximum labeling obtained.
[b] b = Molar F/P ratio of conjugate.

offered, and the reaction is essentially complete within 30 min at 0°–2°C (122). According to the same authors, conjugation with DANS is 75% complete within 2 hr and 100% after 6 hr.

II. PHYSICAL PROPERTIES OF CONJUGATES

The most obvious physical change that serum proteins undergo upon conjugation with fluorescein or rhodamine derivatives is the acquisition of color. DANS conjugates are essentially colorless because their absorption is primarily in the far ultraviolet. Grossly, color and fluorescence of conjugates are similar to that of the free dye, but absorption and emission spectra may differ in details. Reliable, quantitative spectral data are not easily obtained, and information in the literature is often not directly comparable. Intrinsic deficiencies of spectrophotometers and spectrofluorometers include uneven output of light sources and uneven response of of photodetector tubes. As a result, uncorrected spectra are difficult to compare except within the same laboratory. For this reason, too, one sometimes encounters absorption maxima given as different from excitation maxima, although according to fluorescence theory the two should be the same. The sensitivity of some dyes to pH, in particular, introduces an additional difficulty in comparing reports from different authors.

A. Fluorescein

Absorption spectra for FITC, globulin, and FITC-labeled globulin at pH 7.2 are shown in Fig. 28. Spectra for free sodium fluorescein and FIC conjugates at the same pH are the same within experimental limits (955). The spectra show a major fluorescein peak in the visible at 490 mμ (489–495 mμ according to other reports), minor ones around 280 and 321, and a protein peak around 280 mμ. The conjugate shows maxima in both regions. Some authors (386, 419, 955) find that the visible maximum of fluorescein conjugates shifts to a slightly longer wavelength compared to the free dye. A shift of this sort has no significance for qualitative work, but it may introduce a 10–15% error into quantitative determinations based on the maximum for the free dye only. Although the shape of the absorption curve for FITC does not change upon conjugation, the extinction

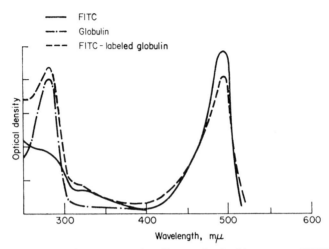

FIG. 28. Absorption spectra for fluorescein isothiocyanate (FITC), un-labeled globulin, and FITC-labeled globulin in alkaline solution [after Hinuma *et al.* (444)].

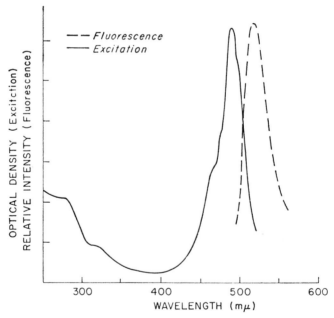

FIG. 29. Excitation and fluorescence spectra of FITC-labeled globulin in alkaline, aqueous solution [after Hansen (419)].

coefficient (optical density of 1 μg/ml in a 1-cm cell at 489 mμ) was found by McKinney *et al.* (711) to be reduced from 0.219 to 0.183 in 0.1*N* NaOH solution.

Excitation and fluorescence spectra for FITC conjugates are similar in shape to those for free dye (Fig. 29), with an emission peak at 517 mμ, but fluorescence efficiency decreases upon binding to protein as the fluorescein load increases (1003) (Fig. 30). Globulin labeled with an average of 23.8 fluorescein residues per protein molecule was only 10% as fluorescent as free dye (375); with half that load,

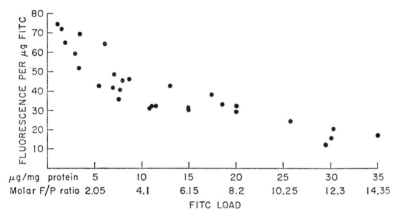

Fig. 30. Decreasing fluorescence emission per microgram of fluorescein in proteins carrying increasing loads of FITC.

efficiency was about 20% of free dye (unpublished data). Both absorbance and emission of FITC conjugates increase about 30% with increasing pH from 6 to 9 (282, 568, 1017).

Fluorescein–globulin conjugates show decreased solubility compared to native protein, proportional to the load of dye. Protein solutions that have remained in solution during conjugation, when the pH is high, sometimes develop precipitate upon dialysis against buffer of pH 7.0–7.5. There are indications that this may result from excessive labeling (335, 337, 706, 1003), and can be avoided by cutting back the amount of dye used per unit of protein in the labeling reaction. Clarified conjugates which develop a fine sediment upon storage at 5°C do not suffer any noticeable reduction in staining titer compared to the original solution.

There are no critical studies concerning stability of globulins labeled with fluorescein, but the practical experience is one of long-term immunological activity with retention of most of the label for years upon storage at 5°C or lower. Slow disassociation of fluorescein may occur upon prolonged storage (257), so that repurification to remove free dye before staining with old conjugates is desirable.

Schiller et al. (955) found that bovine serum albumins carrying an estimated load of 1.4–1.9 molecules of FIC per molecule of protein, showed either identical or only slightly different viscosity and sedimentation patterns compared to native albumins. Hinuma et al. (444) also found no difference in the sedimentation pattern of globulin labeled with FITC at a molar ratio of 4.4. These results indicate that there was no essential change in molecular configuration of the proteins at these levels of conjugation.

Each fluorescein radical introduced into a protein molecule replaces a positively charged amino group on a lysine residue with a negatively charged carboxyl group on the fluorescein molecule. This net increase of two negative charges produces marked changes in the behavior of conjugates with regard to phenomena dependent upon electric charge. Curtain (212) found that labeled γ-globulin with a molar F/P ratio of between 3 and 4 showed greater electrophoretic mobility toward the positive pole than native protein. Goldstein et al. (381) confirmed this and showed that sheep globulin, carrying 15 moles of fluorescein per mole of protein, migrated faster than another sample of the same globulin with a molar ratio of only 7.6. Both authors found that in fractionating conjugates by electrophoresis convection, the faster moving fractions invariably had higher F/P ratios than slower fractions from the same conjugates.

Fluorescein-labeled globulins exhibit stronger attachment to the anion exchange adsorbent, DEAE-cellulose, than native globulins and require higher salt concentrations for elution (907). Elution with increasing molarities of salt yield fractions with increasing F/P ratios (214, 381).

B. Rhodamine

Absorption spectra for aqueous solutions of RB 200, bovine albumin and RB 200-labeled albumin are shown in Fig. 31. They show a major RB 200 peak in the visible at about 550 mμ [564 mμ according to Hansen (419)], the usual protein peak around 280 mμ, and a slight shift toward a longer wavelength in the visible maximum for the conjugated albumin. The same shift was noted by Hansen, who also found a minor absorption peak at 352–355 mμ for both free dye and conjugate.

Excitation and emission spectra for RB 200–globulin conjugates are shown in Fig. 32. Spectra for free dye are similar except for a slight shift toward the blue. Maximum emission for conjugate is at 597 mμ, and for free dye 586 mμ. Chadwick *et al.* (124) list both

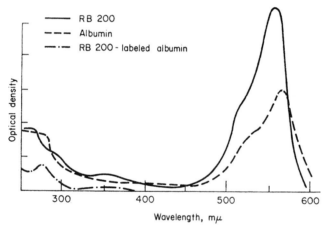

FIG. 31. Absorption spectra for lissamine rhodamine B 200 (RB 200), unlabeled albumin, and RB 200-labeled albumin [after Chadwick *et al.* (124)].

at 610 mμ. Fluorescence efficiency decreases with increasing degree of conjugation (321). At a molar ratio of RB 200 to protein of 3.4, emission is only about 30% that of free dye; at a ratio of 6.8, emission is about 20%. Fluorescence of RB 200 conjugates shows little change with pH around neutrality (321, 446).

To the extent that physical characteristics of RB 200 conjugates have been described, primarily by Fothergill (321), they appear to be similar to those found for proteins coupled with fluorescein.

Absorption and emission spectra for tetramethylrhodamine isothiocyanate (MRITC) conjugates are similar to those of RB 200, with the slight difference that the major absorption and emission peaks are shifted about 20 mμ toward the blue for MRITC (419).

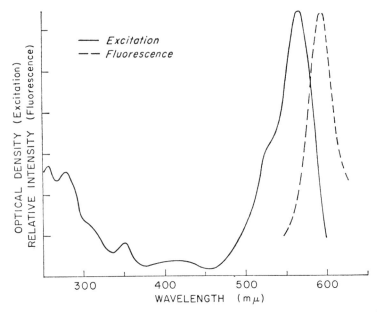

FIG. 32.   Excitation and fluorescence spectra of lissamine rhodamine B 200-globulin conjugate in alkaline, aqueous solution [after Hansen (419)].

Upon exposure to intense radiation, the fluorescence of rhodamine conjugates shifts from orange to yellow.

C. DANS

Absorption spectra for free DANS and DANS–globulin conjugate are shown in Fig. 33. Two maxima are apparent, both in or close to the far ultraviolet, with the entire spectrum for the conjugate, compared to free dye, shifted toward longer wavelengths. The short wavelength maximum, around 250 mµ, is entirely inaccessible in ordinary fluorescence microscopy; it is only the longer wavelength absorption which makes DANS useful in fluorescent antibody work. The maximum in this region is given by various authors as from 320 to 360 mµ depending upon the protein, degree of labeling, and other factors. In any case, the absorption band is broad and extends from about 300 to 420 mµ.

Excitation and emission spectra for DANS-globulin conjugates are shown in Fig. 34. As in the case of RB 200, corresponding spectra for free dye are shifted slightly to the left. Maximum emission is in the same region as for fluorescein, 528 mμ for conjugate and 511 for free DANS. Intensity of emission is relatively uniform with changing pH, increasing less than 10% between pH 6–11 (446, 1017).

Weber (1109) and Hartley and Massey (423) have provided information concerning characteristics of enzymes conjugated with DANS. If, as is likely, these attributes are applicable also to labeled antisera, then it appears that labeling at a ratio of less than 3 moles

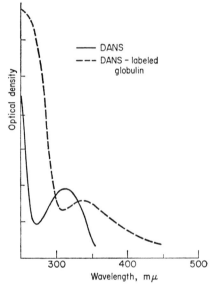

FIG. 33. Absorption spectra for dimethylaminonaphthalene-5-sulfonic acid (DANS) and DANS-labeled globulin [after Hansen (419)].

of DANS per mole of protein causes little or no change in the solubility or sedimentation properties of native sera. The bond formed by reaction of the sulfonyl chloride group of the dye with α- or ε-amino groups of amino acids is very stable, resisting hydrolysis in the presence of $2N$ NaOH or $4N$ HCl for 2–3 days (423).

Each amino group replaced by DANS results in a net charge difference on the protein molecule of −1, compared to −2 for fluorescein or rhodamine. However, there is no comparative information concerning behavior on chromatographic columns or in electric fields of the three types of conjugates.

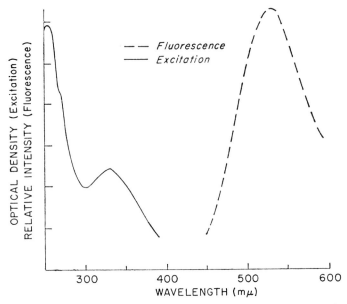

FIG. 34.   Excitation and fluorescence spectra of dimethylaminonaphthalene-5-sulfonic acid-globulin in neutral, aqueous solution [after Hansen (419)].

III. IMMUNOLOGICAL AND BIOLOGICAL PROPERTIES OF CONJUGATES

In this section we are concerned with the extent to which specific biological characteristics, such as immunological or enzymatic activity, are influenced by the labeling process. Rigorous evaluation of these parameters would require information on the possible loss of active protein by denaturation during labeling, as well as on changes in activity based upon comparable protein concentrations of conjugated and native proteins. Unfortunately, such data are rare in the literature. It is common to read that a precipitin titer was reduced, say, 4- or 8-fold after conjugation; but since a drop of this magnitude is easily accounted for by incomplete globulin removal from the original serum, and by dilution during labeling, dialysis or fractionation, such statements do not per se support the view that labeling is harmful to the protein.

First, there is considerable testimony in the literature to the fact that antibody globulins, after labeling, remain active immunologically in conventional serological procedures like hemagglutination, complement fixation, precipitin reactions, and others. Furthermore, Rossi *et al.* (923) have shown that the immunoelectrophoretic patterns of native and labeled rabbit antihuman serum albumin are identical.

Second, it appears that when titers in conventional tests with labeled and native proteins are compared on the basis of protein concentration, no evidence of selective antibody inactivation can be demonstrated (187, 188, 486, 551, 1003). This is true for FIC, FITC, RB 200, and DANS conjugates. Although only in the papers by Coons and his associates is the molar F/P ratio given, about 2, this general finding probably applies to all conjugates in the low to medium F/P range. Redetzki (895) found, too, that DANS globulin conjugates with a molar F/P ratio of 3–4, showed the same rate of antigen–antibody complex formation, and formed the same amount of precipitate as unlabeled antibody. However, Fothergill (321) found that anti-BSA labeled with RB 200 (molar $F/P = 3$) formed 30% less precipitate with bovine serum albumin (BSA) in a quantitative precipitin reaction than native anti-BSA.

With regard to other biological characteristics, specific effects of labeling appear to depend upon the activities involved, and are not readily predictable. For example, Pappenhagen *et al.* (826) found that the clotting properties of human fibrinogen were not affected by FITC labeling at a level of 16 moles of dye per mole of fibrinogen (molecular weight 400,000); at higher ratios the conjugated fibrinogen became unstable and tended to clot spontaneously. Guinea pig whole serum labeled with FIC (F/P ratio 1–2) and inoculated into guinea pigs, induced a state of sensitization to a shocking dose 3 weeks later, but labeled guinea pig albumin did not show this effect (955). Proteins conjugated with fluorescein do not show toxicity upon intravenous inoculation into rabbits, rats, and guinea pigs (775).

In contrast to the relatively mild effects of labeling cited above, Hartley and Massey (423) found that as little as one molecule of DANS per molecule of α-chymotrypsin inhibited the enzymatic activity of the protein. Halikis and Arquilla (411) found that FITC-labeled insulin was less active in reducing blood sugar in rats than native insulin. They also reported that in an insulin–anti-insulin hemagglutination system, cells sensitized with labeled insulin were less active as antigen than cells sensitized with the native hormone.

Lipase conjugated with fluorescein or with RB 200 shows an activity only 50% that of native enzyme (193). DeBarbieri and Scevola (243) found that trypsin and chymotrypsin were completely inactivated, cytochrome lost 23.5% and ribonuclease 63% of initial activity upon reaction with FIC. The antistreptolysin 0 activity of a human serum, expressed in units per milligram of protein, decreased with increasing load of FITC (1141).

Hormonal action of thyrotropin was reduced 12–34% after reaction with RB 200, reduction being proportional to degree of labeling (679). Protamine labeled with DANS showed a slightly increased latency in inducing contractions of the isolated and perfused uterus (566). Polymixin retained its antibiotic activity after conjugation with DANS (790).

Although it is generally true that antisera with high titers in conventional serology also show good staining qualities when labeled, Lewis et al. (628) obtained poor correlation between these two attributes in comparing serum fractions obtained from the same anti-Klebsiella serum by various fractionation procedures. Karakawa et al. (527) also indicated that staining titers did not necessarily parallel precipitin titers with anti-Streptococcus sera.

Chapter Nine

CYTOLOGICAL AND HISTOLOGICAL METHODS

I. FIXATION

Because of the well-known variation in sensitivity that exists among antigens with regard to different physical and chemical conditions, it might be anticipated that many different fixation methods would be necessary for staining different antigens. In point of fact, however, trial and error has demonstrated that a relatively few procedures may be drawn upon to cover essentially all the needs of fluorescent antibody technology. The methods are simplest for bacteria, fungi, and viruses in smear preparations, but are more demanding for agents and soluble antigens located in tissues.

A. Bacteria and Fungi

In this section we are concerned with fixing and staining intact or particulate agents. The staining of soluble products or extracts of microbial agents presents problems similar to those of staining indigenous antigens and will be covered in Section I, D.

A number of common fixatives have been used for smears of bacteria or fungi derived from cultures or infected tissue. These include reagents such as ethanol, methanol, acetone, formalin, phenol, dioxane, and Bouin's. However, comparisons between such reagents and simple heat fixation for *C. diphtherae* (11), *Mycoplasma* (144), *P. tularensis* (490), *P. pestis* (1136), *M. pseudomallei* (747), and *Streptococcus* (746) indicate that ordinary gentle heat fixation as commonly practiced for conventional staining is as good for fluorescent antibody work as chemical fixation. In addition to the species just indicated, a large variety of bacteria and fungi, including *B. anthracis, Leptospira, Treponema, Staphylococcus, Hemophilus, Escherichia, Salmonella, Vibrio, Candida, Histoplasma, Sporotrichium, Saccharomyces, Aspergillus, Actinomyces, Cryptococcus,* and *Blastomy-*

cosis, have been stained with specific antibody after heat fixation as the only method used. Thus, we can conclude that in this general group of agents the usual type of air-dried, heat-fixed smear is entirely adequate for fluorescent staining. This is not to deny the possibility that refined fluorimetric techniques may reveal quantitative differences between different fixation methods. But, as a practical matter it is clear that ordinary heat fixation is adequate.

It is equally clear that antigens of many bacterial and fungal agents resist denaturation by formalin and can be stained in paraffin sections of formalin-fixed tissues. This has been demonstrated for *B. anthracis* (133), *Pasteurella* (690), and *Histoplasma* (870). Information is meager on the survival time of different antigens in formalinized tissues, but in some instances organisms have been demonstrated after fixation periods of 1 year or more (133). Maestrone (665) found that treating frozen sections of formalin-fixed tissues containing *Leptospira* with 1% NH_4OH and 3% Tween-80 for a few minutes each, greatly enhanced the brightness of fluorescence following exposure to labeled antibody. The mechanism for this enhancement is not known.

In view of the uncertainty that exists concerning retention of antigenicity in the face of prolonged fixation and paraffin embedding, negative staining results in paraffin sections of suspected tissues should not be accepted as final. Frozen sections of unfixed blocks offer the best possibility of demonstrating the infectious agent with labeled antibody. Since this procedure is so widely used in connection with soluble and other antigens in tissues, the method is discussed in greater detail in the latter portion of this chapter.

Fresh or lyophilized *Treponema* dried onto slides are employed as antigen in a fluorescent antibody serologic test for syphilis. In the original procedure dried smears were heat-fixed (236). Subsequent workers have fixed dried smears in acetone for 10 min at room temperature (277, 306, 795). In such cases, where standardized procedures are important in maintaining comparability among different laboratories, it is important to follow the recommended fixation method even though other methods may appear to be qualitatively equal.

B. Viruses

Fixation of virus in tissue cultures, smears, or frozen sections is almost universally accomplished by means of acetone. Dried preparations have been stained successfully after having been dipped in acetone at temperatures ranging from 37° to −50°C, and left there from 10 min to several days before exposure to labeled antibody. There is little comparative information about the possible significance of temperature and time in the preservation of acetone-fixed viruses. Kundin and Liu (591) found undiminished antigenicity in sections containing West Nile virus that were left in acetone at room temperature for as long as 4 days. On the basis of the number of viruses studied successfully following a variety of fixation schedules using acetone, it is safe to conclude that immersion of smears or frozen sections in acetone at room temperature for 10–15 min provides adequate fixation in practically all instances. It should be pointed out, however, that such treatment may not totally destroy infectivity of some agents. Formalin (10%) has been found to be more destructive of antigenicity than acetone for rickettsia and mumps virus (191, 387), but was as good as acetone for Venezuelan equine encephalitis virus (728). Dried, unfixed preparations are also readily stained, but in such cases the hazards of accidental laboratory infections must be taken into consideration.

Most studies of virus in tissues have been carried out with frozen sections of unfixed blocks. Nevertheless, the viruses listed below have been demonstrated in conventional paraffin sections following fixation in the indicated conventional fixatives: herpes simplex, formalin or alcohol (931); poliovirus type III, formol–saline (580); tick-borne encephalitis virus, ethanol–acetic acid (1005); Newcastle disease virus, cold ethanol (1133); and neurotropic viruses in brain, Carnoy's (5). This list is extensive enough to suggest that brief exposure to one of the above fixatives, followed by dehydration in cold reagents and rapid embedding in paraffin, or embedding in water-soluble polymers such as Carbowax, may result in sufficient antigen retention for good staining of many other viruses than the ones indicated.

C. Protozoans and Helminths

Protozoans show greater diversity in their reaction to fixatives than bacteria. The problem is further complicated by the tendency for non-specific and autofluorescence to be enhanced by fixatives that are quite satisfactory otherwise, a problem that does not arise with bacteria.

Free-living amebas and paramecia have been studied in the living condition, or following fixation with 1% osmium tetroxide or formalin (39, 1140). By far the greater amount of work has been done with parasitic protozoans. Among the latter, those that can be prepared as dried smears from blood or other body fluids, e.g., malaria parasites, hemoflagellates and *Toxoplasma,* have frequently been fixed briefly in acetone, ethanol, or 1–10% formalin before staining. In the case of blood smears of malaria, Voller and Bray (1094) found formalin and methanol inferior to acetone. For dehemoglobinization of blood smears, 0.1% HCl may be used after fixation. If autofluorescence is a problem, as with smears of trypanosomes, the addition of one part of rhodamine–bovine serum albumin (BSA) to 19 parts of 5% formalin may mask unwanted fluorescence (1132). Organisms that occur in proteinaceous culture or tissue fluids, such as amebas or *Toxoplasma,* may be washed in 1–10% formalin–saline before being stained in suspension or dried on slides (365, 371). Unlike protein-precipitating fixatives, such as ethanol or acetone, formalin does not produce a disturbing floc of coagulated protein to obscure the parasites. Although prolonged fixation in formalin frequently destroys a considerable percentage of antigenicity in protozoans, exposure for up to about 1 hr appears to be well tolerated.

Immature stages of helminths, such as microfilariae, schistosome cercariae, or *Trichinella* larvae, have first been stained lightly with rhodamine–BSA and then fixed in 10% formalin. This procedure was found to be most effective in reducing excessive non-specific fluorescence (937, 938). Adult worms, or eggs containing embryos, may be incubated live in labeled antisera, in order to demonstrate staining of excretory products precipitating at body orifices or on the eggshell.

Antigenicity of parasites in tissues has been demonstrated for the most part in frozen sections of unfixed material, briefly fixed in acetone to prevent diffusion and leaching of soluble products. Blocks containing *Toxoplasma* may be fixed in 95% ethanol (1069), or in acetic acid–ethanol (120) before being embedded in paraffin in the usual manner.

D. Indigenous and Injected Antigens in Tissues

Antigens occurring in tissues are generally fixed in 95% ethanol or acetone for 10–30 min following the cutting of frozen sections from an unfixed tissue block. This applies to native antigens such as thyroid components, plasma proteins, basement membranes, and fibrin, as well as to injected antigens such as ovalbumin or bacterial toxins. Dried sections, cut from frozen, unfixed tissue have also been stained without fixation or following brief treatment with 10% formalin.

In approaching the study of a new antigen, if a cryostat is available, it would be reasonable to attempt the staining of dried, unfixed sections, since these offer the nearest thing to native antigens. Should the quality of tissue architecture, or loss of antigen by diffusion, be objectionable, dried sections may be fixed in 95% ethanol or acetone for 30 min at room temperature. These reagents have been found superior to formalin for thyroglobulin (981) and muscle phosphory-lase (271), and the general literature supports these findings.

Formalin-fixation, followed by routine paraffin embedding, has been used to demonstrate mucin (547), blood group antigens (549), human growth hormone (629), and human chorionic gonadotropin (732).

Bacterial polysaccharides tolerate fixation in the tissue block with Rossman's glycogen fixative* followed by routine paraffin embedding (441). Sainte-Marie (942) described an ethanol fixation–paraffin embedding method that was suitable for bovine serum albumin, γ-globulin, horse ferritin, influenza A, and diphtheria and tetanus toxoids, but was not suitable for ovalbumin. Essentially, the method consisted of fixation for 24 hr in cold 95% ethanol, followed by dehydration and clearing in cold reagents. Embedding in paraffin was at 56°C.

Paraffin and other embedding methods which can be used for unfixed tissues, and which therefore bear directly on the problem of demonstrating antigens in tissues blocks, are described in Section II.

II. TISSUE SECTIONING PROCEDURES

Sectioning methods described below are widely used in general histochemistry, and detailed discussions, descriptions, and bibliographies are available in histochemical texts (see bibliography at the end

* One part of neutral commercial formalin in 9 parts of saturated solution of picric acid in absolute ethanol (924).

of this chapter). Here we can only present the general rationale for each method, the type of equipment needed, and some evaluation of results. A consideration that applies across the board is that practical experience with the particular gear available in one's own laboratory offers the best route to good results, regardless of the method used.

A. Preparation of Frozen Sections

Sectioning unfixed, frozen tissue offers an attractively straightforward means of studying antigens in their native state. Fresh tissue blocks may be frozen on the chuck of a carbon dioxide freezing microtome mounted on the workbench, and the sections transferred to slides for drying and staining. This approach is not likely to be too satisfactory because the poor temperature control does not allow reproducible cutting of thin sections of satisfactory quality. Embedding the tissue in gelatin has been proposed for overcoming some of these objections (104). In the long run, a cryostat (refrigerated box containing a microtome), is likely to be the cheapest means for obtaining good sections, even though the initial cost is greater than that of a bench-model freezing microtome.

The general procedure, when a cryostat is available, is as follows: Tissue blocks, no more than a few millimeters in any dimension, are quick-frozen in a vial containing isopentane immersed in a dry ice–ethanol mixture or liquid nitrogen, or by placing the tissue directly onto the microtome chuck precooled in the same manner. The tissue is frozen to the chuck with a few drops of water and then transferred to the microtome in the cryostat chamber maintained at about $-20°C$. Under favorable conditions of temperature, knife sharpness, type of tissue, and other similar variables, sections may be cut as thin as 2–4 μ. Rolling of sections during cutting may be prevented by means of an antiroll device mounted on the knife, available with most cryostats, or manually with a fine brush. Sections are transferred to slides kept in the cryostat chamber, flattened gently, if necessary, by means of a brush, and withdrawn from the cryostat in order to thaw and dry. They are then immersed in acetone or ethanol for some minutes and removed for staining or storage. Serial sections may be obtained by embedding the block in egg albumin before freezing (876). Blocks may be stored in sealed plastic bags at temperatures of $-20°C$ or less.

Disadvantages of the cryostat method are the diffusion artifacts and degradation of tissue architecture that may occur during thawing of the section, and the greater level of non-specific fluorescence developed during staining, compared to freeze-dried or freeze-substituted tissues. Nevertheless, this method has been by far the most popular in fluorescent antibody work involving tissues.

B. Freeze-Drying

This method takes advantage of the fact that tissues dehydrated from the frozen state retain structural and antigenic integrity sufficient to permit embedding in paraffin and sectioning in the usual manner. The method has much to commend it, but in the past the rather demanding and expensive equipment needed to do a good job has limited its use (286, 330).

Small tissue blocks are frozen rapidly by plunging them into isopentane cooled to $-160°C$, with liquid nitrogen. The tissues are transferred, still frozen, to a vacuum drying tube maintained at a temperature of about $-30°C$, and the evacuation is started. Dehydration at $-30°C$ takes place over a period of hours or days, depending upon design of the apparatus and the tissue involved, under a vacuum of 10^{-3} to 10^{-4} mm of Hg. When the tissue is completely dry the temperature is allowed to rise, and the block is embedded in paraffin, polyethylene glycol, or polyester wax. Embedding may be accomplished by devices built into the evacuation system, or by transfer of the dried tissue to a separate oven. In any case, infiltration is done under vacuum. Sections are cut in the usual manner for paraffin but they should not be floated on water to remove wrinkles due to the possible leaching of unfixed cell components that retain their native solubility. The dry sections are mounted and flattened on slides with the aid of finger pressure or a brush, and the slide is warmed just enough to melt the paraffin and cause it to adhere well. Dewaxing is accomplished by means of xylene or other appropriate solvents and the sections may then be air dried. Depending upon the antigen under investigation, postfixation in alcohol or acetone may or may not be applicable before the staining procedure.

According to Rossi *et al.* (923), freshly sectioned lyophilized tissues show a diffuse yellow autofluorescence that, however, disappears by 48 hr. Cellular structure is well preserved, diffusion artifacts are kept at a minimum, and non-specific staining is said to be significantly reduced in this technique. Mayersbach (698) has provided a detailed evaluation of the method for immunohistological work. Although in general the equipment prescribed for freeze-drying of tissues is rather elaborate, Freed (330) and Lacy and Davies (606) have described a simple apparatus assembled in the laboratory to prepare sections for cytochemical and immunochemical staining. A rather simple and inexpensive freeze-drier is available commercially (Aloe).

C. Freeze-Substitution

Tissues kept at low temperatures may be dehydrated by organic solvents without suffering the denaturation which occurs in the same solvents at higher temperatures. Once dehydrated, tissue components retain much of their original antigenic nature even when embedded in wax in the usual manner. Thus, freeze-substitution offers some of the advantages of freeze-drying without the use of high-vacuum equipment. The method for general histochemistry is reviewed in detail by Feder and Sidman (300), and Patten and Brown (835). Balfour (28) has analyzed the procedure with specific reference to immunochemical staining.

As in the case of freeze-drying, small tissue blocks are "quenched" rapidly by being plunged into propane or isopentane cooled to $-160°C$ by liquid nitrogen. They are then transferred quickly to absolute ethanol at $-70°C$ and left to dehydrate at that temperature for several days. When substitution of tissue water by solvent is complete, the container is allowed to come to room temperature and the tissue is embedded in paraffin, polyethylene glycol, or polyester wax. The same problems of avoiding loss of soluble antigens by post-sectioning procedures that apply in freeze-drying apply in freeze-substituted sections. Balfour (28) found that antibody in plasma cells was well preserved in sections floated on 18% Na_2SO_4 in water but not when floated on alcohol. The reverse was true for injected albumins. Whether sections are floated or mounted dry, postfixation in ethanol after removal of wax may be indicated to reduce solubility of some antigens. Chemical fixatives such as mercuric chloride or picric acid may be added to the substitution fluid in a concentration of 1% to provide fixation as well as dehydration during the substitution period. In that case the tissues are washed in several changes of pure solvent at about 0°C, several hours per change, before embedding.

It should be obvious that specific details of technique are subject to great flexibility in the method just described, e.g., acetone, ether, chloroform, butyl alcohol, and other organic solvents may be used instead of ethanol for dehydration; metallic or other fixatives may or may not be added; and flotation with postfixation of sections may be accomplished with various alcohols or salt solutions. At present, the approach for any particular antigen must be empirical since there are only a few instances where the method has been used for fluorescent antibody studies (29, 86, 981, 1031).

III. MISCELLANEOUS PROCEDURES

The general preparation of slides for smears or tissue sections is the same for fluorescent antibody work as for general staining. Variations on general procedures derive from the facts that immunochemical staining is almost always performed by adding a few drops of reagent to the preparation, rather than by immersing the entire slide; and that non-fluorescent mounting media are necessary rather than the usual fluorescent, xylol-soluble resins. Although technical problems raised by these requirements are relatively trivial in comparison with other aspects of fluorescent antibody methods, it saves time to take advantage of techniques others have developed to solve their problems. The following pages present some methods that have been found helpful.

A. Preparing Slides

Slides should be selected that are of proper thickness, if a dark-field condenser is to be used. Generally, this means 1.0–1.2 mm. For purposes of titration or other comparative staining, 50 × 75 mm slides are very useful, although multiple smears can also be applied to ordinary 25 × 75 mm slides. The slides should be washed thoroughly with detergent, and rinsed with distilled water and alcohol; smears of bacteria, fungi, blood, or tissue are made as usual.

Smears may be circled with a line scribed by a diamond point pencil. This provides minimal protection against running together of drops of serum or conjugate. In addition, since smears are frequently transparent and colorless, the line provides reference points for focusing both condenser and objective in the plane of the smear.

Better protection against running is obtained by ringing preparations with a substance such as Marktex ink or paint (Mark-Tex Corp.). This is delivered by a penlike device, and adheres well to clean glass even after hours of exposure to serum or wash solutions.

When many slides need to be prepared in advance, for example for routine serologic testing, it may be easier to coat slides completely

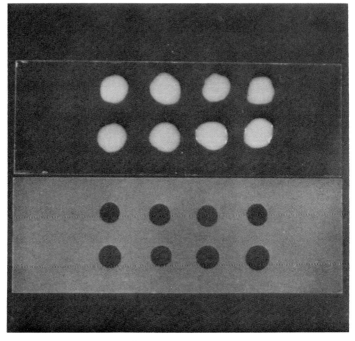

FIG. 35.   Appearance of slides before and after spraying to prevent running of reagent drops. See text for details.

with a water-repellant substance except for areas left clear for making smears. The simplest way to do this, the author has found, is to apply glycerol, undiluted or about 50% in water, in the form of drops over the areas to be protected on a number of slides lined up on the workbench. The entire group is then sprayed with a Teflon-like compound (Fluoro-Glide, Chemplast, Inc.), and a few moments later the glycerol is rinsed off each slide individually under the tap. The slides, placed in a rack, may then be dipped briefly in distilled water and set up on end to dry. By this means, slides acquire a ground-glasslike appearance except for clear areas protected by the glycerol (Fig. 35). The coating provides excellent protection against running together of drops, smears are easy to locate even in a darkened room, and it is easy to write and to focus on the sprayed surface.

Niel and Fribourg-Blanc (795) have described a method of preparing siliconized slides with clear wells for smears. Cosmetic nail polish is used to protect the desired areas during exposure to the silicone solution. Polish is removed with acetone and the slides rinsed with ether–acetone and then water.

To prevent loss of organisms during staining, Saslaw *et al.* (949) used slides coated with 0.75% gelatin in water, containing 0.5% phenol as preservative. Clean slides are dipped into the solution, and set on end to drain and dry. Gelatinized slides are also sometimes used to keep tissue sections from washing away during handling.

B. Mounting Media

The simplest and most commonly used mountant is the one first described by Coons, 9 parts glycerol and 1 part phosphate-buffered saline, pH 7.2–7.5. The mixture exerts a clearing effect on stained preparations and, being hygroscopic, does not dry out even upon prolonged storage.

The pH of this mountant may be manipulated to achieve more intense fluorescence, or to emphasize one color over another when more than one fluorescent label is involved in the same preparation. Pital and Janowitz (851) mounted bacterial smears in glycerol adjusted to pH 9.0 with carbonate–bicarbonate buffer (apparently $0.5M$). They obtained 3–4+ fluorescence with smears rated only 1–2+ when mounted under pH 7.2 glycerol. Hiramoto and Hamlin (449) demonstrated both rhodamine- and fluorescein-labeled antibody in the same cells by mounting doubly stained sections first in pH 4.0 and then pH 10.0 glycerol. The green fluorescence of fluorescein was quenched at the lower pH, permitting visualization of the orange fluorescence of rhodamine; at the higher pH, both dyes fluoresced to produce a yellow color. The glycerol mountants were prepared as 1:1 mixtures of glycerol and commercial buffers. Before mounting, sections were rinsed in buffer of the same pH as the mountant.

The cover-slip of a glycerol-mounted preparation may be immobilized and sealed by ringing with nail polish or resins of the type used for permanent mounting of conventionally stained sections. Such slides keep for months at 5°C or in a freezer, although there are conflicting reports on the extent to which fluorescence may be retained under these conditions. Differences may exist among different antigen–antibody systems in this respect. A semipermanent mounting medium may be prepared with the water-soluble resin, polyvinyl alcohol (918). Twenty grams of polyvinyl alcohol (Evanol 51–05, E. I. du Pont de Nemours and Co.) are dispersed in 80 ml of cold saline buffered at pH 7.2. The suspension should be heated to about 70°C in a water bath to dissolve the resin and, when cool, 40 ml of glycerol are added. The final pH is between 6.0 and 7.0. This medium is non-fluorescent and sets as a semisolid gel when mounted under a cover slip. McCurdy and Burstone (705) have described a 20% solution of polyvinyl alcohol, Vinol 325, from Air Reduction Chemical and Carbide Co., as a mountant for enzyme stains. It may serve equally well for fluorescent preparations. A permanent mounting resin that is soluble in xylene was used by Chadwick et al. (124). It is marketed under the name of Fluormount by Edward Gurr, Ltd.

C. Immersion Media

As stated in Chapter 5, the transmission of all substage condensers is increased when they are "immersed," and immersion is absolutely necessary for paraboloid and cardioid dark-field condensers. At the present time this is almost always accomplished with mineral immersion oils that show lower autofluorescence than the cedar-wood oil used in the past. The refractive index of immersion oils is around 1.515.

Niel and Fribourg-Blanc (795) use an aqueous immersion medium that is less viscous than oil, non-fluorescent, and easily washed off slides that are to be reused. The composition is: propylene glycol, 7 ml; ethylene glycol, 3 ml; glycerol, 1 ml; and water, 2 ml.

When bright-field illumination is used to stimulate fluorescence, autofluorescence of objectives and oculars can produce a disturbing background glow that may cause loss of contrast. This difficulty can be eliminated in the case of immersion objectives by use of an "immersion filter" containing a yellow dye (682, 819). Crystalline phenol, 6.5 gm, is dissolved in glycerol, 3.9 ml. The solution is saturated with Naphthol Yellow S (C.I. 10) at 100°C, cooled, and centrifuged to remove undissolved dye. The refractive index of this medium is 1.515 and it is said to be harmless to microscope objectives. Since blue excitation light is absorbed by this "filter" before entering the objective, no autofluorescence can be excited above that point, although a small amount of background glow may persist due to autofluorescence of the condenser and microscope slide.

BIBLIOGRAPHY

Barka, T., and Anderson, P. J. (1963). "Histochemistry: Theory, Practice and Bibliography." Harper (Hoeber), New York.

Burstone, M. S. (1962). "Enzyme Histochemistry." Academic Press, New York.

Glick, D. (1961). "Quantitative Chemical Techniques of Histo- and Cytochemistry." Wiley (Interscience), New York.

Pearse, E. (1960). "Histochemistry, Theoretical and Applied." Little, Brown, Boston, Massachusetts.

Steedman, H. F. (1961). "Section Cutting in Microscopy." Thomas, Springfield, Illinois.

Chapter Ten

STAINING METHODS

I. GENERAL COMMENTS

Manipulations involved in all staining reactions are the ultimate in simplicity. Drops of labeled or unlabeled sera are pipetted onto slides or into tubes containing the materials to be stained, and these are then incubated for varying periods of time. Despite this simplicity, rather sophisticated immunological reactions may be carried out with such manipulations, and equally sophisticated controls are necessary before staining results can be evaluated.

Information about either antigen or antibody is obtained by means of the same basic procedures. Thus, for example, if a fluorescent antiserum of known specificity yields a fluorescent product with an unknown antigen, we can conclude that the antigen was homologous to the antibody. Conversely, if the antigen is known it is possible to determine the nature of unknown antibody.

In this chapter, staining methods and controls are grouped according to whether information is being sought about antigen or antibody. This arrangement may be of some assistance in deciding which one of several possible methods is best suited to the problem on hand.

II. STAINING ANTIGEN WITH KNOWN ANTIBODY

There are two primary reasons for staining antigen: to identify unknown antigen occurring either alone or in mixtures with other antigens—this is frequently a diagnostic application; and to determine the distribution of known antigen in tissues or cells. Naturally, each of these fundamental applications is subject to considerable elaboration and refinement.

Staining can be accomplished either directly, with labeled specific antiserum, or indirectly by one of the layering or "sandwich" techniques. The techniques, their particular advantages, and controls necessary to establish specificity are described below.

A. Direct Method

1. TECHNIQUE

This is the simplest of staining reactions (Fig. 36). A few drops of appropriately diluted labeled antibody are applied to the antigen, generally on slides, and the slides are incubated in a wet chamber for a period of 10 min to 1 hr. Reactions have been carried out at temperatures ranging from 5° to 45°C, but mostly at room (25°C)

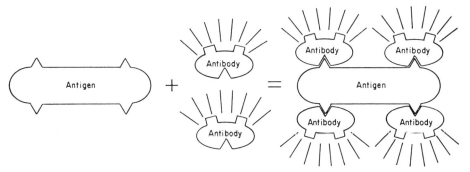

FIG. 36.   Schematic representation of direct staining reaction. (In this, and subsequent figures, radiating lines indicate fluorescence.)

or incubator (37°C) temperatures. In exceptional cases involving for example, whole teased muscle fibers, staining has been carried out for as long as several days (309).

The incubation chambers needed to prevent drying of conjugate are easily prepared by adding wet paper toweling or the like to petri dishes, covered trays, and desiccator jars, depending upon the number of slides stained. Following incubation, the drops of conjugate are shaken off and the slides immersed in saline, with occasional agitation, for 10 min. They are then rinsed in tap or distilled water to avoid development of a film from salts of the wash liquid, dried, and mounted. There are no critical studies on the significance of these details. For example, washing may be carried out for 30 min in buffer, and smears may be mounted while still wet, without apparently affecting results to any noticeable degree. Organisms are sometimes stained while in suspension in test tubes. Washing is then accomplished by centrifugation and decantation; buffered glycerol mountant is added to the last sediment.

Kellogg and Deacon (545) stained *Neisseria* and *Treponema* by allowing small drops of conjugate to dry within a few seconds on smears kept at 45°C. The smears were then washed and rinsed for a few more seconds and mounted as usual. This method is claimed to yield even more specific results than the usual staining procedure, in addition to being much more rapid.

In working with new antisera, it is generally necessary to run preliminary titrations to determine optimal concentrations of conjugate. This is done by staining a series of preparations with twofold dilutions of conjugate in saline or buffer. The highest dilutions yielding acceptably bright fluorescence, and meeting the tests for specificity given below, are then taken for actual work.

2. ADVANTAGES

The main advantage of the direct method is that only a single staining reagent is used. Once an antiserum has been labeled, titrated, and evaluated, staining reactions are straightforward and require only a minimum of control reactions to establish specificity. A less important advantage, which may acquire significance when large numbers of reactions are being run for diagnostic purposes, is that staining manipulations are simpler than for any of the indirect procedures.

3. CONTROLS

Immunological specificity of the fluorescence that is observed after any staining procedure must be established by appropriate controls. The nature of the antigen under investigation may not always permit use of all controls theoretically possible, but, obviously, the more controls used, the more confidence in the results.

a. Antigen should remain unstained upon exposure to "normal" conjugate applied at the same concentration as the specific reagent. ("Normal" is used here to mean a serum containing no known antibody to the antigen under investigation.) When antigen stains brightly with a high dilution of antibody conjugate, it is generally no problem to demonstrate lack of staining with a comparable dilution of normal conjugate. However, when antibody titer is low, and non-specific staining is more likely to occur as a result of the higher concentration of conjugate used, it is desirable to compare labeled sera on the basis of their *dye*, as well as protein, concentrations. This helps avoid artifacts that might arise from grossly different concentrations of dye in the conjugates being compared.

b. It should be possible to remove or greatly reduce the staining capacity of an antibody conjugate by absorbing it with homologous antigen suspensions or solutions. Aliquots of the same conjugate which are exposed to the same volumes of heterologous materials, or saline, under the same conditions, should continue to stain the homologous antigen. It is not uncommon for staining titer to be reduced as a result of dilution or non-specific loss even when heterologous absorbants are used. Nevertheless, homologous absorption should result in distinctly greater reduction in staining titer.

Sometimes, as in the case of rabies studies, this control is employed whenever a diagnostic determination is attempted (385). Thus, suspensions of normal and rabies-infected mouse brain are added to aliquots of the specific conjugate, and duplicate smears are stained with these mixtures. Smears are considered positive for rabies virus only when characteristic fluorescence is observed after exposure to the normal brain mixture and is absent in the other smear.

c. It should be possible to block or inhibit a homologous staining reaction by exposing the antigen to homologous *unlabeled* antibody before or at the same time the *labeled* antibody is added. By this means, antigenic sites become occupied with unlabeled molecules, resulting in reduced or eliminated fluorescence compared to the same reaction carried out with unlabeled *normal* serum. (Details of this reaction are described in Section IV.)

Unlabeled antibody precipitated onto the antigen in the first step of a two-step inhibition reaction may be replaced by labeled antibody in the second step owing to equilibrium considerations. To enhance the likelihood of demonstrating clear-cut inhibition, it is common, therefore, to expose antigen to unlabeled serum for perhaps two or three times as long as the exposure to labeled serum. This particular complication of the two-step procedure is avoided in the one-step method in which bound antibody is in equilibrium with both labeled and unlabeled antibody at the same time. However, inhibition may be difficult to recognize if labeled antibody is present in the mixture in much higher concentration than unlabeled. In general, a mixture of equal volumes of original, unlabeled antiserum and a suitable dilution of its derived conjugate will show good inhibition. The proper conjugate dilution to use can be determined by preliminary titrations.

This control, particularly in the one-step form, is easy to perform whenever staining is attempted. Parallel reactions can be run with specific conjugate mixed with either normal or antiserum to provide an immediate comparison of results.

d. Specific conjugate should not stain heterologous antigen. The choice of "heterologous" antigen may involve some difficulty. Thus, species that are closely related taxonomically may share common antigens and thus yield true reactions that may be misinterpreted as non-specific staining. On the other hand, widely different organisms may possess such different affinities for non-specific staining that, again, results may be misinterpreted. This problem applies, as well, to antigen extracts or tissue antigens. A guide to the immunological suitability of a control antigen may be obtained from other types of serologic data which may be available; non-specific tendencies can be evaluated by comparison with staining produced by known normal conjugates.

B. Antiglobulin Method

1. TECHNIQUE

This procedure is frequently referred to as the "indirect" method. The substance actually rendered fluorescent is not the antigen under consideration, but rather an intermediate material whose distribution corresponds precisely to that of the antigen being studied. This important method, shown schematically in Fig. 37, was first described in detail by Weller and Coons (1114) although, as mentioned in Chapter 1, others were working along similar lines simultaneously.

The technique takes advantage of the fact that antibody molecules, in addition to reacting with antigens, are themselves capable of serving as antigen which can be demonstrated by fluorescent antibodies. Thus, antiserum that has been prepared in a goat against rabbit globulin, as an example, and then labeled with fluorescein, will react with rabbit antibody even when the latter is combined in an antigen–antibody complex with, say, a bacterial cell. By this means, antigen may be rendered fluorescent even though the primary antiserum is itself not labeled.

The procedure is as follows: A few drops of unlabeled specific antiserum are layered over the antigen in the first step, and incubated as in the direct method for between 15 and 60 min. The slides are then washed for 10 min in saline, rinsed in water, and dried. In step 2, fluorescent antiglobulin, corresponding to the animal species that provided the unlabeled serum used in step 1, is applied to the antigen for a period similar to that of the first step. Washing and mounting

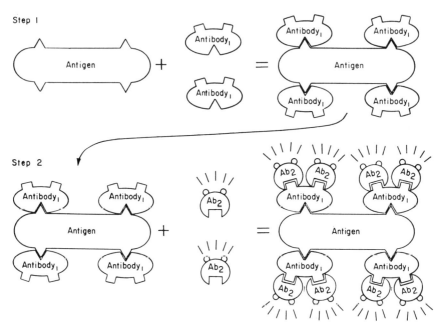

FIG. 37. Schematic representation of antiglobulin (indirect) staining reaction. In step 1, non-fluorescent antibody$_1$ is bound to the primary antigen. In step 2, fluorescent antiglobulin (Ab$_2$) binds to antibody$_1$ acting as a secondary antigen.

are carried out as described under direct staining. The microscopic appearance of antigen stained by this method is quite indistinguishable from that stained by the direct technique.

Block titrations of antiserum and conjugated antiglobulin should be run to determine optimum concentrations for each reagent. These may vary from undiluted to as much as 1:100 for each reagent, depending upon the particular system.

2. ADVANTAGES

There are two important advantages to this method. In any one laboratory, it is common to find the bulk of anti-agent sera derived from just a few animal species. By acquiring the necessary antispecies conjugates, all available samples of antiserum can be used for staining purposes without having to label each one separately.

The second advantage is the distinct increase in sensitivity that the indirect method provides. Since the molecular combining ratio of antibody to antigen is always greater than 1, and may be as much as 10 or more, the intermediate layer of unlabeled antibody in effect multiplies the number of sites to which fluorescent markers can be attached. Furthermore, whereas anti-agent sera may be limited in titer due to technical difficulties in antibody preparation, it is relatively simple to develop high-titered antiglobulin sera. Because of the variable nature of both these sources of increased sensitivity, it is difficult to assign a figure to the enhancement of fluorescence for any particular system. Nevertheless, some workers have found that antigens not detectable at all by direct staining have been rendered brightly fluorescent by the antiglobulin technique.

3. CONTROLS

The greater complexity of the antiglobulin method and its greater sensitivity increase the number of controls needed, since non-specific fluorescence tends to become more prominent under such conditions. Suggested control reactions are indicated on Table XIX.

It is desirable to try several sera in the normal serum control, because there may be variation in the degree to which different sera

TABLE XIX
CONTROLS FOR ESTABLISHING SPECIFICITY OF STAINING
BY THE ANTIGLOBULIN METHOD

Antigen	Reagent for step 1	Reagent for step 2	Result
Homologous	None or saline	Labeled antiglobulin	No fluorescence
	Normal serum	Labeled antiglobulin	No fluorescence
	Absorbed specific antiserum	Labeled antiglobulin	No fluorescence
	Specific antiserum	Labeled normal serum	No fluorescence
Heterologous	Specific antiserum	Labeled antiglobulin	No fluorescence

may be taken up by antigen non-specifically. Sometimes, specific anti-agent serum, from a different species than that against which the antiglobulin is directed, is substituted for normal serum. Positive results may be obtained in such cases as a result of cross-reactions among globulins from different animals (431).

In performing the control reactions, labeled and unlabeled sera should be taken in the same concentrations as for the expected specific reaction, in order to avoid spurious results on both the positive and negative sides. The proper choice of heterologous antigen presents the same problems here as in the comparable control for direct staining.

C. Anticomplement Method

1.   TECHNIQUE

Antigen–antibody complexes incorporate complement if the latter is present in the reaction mix. Goldwasser and Shepard (386) were able to show that complement itself was antigenic and capable of reacting with fluorescent anticomplement. They stained rickettsiae by first reacting the organisms with a mixture of unlabeled specific antiserum plus unlabeled, normal guinea pig complement. This was followed by labeled anticomplement (actually antifresh guinea pig globulin) to yield fluorescent rickettsial bodies. The demonstration of antigen by this method, therefore, is indirect, as in the antiglobulin procedure described above, except that in this case there are two unlabeled intermediate substances: specific antiserum and complement (Fig. 38).

In step 1, equal volumes of inactivated specific antiserum (rabbit, human, goat, etc.) and active guinea pig complement are mixed in a tube, and the mixture overlaid on the antigen. After incubation for about 30 min the smears are rinsed and dried. For the second step, labeled antiguinea pig complement is added for another 30 min. Washing and mounting are as described for direct staining.

The concentration at which each reagent should be used may have to be determined by titration. In that case, serial dilutions of complement should be added to tubes containing about a 1:10 dilution of antiserum for step 1 of the procedure, and staining should be accomplished in step 2 with perhaps a 1:4 dilution of conjugate. Having determined the minimum amount of complement needed, the other reagents can be titrated in the usual manner. Hinuma *et al.* (444) used 5–7 hemolytic units of complement, amounting to a 1:10 dilution of fresh guinea pig serum. Antibody dilutions of as much as 1:100 may be usable, and anticomplement conjugate may go out to 1:50. Sizable variations from these guideline concentrations may occur, depending upon the system. Serum inactivation is carried out as usual at 56°C for 30 min.

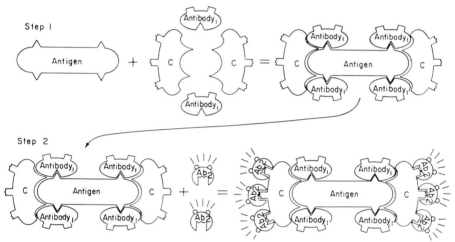

FIG. 38. Schematic representation of anticomplement staining reaction. In step 1, non-fluorescent complement (C) becomes bound to the reaction product of the primary antigen and its non-fluorescent antibody₁. In step 2, fluorescent anticomplement (Ab₂) attaches to C acting as a secondary antigen.

2. ADVANTAGES

The anticomplement system possesses the advantage over the antiglobulin system in that all antisera, regardless of the source species, can be used for staining purposes with the aid of but a single labeled anticomplement serum. The only requirement is that the antigen–antibody system involved bind complement.

The sensitivity of complement staining has been reported as higher than that of the indirect method (205, 386, 444), but whether this resulted from intrinsically greater sensitivity or simply from higher titers in the anticomplement sera, compared to the antiglobulins used, is not clear. In any case, since the amount of complement fixed by an antigen–antibody complex is about equal to the amount of antibody reacting, the anticomplement method is a more sensitive detector of antigens than direct staining.

In spite of these advantages, this method has not enjoyed nearly as much popularity as the antiglobulin technique. Probably this is a result of the wide use of relatively few species for antiserum production, and of the ready availability of antiglobulins directed against these common species. This situation makes it less attractive to complicate the staining procedure with an additional reactant, and with the extra titrations and controls that become necessary as a result.

3. CONTROLS

The number of controls needed for the anticomplement method is even greater than that necessary in the antiglobulin technique, since the additional reactant introduces an additional potential source of

TABLE XX

CONTROLS FOR ESTABLISHING SPECIFICITY OF STAINING
BY THE ANTICOMPLEMENT METHOD

Antigen	Reagent for step 1[a]	Reagent for step 2	Result
Homologous	None or saline	Labeled anti-complement	No fluorescence
	Normal serum	Labeled anti-complement	No fluorescence
	Specific antiserum	Labeled anti-complement	No fluorescence
	Active complement	Labeled anti-complement	No fluorescence
	Normal serum + active complement	Labeled anti-complement	No fluorescence
	Specific antiserum + inactivated complement	Labeled anti-complement	No fluorescence
	Specific antiserum + active complement	Labeled normal serum	No fluorescence
Heterologous	Specific antiserum + active complement	Labeled anti-complement	No fluorescence

[a] All sera should be heated at 56°C for 30 min to inactivate endogenous complement.

non-specificity. Thus, Goldwasser and Shepard in their original description of the anticomplement method referred to staining induced by some "normal" complement donors in the absence of added immune serum.

Table XX presents the various combinations of reagents to use in each step in order to prove the specificity of staining observed. It is desirable to inactivate all sera before use in order that the only active complement present be that which has been added in known concentration. Remarks made above under the other staining methods relative to concentration of reagents and choice of heterologous antigen, apply equally well here.

D. Double Staining Methods

Sections or smears may be stained with antisera labeled with different dyes to provide information on multiple antigens on the same preparation or even within the same cells (105, 121, 138, 215, 449, 718, 961). Such staining has been carried out by the direct method. Although the antiglobulin technique is not ruled out as a theoretical possibility, practical considerations make it much less attractive for double staining.

Staining can be done either in sequence, one labeled antiserum at a time with the usual washings in between, or in one step, with mixtures of conjugates labeled with different dyes. So far, the dyes employed have been FITC and rhodamine derivatives. Each conjugate should be titrated separately to determine optimum dilutions, and mixtures can then be made up correspondingly. The usual controls for direct staining apply, and it should be possible, for example, to inhibit each component of a mixture independently.

The usual filter systems readily permit visualization and differentiation of pure fluorescein and rhodamine fluorescence. Special techniques have sometimes been used to allow more objective analysis of yellowish intermediate colors appearing as a result of multiple antigens occurring in the same structure. The method of Hiramoto and Hamlin (449) of mounting specimens first at pH 4.0, in order to quench the fluorescein, and then at pH 10 to reactivate it, has already been mentioned in Chapter 9, Section III, B. Cebra and Goldstein (121) examined their specimens with a sequence of ocular filters: Wratten K2 (yellow) for the overall picture, Wratten 23 A (red) for rhodamine, and Wratten 57 A (green) for fluorescein. Mellors and Korngold (718) used an eyepiece spectroscope to examine the emission spectra of stained cells.

III. STAINING ANTIBODY *IN SITU*

In this section, we are concerned with the problem of demonstrating that an immunoglobulin present in a tissue section is a specific antibody against a particular antigen. This problem has received relatively little attention compared to other investigations involving fluorescent antibody methods. Both direct and indirect staining techniques have been used, as described below.

A. Direct Method

For this procedure labeled antigen is used as an immunohistochemical staining agent for its specific antibody. The method was used by Mellors *et al.* to demonstrate the presence of rheumatoid factors in certain cells (717, 720). Antigens consisted of a labeled, soluble, immune complex formed between fluorescent bovine serum albumin and specific rabbit antiserum, and of a labeled human γ-globulin aggregated by heat. Eveland (298) has used labeled bacterial antigen to stain antibody-producing cells in tissue cultures.

A few drops of labeled antigen are delivered onto the section containing antibody, and the slide is incubated for 0.5–1 hr. Washing and mounting are carried out as usual. The process is entirely comparable to its obverse, direct staining of antigen.

The obvious advantages of this method are its directness and simplicity. Nevertheless, antigens vary so greatly in susceptibility to denaturation that the usefulness of this approach may be limited by the physical and chemical conditions necessary for labeling.

Controls for this method are comparable to those used in direct staining for antigen. Briefly, antibody-containing sections should not stain following exposure to: (1) labeled heterologous antigen; (2) labeled homologous antigen absorbed with antibody; and (3) labeled homologous antigen plus unlabeled homologous antigen. Conversely, sections of "normal" tissue should remain unstained following exposure to labeled antigen.

B. Indirect Method

This method circumvents the problem of possible denaturation of antigen during labeling by employing unlabeled antigen as the primary reagent. The unstained antigen–antibody complex thus formed is then rendered visible by use of the usual type of labeled antibody prepared in the same or another animal (Fig. 39). Coons *et al.* (189) em-

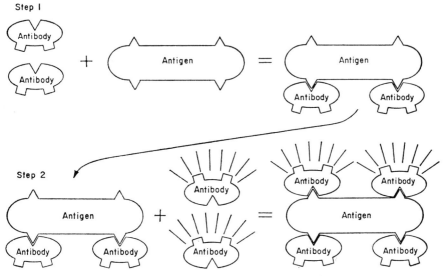

Fig. 39. Schematic representation of staining antibody in tissue sections by the indirect method. In step 1, non-fluorescent antigen is fixed in space by reaction with antibody *in situ*. In step 2, fluorescent antibody attaches to the antigen precipitated during step 1.

ployed this method to locate antibody against γ-globulin and oval-bumin in rabbits.

In the first step, a few drops of diluted, unlabeled antigen are pipetted onto the sections to be stained. (Coons *et al.* used a 1:2000 dilution of antigen, perhaps to avoid entering the zone of antigen excess.) After incubation for 30 min the slides are washed and rinsed in the usual manner. In step 2, a few drops of specific labeled anti-serum, directed against the antigen used in the first step, are overlaid on the sections and incubation is repeated for an additional 30 min. Washing and mounting are as usual.

The main advantage of this indirect method is as indicated above; native antigen can be employed to detect the cellular antibody. Coons also found the technique to be more sensitive than the direct procedure. An important disadvantage is that labeled antibody used in the second step may stain original antigen employed to immunize the animal, if any is present. With proper controls, however, this contingency can be detected and evaluated in the overall staining picture.

Controls are needed to establish the specificities of reactions occurring in both steps of the procedure. Table XXI indicates some of

TABLE XXI

CONTROLS FOR ESTABLISHING SPECIFICITY OF ANTIBODY STAINING BY THE INDIRECT METHOD

Substrate section containing	Reagent for step 1	Reagent for step 2	Result
Homologous antibody	None or saline	Labeled homologous antibody	No staining
	Heterologous antigen	Labeled homologous antibody	No staining
	Homologous antigen	Heterologous, labeled antibody	No staining
Heterologous or no antibody	Homologous antigen	Homologous, labeled antibody	No staining
Homologous antibody	Homologous antigen	Homologous, labeled plus homologous un- labeled antibody	No staining

the basic control reactions. Others, involving absorption of the antigen and labeled antibody reagents are also possible, and may be desirable under specific circumstances.

IV. IDENTIFICATION OF ANTIBODY IN SERUM

Although the fluorescent antibody method is primarily a staining technique, the fact that antiserum enters into the reaction has always meant that some sort of serologic testing procedure was implicit in the method. This potential has been exploited by appropriate adaptations of the three staining techniques in which unlabeled serum participates: the antiglobulin method, the inhibition control, and the anticomplement technique. Each of these methods, with their particular advantages, is described below.

By and large, fluorescent antibody serology offers major advantages over conventional serologic techniques whenever the preparation of conventional antigens (usually soluble extracts) is difficult or unreliable. The cytochemical nature of the fluorescence method means that whole cells or organisms can be used as antigen, and that contaminant antigens need not interfere with the specific reaction being sought. Beyond this advantage, there is no indication that serologic results by fluorescent antibody are superior to or more revealing than conventional techniques. Sensitivity levels tend to be lower than indirect hemagglutination tests and higher than complement fixation, but are subject to many variables.

At present, the single most important diagnostic application of fluorescent antibody serology is probably the test for syphilis. A test for malaria antibodies has also had significant research results, since it is the first dependable serologic procedure for that infection. Methods have been published for a considerable number of other diseases, but practical and routine use of these tests has tended to lag. The difficulty of controlling and standardizing a host of technical details has no doubt influenced the slow rate at which diagnostic fluorescent antibody serology has spread.

A. Antiglobulin Method

1. TECHNIQUE

In this method, known, standardized antigen and standardized fluorescent antiglobulin are used to determine the presence or absence of antibody in an unknown, unlabeled serum. The technique is the same as for indirect staining of antigen, being performed in two steps.

Serum to be tested is diluted serially in saline or buffer, and a few drops of each dilution are delivered onto smears of known antigen. After an appropriate incubation period, 0.5–1 hr, the smears are washed in saline for 10 min, rinsed in water, and dried. A few drops of an appropriate dilution of labeled antiglobulin, corresponding to the species providing the test serum, are then applied to all smears, and the slides are again incubated for 0.5–1 hr. Washing and mounting are as usual. Known positive and negative control sera which have previously been titrated and checked for specificity according to the methods described in Section II, B above, should be included in the run whenever unknown sera are tested.

Positive test serum should cause the antigen to fluoresce, particularly in the higher serum concentrations. Brightness should diminish with dilution to permit determination of a staining titer. Evaluation of minimum titers to be considered "positive" must be made on the basis of known control sera. For example, it may be necessary to disregard reactions occurring at dilutions lower than, say, 1:16, if normal sera cause fluorescence at 1:8.

Testing by the above method for the presence of antibody in an odd serum produced in the laboratory is not difficult. On the other hand, titration of many diagnostic sera to reproducible end points demands a rather high degree of standardization of procedures and reagents. Prepared antigen and diluted antiglobulin may lose titer on storage; incubation periods during the staining reaction should be long enough so that the time lag between delivering the first and last test sera to their smears does not become a significant percentage of the incubation period; readings should be made in a darkroom after a certain minimum degree of dark adaptation has occurred; allowance should be made for possible fading of fluorescence during examination of smears and exposure to the excitation beam.

Evaluation of end points by eye is at best a subjective process, but use of objective criteria can help improve reproducibility. Morphologic distribution of fluorescence in cellular antigens, brightness, relationship of specific fluorescence to non-specific counterstain, percentage of cells showing a certain level of fluorescence, are all criteria that can be employed to standardize the reading of titration end points.

2.   ADVANTAGES

The antiglobulin method is a relatively simple procedure to institute since, in many cases, high-titered, antispecies sera can be purchased already labeled, ready for use. Sensitivity is such that serum titers of 1:1000 are not uncommon. A limitation on the method is that serum from only one species can be tested with any particular labeled antiglobulin. In broad, epidemiological surveys, separate antiglobulins would be necessary if testing extended to the animal population of an area.

B. Inhibition Method

1. TECHNIQUE

The basic reagents for this technique are known antigen and specific, labeled antibody. The degree to which an unknown serum blocks or inhibits the reaction between the basic reagents is taken as a measure of its antibody content. Although this procedure is often performed in two steps as a control for direct staining, the one-step

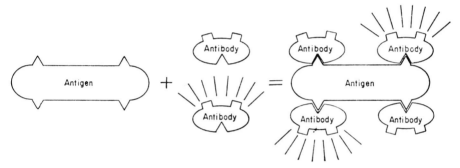

FIG. 40. Schematic representation of the one-step inhibition reaction. Antigen exposed to a mixture of fluorescent and non-fluorescent antibody binds fewer fluorescent particles and shows reduced fluorescence.

method shown schematically in Fig. 40 has been preferred for serologic testing.

Serial dilutions of test serum are delivered to a set of tubes (0.1–ml volumes are convenient). An equal volume of appropriately diluted (see below) conjugated antiserum is pipetted into each tube, and a few drops from each mixture are deposited on smears of antigen. After 1 hr of incubation the slides are washed and mounted as usual. Previously titrated positive and negative control sera should be included in each test.

In this test, presence of antibody in the test serum is indicated by *absence* or *reduction* of fluorescence at the higher serum concentrations. With increasing serum dilution, fluorescence should become brighter until it reaches the level seen in the normal serum control.

Sensitivity and readability of the test is improved by taking the conjugated antiserum in a dilution which yields a medium or low level of fluorescence with normal serum. Reduction in brightness caused by positive serum is more easily recognized under those conditions, and the sudden increase in brightness at the end point is more apparent.

The proper concentration of conjugate to use can be determined by titration. Twofold dilutions of conjugated antiserum are delivered into duplicate sets of tubes. To one set is added equal volumes of a 1:2 or 1:4 dilution of normal serum, and to the other is added the same dilution of known antiserum. The various mixtures are added to separate smears of antigen. The highest dilution of conjugate showing the clearest distinction between positive and negative controls is taken to be the proper concentration for diagnostic testing.

Precautions concerning standardization of reagents and techniques, indicated above in the antiglobulin method, apply here too.

2.   ADVANTAGES

If specific, labeled antiserum has been used in the laboratory for direct staining, it is simple to set up the inhibition test since no additional reagents are needed. Furthermore, serum from any source can be tested with the same labeled antiserum, thus avoiding this particular limitation of the antiglobulin technique. These advantages appear to be of minor significance, however, and the inhibition technique has not enjoyed the popularity of the antiglobulin method for serologic testing.

In one respect, however, the inhibition reaction may offer important advantages over the indirect methods. If it is necessary to distinguish between antibodies to closely related antigens, the conjugated antibody reagent can be absorbed with the unwanted antigen to yield a reagent specific only for a very narrow range of antigens. Inhibition would then be caused only by an equally narrow range of unlabeled antibody in the test serum. Similar results could be achieved in the antiglobulin method only by the laborious process of absorbing each individual test serum separately.

From the rather limited information available, the inhibition method appears to be severalfold less sensitive than the antiglobulin technique.

C. Anticomplement Method

1. TECHNIQUE

This method has only rarely been employed for serologic testing (205) but it would appear to be widely applicable for that purpose. Reagents needed are known antigen, titrated complement and titrated, labeled anticomplement. The procedure is similar to that followed in the antiglobulin test described earlier in this chapter.

Test serum is inactivated and dilutions are delivered into tubes containing a constant amount of active guinea pig complement. Drops of each mixture are pipetted onto smears of antigen and the slides are incubated for 30 min or 1 hr. After washing and drying, labeled anticomplement is added for an additional, equal incubation period. Washing and mounting are as usual.

Results are read as in the indirect method, i.e., the presence of antibody in the unknown serum is indicated by bright fluorescence, diminishing with increased dilution of the serum. Positive and negative controls provide baseline fluorescence against which the serum titration is evaluated.

2. ADVANTAGES

In the absence of evaluations of this procedure as a diagnostic serological test, it is only possible to discuss its usefulness in terms of potential. The method would appear to combine the sensitivity of the antiglobulin technique with the unrestricted range of the inhibition procedure, so far as source of test serum is concerned. The main drawbacks to the anticomplement test would be the need for two new, carefully controlled reagents, complement and labeled anticomplement.

D. Soluble Antigen Method

Serologic methods, using fluorescent antibody as the indicator, have been devised for antigens consisting of soluble extracts of helminths or various body tissues (207, 333, 827, 1064, 1066). The methods all have in common the preparation of more or less purified extracts which are applied to glass, paper, or agar substrates, and are then stained by direct or indirect means with fluorescent antiserum. In another approach, viruses and other soluble antigens were reacted with labeled antisera and the resulting precipitates collected on membrane filters. The fluorescent precipitates were then read directly on a fluorometer (788, 789).

Although these techniques may offer certain advantages in special circumstances, it is difficult to conceive of them having any broad application. Compared to conventional serological tests with soluble extracts, these methods are generally less sensitive and not as well standardized, although the membrane filtration method appears more sensitive than the other techniques. The most ambitious effort in the direction of standardization and quantitation (1065), in which a macrofluorometer was employed to measure fluorescence, resulted only in identification of sera diluted 1:2 as either "reactive," "non-reactive" or "weakly reactive." Under the best of circumstances it is unlikely that fluorescent antibody serology with extract antigens of the type now known, could offer any significant advantages over the well-established conventional techniques.

Chapter Eleven

UNWANTED FLUORESCENCE

It is a rare fluorescence image in which background is completely black and only the object of interest is visible. More commonly, the image shows about three levels of brightness. At bottom is the background glow contributed by autofluorescence and light scatter from optical elements, immersion media, and filters. Brighter than this, but still generally dull, is the diffuse fluorescence of biological origin— tissues, microorganisms, cellular constituents, and debris. At the brightest level the clear fluorescence of specifically stained objects is seen.

Control of the lowest level is achieved by appropriate choice of filters, lighting techniques, and other physical constituents of the microscope system. Control of the highest level is, of course, a function of conjugate titers, labeling efficiencies, and all the other factors entering into staining with fluorescent antibody. This chapter is concerned with problems encountered in the middle brightness range, involving biological elements. Fluorescence from this source is called "unwanted" because, at best, it serves only to orient the viewer in the microscope field, a function which could be accomplished by other means, if necessary; at worst, it may be bright enough to interfere with recognition of specific fluorescence. The three major sources of this fluorescence, and suggestions for control, are discussed below.

I. AUTOFLUORESCENCE

Autofluorescence, to some degree, is practically universal in biological materials. Thus, unstained freshly cut sections, intact microorganisms, tissue culture monolayers, and the like all show bluish-gray autofluorescence upon excitation with either ultraviolet or blue light. The emission spectrum is broad enough for the fluorescence to appear a dull, nondescript greenish-yellowish-brownish color when viewed with a light yellow barrier filter. By and large, such low intensity, primary fluorescence is rarely confused with the brighter, cleaner, and sharper appearance of objects secondarily stained with fluorescent dyes. Nevertheless, the problem is complicated by the fact that autofluorescence of tissues may be enhanced by fixation, storage, and other factors; different tissues and microorganisms may show different degrees of fluorescence under the same conditions; and last, superimposed upon this universal fluorescence, certain tissues and microorganisms may show strong fluorescence of particular colors due to specific compounds they may possess.

Brief fixation in formalin or other simple fixatives does not unduly increase autofluorescence, but fixation in formalin for several months may increase the fluorescence of red blood cells and fats (415). Jackson (488) found greater fluorescence in sections cut from embedded, frozen-dried tissues than from those cut on a cryostat without embedding. Liver and brain embedded in polyester wax after freeze-substitution showed minimal fluorescence (1095), but Balfour (28) states that autofluorescence increases in such tissues after 3 months storage at room temperature. Autofluorescence of paraffin-embedded tissue increased more rapidly in cut sections than in the uncut block, but blocks 6 months old still yielded usable sections (120). It is worth noting that autofluorescence may reach such high levels in old blocks or sections that specific staining may be impossible to recognize.

Hicks and Matthaei (439) have described the normal autofluorescence appearance of various human tissues and substances. For the most part, the appearance is bluish-white with ultraviolet irradiation and a colorless eyepiece filter, and more intense greenish to yellowish with blue light irradiation and a light yellow ocular filter. Nuclei in general, connective tissue, mucus, lipids, and red and white blood cells, show minimal or no fluorescence. At the other extreme, elastic tissue exhibits bright blue or yellow fluorescence, depending upon the ocular filter. Exoskeleton and other chitinous components of arthropods fluoresce bright yellow or yellow–brown (101, 977).

Out of 36 common species of bacteria and fungi studied, 30 were yellow–green and 6 showed some reddish fluorescence in addition to the yellow–green (1008). The low level of autofluorescence in these species does not complicate their study with fluorescent antibody. Among fungi of medical interest, the yeast phases of *Candida albi-*

cans, Cryptococcus neoformans, Histoplasma capsulatum, and Blasto-myces dermatitidis appear a dull bluish-gray to -green when unstained (1088). *Trichophyton rubrum, T. interdigitale, Penicillium expansum, Aspergillus fumigatus,* and *Nocardia asteroides* show weak and negligible autofluorescence (741). On the other hand, *Coccidioides immitis* spherules, endospores, and arthrospores, as well as tuberculate spores of *Histoplasma capsulatum* and spores of *Sepedonium* show brilliant autofluorescence of greenish-yellow or orange color when viewed with a yellow secondary filter (389). In addition, *Epidermophyton floccasum* and *Microsporum japonicum* are a brilliant pale blue color before being stained (741). Darken (233) has reviewed some of the literature on autofluorescence of actinomycetes.

Fluorescence colors of a few inorganic and organic substances found in tissues are as follows: iron, brown; calcium, bright yellow; melanin, brown; lipofuscin, very bright yellow; porphyrins, red; riboflavin, yellow–green; vitamin A, bright yellow; chlorophyll, red (279, 439). References to the literature on this subject can be found in the review by Price and Schwartz (866).

General tissue autofluorescence may be kept low by prompt use of cut sections and blocks. If the latter are to be stored for any length of time, temperatures of −20°C and below should be used. Some autofluorescent pigments and fat-soluble compounds may be extracted with suitable solvents. Autofluorescence of microorganisms is often influenced by the culture medium on which they are grown, providing a parameter which may be manipulated to advantage. No solutions have been offered for avoiding the bright autofluorescence of certain fungi. Sometimes, the difference in distribution of fluorescence and in hue between control and test material provides sufficient basis for recognizing specific staining. In the overall picture, autofluorescence can generally be kept sufficiently low for most work.

II. CROSS-REACTIONS

By cross-reactions we refer to true immunologic reactions occurring between labeled antisera and antigens found in organisms other than the one under investigation. This phenomenon is so widespread in immunology that no purpose will be served by listing the many examples encountered in fluorescent antibody studies. The brightness of staining reactions with heterologous species or strains may be entirely comparable to that found with homologous forms, or may be noticeably less intense, though still clearly "positive."

Control of such unwanted fluorescence follows classic immunological techniques: fractionation and purification of immunizing antigens; absorption of antisera with heterologous, cross-reacting antigens; and purification of test antigens, if possible.

Antisera are frequently absorbed with equal volumes of packed cells in order to effect complete removal of antibody activity. Since labeled globulins are almost always more dilute than original serum, and since they are generally taken for staining in the form of a dilution of the full strength conjugate, absorptions may often be performed with considerably fewer organisms than needed for whole serum. This consideration may be important in working with hard-to-grow organisms.

An ingenious adaptation of the one-step inhibition staining control has been used by Redys *et al.* (898) as a device for blocking cross-reactions. Having found in staining Group A streptococci that absorption with cross-reacting Group C organisms did not completely remove the cross-reacting antibody, a small amount of unlabeled Group C antiserum was added to labeled Group A conjugate. This rendered the resultant mixture completely specific for Group A only. This approach may be especially useful in instances where antiserum, as from patients, may be more available than large numbers of organisms for eliminating cross-reactions.

III. NON-SPECIFIC STAINING

A. General Comments

Non-specific staining is distinguished from autofluorescence by the fact that the fluorescence appears only after incubation with labeled serum; and from cross-reactions by the fact that the fluorescence is not influenced by controls for specificity. The term is applied here only to induced fluorescence which is not the result of antigen–antibody interaction. Fortunately, this type of unwanted fluorescence is entirely lacking, or of minimal importance, in dealing with bacteria or fungi. On the other hand, most protozoans and tissue cells exhibit non-specific staining to a degree that makes this the most important source of unwanted fluorescence.

The extent to which cells take up labeled sera non-specifically varies widely. It is influenced by the organ or tissue involved, the source species, sectioning technique, and other poorly defined factors which cause variation even between individual animals of the same species. The basis for this type of staining was for a time considered to be immunological, resulting perhaps from a hypothetical, common, widely distributed antigen. The investigations of Hughes (475), Mayersbach and Schubert (701), and Nairn *et al.* (779, 781) on the staining of tissue sections treated in various ways, and of Riggs *et al.* (907), Curtain (214), Goldstein *et al.* (381), and McDevitt *et al.* (706) on the staining properties of fractionated conjugates, has quite thoroughly established the major cause of non-specific staining to be not immunological, but rather a charge effect. That is, relatively basic proteins in cells attract and bind relatively acid proteins from serum, whether the latter are labeled or not. Inasmuch as labeling with the dyes now used always increases the relative acidity of serum proteins by blocking some of the native amino groups on the proteins, non-specific attachment of conjugates tends to be greater than that of native serum.

The evidence for this conclusion has been reviewed by Rossi *et al.* (923). Whether the hypothesis is completely or only partially accurate is not as important for purposes of this chapter as the fact that this view of the problem is consistent with methods available for reducing non-specific staining. Proposed techniques for dealing with the problem involve manipulations of both the material being stained and the conjugate. In the following pages, corrective techniques are listed in order of proximate complexity, with the simplest techniques first. It should be recognized that no method is absolutely effective in the sense of producing a situation in which, regardless of conjugate concentration, absolutely nothing stains except the specific antigen. On the other hand, effective, practical control is often achieved even with relatively simple procedures. The approach in each case must, as yet, be quite empirical.

B. Methods of Control

1. DILUTION

If the serum (in indirect staining techniques), or the conjugate (in both direct and indirect methods), possesses a high enough specific titer, simple dilution will frequently carry the reagent past the point of non-specific staining while still retaining good specific activity. It is difficult to give precise figures here because of the many variables involved, but assuming an average conjugate with a molar F/P ratio of between two and four, and a protein concentration of 20 mg/ml, it would ordinarily be possible to avoid non-specific staining by using a dilution greater than 1:50. Under favorable conditions, specific staining of good intensity may be obtained with protein concentrations of less than 0.5 mg/ml, which is ordinarily past the range of non-specific activity. With heavily labeled conjugates, however, even extreme dilution may not be effective.

2.   CONTROL OF pH

According to Mayersbach and Schubert (701), reduction of the tissue isoelectric point by rinsing stained sections in buffer of pH 8.5 (at most), decreases non-specific retention of dye. This control may be hazardous to specific staining because of the possible dissociation of bound antibody at the elevated pH.

3.   COUNTERSTAINING

Counterstaining with one of the non-specific dyes suggested in Chapter 7 is often a simple and effective remedy for non-specific uptake of fluorescein. Since all of these dyes fluoresce in the orange and red region, they cannot be used with specific rhodamine conjugates. It is important to determine, experimentally, the appropriate concentration at which to take the counterstain without swamping specific fluorescence. Different materials fixed, or otherwise handled, in different ways react differently to the counterstains, and concentrations reported in the literature should be viewed as only a general guide.

4.   ABSORPTION WITH TISSUE PREPARATIONS

The absorption of fluorescein conjugates with acetone-precipitated liver powder (188) was the earliest technique recommended for reducing non-specific staining. Despite objections that the method causes excessive overall loss of protein and specific titer, and that it is not too effective in the first place, this procedure unquestionably works. It may be especially useful in treating volumes of conjugate too small to be processed more elegantly on fractionation columns. The rationale for this technique has not been defined experimentally. However, it would appear likely that tissue particles used for absorption retain their native affinity for relatively acid proteins, and thus behave in bulk the same way they behave in sections. In any case, a large number of publications testify to the reasonable effectiveness of the method, and its simplicity and low cost are advantageous.

Tissue powder may be prepared from any parenchymatous tissue —liver, spleen, kidney, heart, and skeletal muscle all being suitable. Although it is sometimes indicated that the particular organ of the particular species whose sections are to be stained provides the most effective absorbent, there is no critical evidence that these parameters are of more than minor significance. The general procedure for preparing tissue powders is to homogenize the organ or tissue pool in water or saline, filter through cheesecloth to remove coarse particles and then wash with acetone to precipitate, and later to dry, the resulting solids. The precipitated protein should be washed in saline before being dried in order to remove soluble materials that might otherwise contaminate conjugates during the absorption process. The dried powder remains effective for years upon storage at 5°C or lower. Variations on this general method are given by Coons *et al.* (189), Carver and Goldman (120), and Hiramoto *et al.* (456). Kaplan (514) used a thoroughly washed tissue homogenate, rather than dried powder, for absorption. To reduce non-specific staining of human skin, Rappaport (886) prepared a powder from human callouses; bone marrow powder has been used to absorb out non-specific activity against leukocytes (976), and human tissue culture cells were effective in reducing unwanted staining of plant cells harboring viral antigen (771).

The method of using tissue powders is to incubate, two or three times in succession, a mixture of powder and conjugate (50–100 mg/ml). Absorption should be for at least 1 hr each time at room or incubator temperature, with occasional shaking. The conjugate is recovered by centrifugation, preferably at over 3000 rpm. When absorptions are performed with dry powders, and recovery is by centrifugation in ordinary tubes, conjugates acquire a pH of about 5.5 (134), and there is about a 20% loss in volume at each absorption. To avoid these undesirable effects, the required weight of powder should be soaked for 1 hr in buffered saline just before use, and absorptions should be carried out in centrifugal filter bottles, of the

Hemming type (Standard Scientific Corp., New York). By substituting ordinary filter paper for the sterilizing pad used in the Hemming assembly, and centrifuging the absorbed conjugate through the filter at 2000 rpm, the total loss in volume after three absorptions can be kept under 10%.

Hudson (472) mixed one part of liver powder to four parts of Celite and prepared a chromatographic column containing 1 gm of mix for each milliliter of conjugate to be absorbed. Equilibration and elution were carried out with saline buffered at pH 7.2. About 40% of the applied protein was recovered and the reagent was highly specific.

Conventional and fluorescent staining titers tend to drop following tissue powder absorption due to non-specific loss of protein (502, 699, 780). Protein concentration of absorbed conjugates may sometimes show an actual *increase,* concurrent with a reduction in fluorescein content. This apparently results from the leaching of unlabeled serum-soluble proteins from the tissue powder into the conjugate, while, at the same time, labeled protein is being removed by binding to the powder.

5.   COLUMN CHROMATOGRAPHY

Chromatography on diethylaminoethyl-cellulose (DEAE) yields fractions of conjugates with varying ratios of dye to protein. Since fractions carrying a low load of dye are less acid than those with the greater load, less non-specific binding occurs with the lightly loaded fractions. These are eluted from DEAE by low salt concentrations at pH 6.3. The method of performing this fractionation has been described in Chapter 7.

Fractionation on DEAE comes closest, perhaps, to providing a rational, reproducible, and simple method for obtaining conjugate solutions of high specificity. Another chromatographic technique whose complexity limits its use, but which may be highly effective in special cases, is the use of immunoadsorbent columns to isolate essentially pure, specific antibody from serum or globulin. Curtain and O'Dea (217) coupled soluble antigens to cellulose which was then put into a column. Conjugated antiserum was applied to the column at pH 6.8 and eluted at pH 3.2. The eluate protein was over 90% precipitable by antigen. Such conjugates, containing minimal amounts of non-antibody protein, should give bright staining at dilutions far beyond the range where non-specific uptake occurs.

Brooks *et al.* (88) have showed that conjugated 19S globulins contributed to non-specificity, but yielded low specific staining as compared to 7S globulins. Fractionation on columns of Sephadex 200 allowed separation of the two classes of globulins, thus improving specificity.

APPLICATIONS

Chapter Twelve

APPLICATIONS OF FLUORESCENT
ANTIBODY

Fluorescent antibody methods have by now been applied to essentially all aspects of microbiology and pathology. To facilitate access to the considerable literature involved, I have prepared the following annotated bibliography, based upon the list of references to be found at the end of this book. The overwhelming majority of references listed are in English, although a few papers in other Western European languages are also included. I have deliberately refrained from listing reports in Russian, Japanese, Hungarian, and other such esoteric languages for the simple reason that not many readers of this book are likely to be competent in those tongues and, for those who are, reviews of the national literatures are available in national publications. The review articles cited under each broad category below, as well as the more thorough laboratory reports, should provide additional guidance to specific areas of interest to the reader, since the bibliography as it stands does not pretend to be absolutely complete.

In breaking down the applications to specific organisms and disease conditions I have not followed rigorous classification schemes, preferring instead to present simple, alphabetized lists. I think this will make the annotated bibliography more convenient to use. In any case, if the reader will accept these lists as simple guides to be used with some flexibility, the time he will need to spend in tracking down work already performed in specific areas should be shortened materially.

I. GENERAL FLUORESCENT ANTIBODY METHODS
AND APPLICATIONS

8, 54, 77, 134, 175, 177–184, 232, 368, 733, 762, 819, 855, 923, 1012, 1017, 1056, 1126

II. APPLICATIONS IN BACTERIOLOGY

A. Reviews

90, 131, 135, 164, 369, 494, 642, 643, 785, 834, 979, 1127

B. Specific Organisms

1. *Bacillus anthracis* and Related Species
61, 63, 133, 140, 267, 324
2. *Brucella*
62, 902, 1148
3. *Clostridium*
35, 36, 76, 231, 567, 845, 1015
4. *Corynebacterium diphtheriae* and Related Species
11, 510, 744, 748, 754, 871, 950, 1120
5. *Escherichia coli*
52, 64, 79, 126, 127, 136, 141, 196, 199, 229, 230, 246, 298, 318, 347, 634, 672, 688, 693, 787, 818, 900, 952, 970, 1020, 1048, 1049, 1052, 1067, 1121
6. *Hemophilus*
64, 248, 402, 465, 530, 683, 684, 738, 739, 824, 896, 897, 964, 965
7. *Leptospira*
132, 155, 203, 218, 219, 479, 664–667, 759, 848, 976
8. *Mycobacteria*
198, 509, 727, 978
9. *Mycoplasma*
30, 59, 106, 115, 130, 144, 145, 148–150, 173, 220, 276, 497, 633, 639, 641, 645, 673, 686, 760, 999, 1045, 1071, 1080
10. *Neisseria*
52, 223–228, 240, 241, 338, 402, 437, 462, 545, 694, 730, 738, 739, 740, 752, 823, 838, 968, 1124
11. *Pasteurella*
325, 326, 473, 490, 532, 690, 709, 750, 872, 1123, 1135, 1136
12. *Salmonella*
163, 348, 352, 353, 407, 672, 1022, 1038, 1047, 1050, 1051
13. *Shigella*
318, 319, 468, 602, 660, 813, 1040, 1041, 1053

14. *Staphylococcus*
   52, 111, 117, 157–159, 250, 251, 332, 560, 577, 926, 957
15. *Streptococcus*
   27, 52, 141, 165, 262, 284, 285, 296, 358, 408, 409, 413, 512,
   518, 527–529, 609, 685, 746, 749, 768, 842, 865, 892, 898,
   899, 925, 949, 958, 962, 997, 1068, 1138, 1139, 1153, 1154
16. *Treponema*
   48, 96, 236–239, 277, 294, 306, 342, 404, 406, 477, 545, 614,
   652, 729, 781, 795–797, 854, 1018, 1044, 1070, 1131, 1146
17. *Vibrio*
   44, 714, 933
18. Miscellaneous
   52, 60, 65, 118, 128, 187, 195, 197, 234, 297, 315, 401, 403,
   441, 458, 738, 739, 747, 782, 786, 809, 856, 994, 1054, 1087,
   1098

III. APPLICATIONS IN MYCOLOGY

A. Reviews

390

B. Specific Organisms

1. *Blastomyces*
   85, 526, 542, 862, 1088
2. *Candida*
   388, 594, 616, 953, 1088
3. *Cryptococcus*
   73, 533, 1088
4. *Histoplasma*
   85, 113, 389, 537–539, 541–543, 849, 862, 870, 1088, 1145
5. *Sporotrichium*
   524, 525, 596
6. Miscellaneous
   7, 142, 391, 523, 595, 597, 696, 741, 742, 847, 915, 920, 956,
   984, 989, 990, 1033, 1063

IV. APPLICATIONS IN PARASITOLOGY (INCLUDING FREE-LIVING PROTOZOANS)

A. Reviews

14, 15, 368, 369, 934, 945, 1093, 1151

B. Specific Organisms

1. Amebas
363, 364, 367, 370, 371, 373, 377–379, 495, 496, 498, 761, 983, 1140, 1150
2. *Ascaris* and Related Nematodes
204, 488, 489, 603, 737, 937, 1021, 1029, 1030
3. Filarial Worms
108, 657, 659
4. *Leishmania*
86, 172, 270, 434, 811, 972
5. Malaria
1, 75, 166–171, 194, 216, 256, 345, 481, 482, 587, 599–601, 1000, 1001, 1057–1060, 1091–1096
6. *Schistosoma* and Other Trematodes
16–18, 95, 174–176, 252, 308, 341, 350, 351, 487, 511, 630, 839, 874, 935, 936, 938, 939, 941, 1055, 1064, 1065
7. *Toxoplasma gondii*
14, 40, 109, 120, 222, 316, 331, 343, 365, 366, 376, 380, 544, 582, 681, 1013, 1023, 1034, 1069, 1081, 1104
8. *Trypanosoma*
43, 295, 307, 357, 658, 940, 971, 1066, 1113, 1132
9. Miscellaneous
32, 38, 39, 58, 68, 93, 94, 344, 707, 802, 911, 912, 969, 1149

V. APPLICATIONS IN VIROLOGY (INCLUDING RICKETTSIA-LIKE ORGANISMS)

A. Reviews

22, 185, 435, 643, 648, 734, 904, 951, 1110, 1127, 1142

B. DNA Viruses

1. Adenoviruses
   82, 83, 110, 247, 346, 474, 480, 671, 807, 810, 846, 860, 881, 928, 1007
2. Herpes Viruses
   3, 49, 66, 235, 349, 398, 399, 463, 478, 504, 610, 676, 798, 812, 843, 844, 875, 883, 931, 1025, 1073, 1097, 1114
3. Papilloma Viruses
   137, 534, 535, 804, 805, 998
4. Polyoma Viruses
   50, 254, 263, 327, 557, 623, 735, 764, 932, 975, 1078, 1079
5. Pox Viruses
   119, 274, 405, 555, 576, 584, 624, 649, 650, 651, 766, 806, 885, 917, 947, 992, 1004, 1010, 1114
6. Simian Vacuolating Virus (SV40)
   112, 255, 272, 304, 356, 474, 485, 559, 621, 726, 810, 859 877, 878, 881, 882, 928, 974, 1043

C. RNA Viruses

1. Arboviruses
   99, 275, 506, 590, 591, 593, 598, 728, 767, 800, 803, 980, 1005, 1009, 1032
2. ECHO Viruses
   221, 340, 425, 426, 491, 901
3. Hepatitis Viruses
   81, 674, 758, 868
4. Leukemia Viruses (Including Lymphoma and Rous Sarcoma)
   311, 416, 430, 432, 562–564, 675, 719, 821, 822, 833, 879, 1072, 1089, 1090
5. Measles
   26, 161, 631, 646, 647, 695, 799, 825, 880, 884
6. Mumps Virus
   139, 191, 617, 1106, 1107
7. Myxoviruses (Primarily Influenza)
   4, 70, 71, 74, 245, 258, 301, 302, 328, 421, 483, 636–638, 640, 783, 817, 1108

8. Newcastle Disease Virus
499, 501, 668, 669, 670, 869, 894, 919, 1026, 1027, 1117–1119, 1133
9. Paramyxoviruses (Other than Those Listed Separately)
91, 114, 154, 162, 558, 631, 632, 644, 663, 743, 756, 757, 1152
10. Picornaviruses (Primarily Polio)
97, 98, 443, 580, 611, 702, 767, 873, 905, 906, 1007
11. Plant Viruses
445, 771–774, 959, 986–988
12. Rabies Virus
12, 13, 25, 116, 206, 242, 305, 329, 339, 384, 385, 505, 507, 615, 713, 770, 1046, 1130

D. Rickettsia-like Organisms

1. Trachoma—Lymphogranuloma—Psittacosis
34, 53, 100, 362, 410, 418, 493, 536, 753, 765, 792–794, 922, 966, 1061, 1097
2. Rickettsia (Including *Anaplasma*)
10, 20, 84, 101–103, 191, 280, 293, 387, 583, 585, 586, 592, 913, 914, 960

E. Miscellaneous

2, 45–47, 57, 87, 89, 457, 484, 486, 503, 508, 531, 552, 558, 708, 736, 767, 890, 973, 1011, 1014, 1103, 1134

VI. APPLICATIONS IN PATHOLOGY (INCLUDING NORMAL TISSUE ANTIGENS)

A. Reviews

147, 517, 661, 995

B. Specific Organs and Tissues

1. Blood Cells and Plasma Proteins
105, 107, 213, 215, 269, 359, 360, 361, 433, 470, 492, 549, 613, 710, 745, 863, 1006, 1028, 1105, 1122

F. Rheumatic Diseases

19, 33, 265, 436, 704, 717, 720, 721, 893, 982, 1086, 1116

G. Miscellaneous

72, 92, 201, 383, 455, 514, 547, 548, 553, 556, 581, 589, 678, 853, 864, 916, 927, 1036, 1085, 1112

VII. APPLICATIONS IN IMMUNOLOGY

A. Reviews

264, 320

B. Antibody Production and Localization

121, 138, 189, 260, 281, 417, 422, 449, 612, 709, 717, 718, 784, 836, 886, 887, 944, 1076, 1077, 1100–1102, 1125, 1128, 1129, 1137

C. Antigen Localization

188, 190, 191, 317, 441, 519, 943, 967

VIII. NONSTAINING USES OF FLUORESCENT ANTIBODY (TEST TUBE REACTIONS)

323, 427, 459, 662, 769, 788, 789, 1042

APPENDIX A

I. DIRECTORY OF COMMERCIAL SOURCES SPECIFICALLY MENTIONED IN THE TEXT AS SOURCES OF EQUIPMENT AND SUPPLIES

Aloe Scientific Co., 1831 Olive St., St. Louis, Mo. 63103, U.S.

A.E.I. Lamp and Lighting Co., Ltd., Melton Rd., Leicester, England

Agfa AG, Leverkusen, Germany

Air Reduction Chemical and Carbide Co., 150 E. 42nd St., New York, N.Y. 10017, U.S.

American Optical Co., Instrument Division, Buffalo, N.Y. 14215, U.S.

Ansco, Binghamton, N.Y., U.S.

Atlas Powder Co., Wilmington, Del. U.S.

Baker Instruments, Ltd., Purley Way, Croydon, Surrey, England

Baltimore Biological Laboratory, Box 6711, Baltimore, Md. 21204, U.S.

Bausch and Lomb, Rochester, N.Y. 14602, U.S.

British Drug Houses, Ltd., Poole, Dorset, England

Bio-Rad Laboratories, Richmond, Calif., 94804, U.S.

Calbiochem, 3625 Medford St., Los Angles, Calif., U.S.

Chance-Pilkington Optical Works, Smethwick 40, Birmingham, England

Chemplast, Inc., 3 Central Ave., East Newark, N.J., U.S.

Colab Laboratories, 1526 Halsted St., Chicago Heights, Ill. 60411, U.S.

Commercial Solvents Corp., Terre Haute, Ind., U.S.

Cooke, Troughton and Simms, Inc., 91 Waite St., Malden, Mass. 02148, U.S.
(Haxby Rd., York, England)

Corning Glass Works, Optical Sales Dept., Corning, N.Y. 14830, U.S.

Difco Laboratories, 920 Henry St., Detroit, Mich. 48201, U.S.

Dow Chemical Co., Midland, Mich. 48640, U.S.

E.I. DuPont de Nemours & Co., Wilmington, Del. 19898, U.S.

Eastman Kodak Co., Rochester, N.Y., U.S.

Edward Gurr, Ltd., Michrome Laboratories, 42 Upper Richmond Rd., West London, S.W. 14, England

Evans Electroselenium Ltd., St. Andrew's Works, Hallstead, Essex, England

Galileo Corporation of America, 18 E. 53rd St., New York N.Y. 10022, U.S.
    (Officine Galileo S.p.A., Milan, Italy)

General Aniline and Film Corp., 140 W. 51st St., N.Y. 10020, U.S.

General Electric, Outdoor Lighting Dept., Hendersonville, N.C., U.S.

Gevaert Co. of America, 321 W. 54th St., New York, N.Y., U.S.
    (Photo-Produits Gevaert S.A., Mortsel, Antwerp, Belgium)

Hanovia Lamp Division, 100 Chestnut St., Newark, N.J. 07105, U.S.

Ilford, Inc., 37 W. 65th St., New York, N.Y., U.S.
    (Ilford Ltd., Ilford, Essex, England)

Imperial Chemical Industries, Ltd., 488 Madison Ave., New York, N.Y., U.S.
    (Nobel House, Buckingham Gate, London, S.W. 1, England)

E. Leitz, Inc., 468 Park Ave. South, New York, N.Y. 10016, U.S.
    (Ernst Leitz GMBH, Wetzlar, West Germany)

Mark-tex Corp., 161 Coolidge Ave., Englewood, N.J., U.S.

Nikon, Inc., 623 Stewart Ave., Garden City, N.Y. 11533, U.S.
    (Nippon Kogaku K.K., Tokyo, Japan)

Nutritional Biochemicals Corp., 21010 Miles Ave., Cleveland, Ohio 44128, U.S.

Osram G.m.b.H., Berlin, West Germany

PEK Labs., Inc., 825 E. Evelyn Ave., Sunnyvale, Calif., U.S.

Pharmacia Fine Chemicals, Inc., 800 Centennial Ave., Piscataway, N.J. 08854, U.S.
    (Pharmacia, Uppsala, Sweden)

North American Philips Co., Inc., 100 E. 42nd St., New York, N.Y. 10017, U.S.
    (N.V. Philips Gloeilampenfabrieken, Eindhoven, Holland)

Photovolt Corp., 95 Madison Ave., New York, N.Y., U.S.

Polaroid Corp., Box 200 A, Cambridge, Mass. 02139, U.S.

Reichert microscopes, William J. Hacker & Co., Box 646, West Caldwell, N.J., U.S.
   (C. Reichert Optische Werke AG, Vienna 17, Austria)
Carl Schleicher and Schuell Co., Keene, N.H., U.S.
Schoeffel Instrument Co., 15 Douglas St., Westwood, N.J. 07675, U.S.
Schott filters—Fish-Schurman Corp., 70 Portman Rd., New Rochelle, N.Y. 10802, U.S. (Schott and Gen., Mainz, West Germany)
Salford Instruments, Salford, England
Superior Electric Co., Bristol, Conn. 06010, U.S.
Sylvania Electric Products, Burlington Rd., Bedford, Mass. 01730, U.S.
G.K. Turner Associates, 2524 Pulgas Ave., Palo Alto, Calif., U.S.
Union Carbide Chemicals Co., 270 Park Ave., New York, N.Y. 10017, U.S.
W. Watson and Sons, 313 High Holborn, London, W.C. 1, England
Wild Heerbrugg Instrument Co., 564 Smith St., Farmingdale, N.Y. 11735, U.S.
   (Wild Heerbrugg Ltd., Heerbrugg, Switzerland)
Winthrop Laboratories, 90 Park Ave., New York, N.Y. 10016, U.S.
Carl Zeiss, Inc., 444 5th Ave., New York, N.Y. 10018, U.S.
   (Carl Zeiss, Oberkochen, West Germany)

II. DIRECTORY OF COMMERCIAL SOURCES FOR REAGENTS (ANTISERA, CONJUGATES, DYES, ETC.), WHETHER OR NOT THEY ARE SPECIFICALLY MENTIONED IN THE TEXT

Antibodies, Inc., 835 L St., Davis, Calif. 95616, U.S.
Baltimore Biological Laboratory, Box 6711, Baltimore, Md. 21204, U.S.
Brook Microbiologicals—Aloe Scientific Co., Dept. RK, 1831 Olive St., St. Louis, Mo. 63103, U.S.
Case Laboratories, Inc., 515 N. Halsted St., Chicago, Ill., U.S.
Colorado Serum Co., 4950 York St., Denver, Colo., U.S.
Dajac Laboratories, 5000 Langdon St., Philadelphia, Pa., U.S.
Difco Laboratories, 920 Henry St., Detroit, Mich. 48201, U.S.
Hyland Laboratories, 4501 Colorado Blvd., Los Angeles, Calif. 90039, U.S.

Mann Research Laboratories, 136 Liberty St., New York, N.Y.
10006, U.S.
Microbiological Associates, 4813 Bethesda Ave., Bethesda, Md.
20014, U.S.
Nutritional Biochemicals Corp., 21010 Miles Ave., Cleveland, Ohio
44128, U.S.
Pentex Inc., Box 272, Kankakee, Ill. 60901, U.S.
Roboz Surgical Instruments Co., 810 18th St. N.W., Washington,
D.C. 20006, U.S.
Sylvana Chemical Co., Orange, N.J., U.S.

APPENDIX B—BUFFERS

Figures given below for preparing buffer solutions should be taken only as approximations, since various factors influence the precise pH attained with reagents off the shelf. In all cases, the pH should be checked on a meter, if possible, and brought to the desired level by appropriate titration with one or the other of the component reagents.

1. Phosphate-buffered saline, pH 7.5, 0.01M buffer:

Na_2HPO_4 (anhydrous; MW, 141.96)	1.20 gm
$NaH_2PO_4 \cdot H_2O$ (MW, 137.99)	0.22 gm
NaCl (MW, 58.44)	8.50 gm
Distilled water to make	1000.00 ml

2. Phosphate buffer, pH 6.3, 0.0175M (for DEAE chromatography)

   a. Dissolve 2.48 gm of Na_2HPO_4 in 1 liter of distilled water
   b. Dissolve 2.41 gm of NaH_2PO_4 in 1 liter of distilled water
   c. Add 1 part of (a) to 2 parts of (b) and adjust to pH 6.3

3. Saline solutions (for DEAE chromatography)

   a. Prepare 2M stock solution by dissolving 11.69 gm of NaCl in 100 ml of phosphate buffer from (2) above
   b. To prepare 0.125M NaCl, mix 6.25 ml of 2M NaCl with 93.75 ml of phosphate buffer, pH 6.3
   c. To prepare 0.250M NaCl, mix 12.5 ml of 2M NaCl with 87.5 ml of phosphate buffer, pH 6.3

4. Carbonate buffer, pH 9.5, 0.5M

   a. Dissolve 5.3 gm of Na_2CO_3 (anhydrous, MW, 105.99) in 100 ml of 0.85% saline
   b. Dissolve 4.2 gm of $NaHCO_3$ (anhydrous, MW, 84.01) in 100 ml of 0.85% saline
   c. Add 5.8 ml of (a) to 10.0 ml of (b) and adjust to pH 9.5

REFERENCES

1. Abele, D. C., Tobie, J. E., Hill, G. J., Contacos, P. G., and Evans, C. B. (1965). Alterations in serum proteins and 19S antibody production during the course of induced malarial infections in man. *Am. J. Trop. Med. Hyg.* **14**: 191-197.
2. Aiken, J. M., Hoopes, K. H., Stair, E. L., and Rhodes, M. B. (1964). Rapid diagnosis of hog cholera: A tissue-impression fluorescent-antibody technique. *J. Am. Vet. Med. Assoc.* **144**: 1395-1397.
3. Albrecht, P., Blaskovic, D., Jakubik, J., and Lesso, J. (1963). Demonstration of pseudorabies virus in chick embryo cell cultures and infected animals by the fluorescent antibody technique. *Acta Virol.* **7**: 289-296.
4. Albrecht, P., Blaskovic, D., Styk, B., and Koller, M. (1963). Course of A2 influenza in intranasally infected mice examined by the fluorescent-antibody technique. *Acta Virol.* **7**: 405-413.
5. Albrecht, P., Mrenová, M., and Karelová, E. (1966). Paraffin embedding techniques for immunofluorescent demonstration of neurotropic viruses. *Acta Virol.* **10**: 155-160.
6. Albrecht, P., and Sokol, F. (1961). Fluorescent antibody method: Optimal conditions for conjugation of 1-dimethylaminonaphthalene-5-sulphonyl chloride with gamma globulin. *Folia Microbiol. (Prague)* **6**: 49-54.
7. Al-Doory, Y., and Gordon, M. A. (1963). Application of fluorescent-antibody procedures to the study of pathogenic dematiaceous fungi. I. Differentiation of *Cladosporium carrionii* and *Cladosporium bantianum*. *J. Bacteriol.* **86**: 332-338.
8. Alexander, W. R. M. (1958). The application of the fluorescent-antibody technique to haemagglutinating systems. *Immunology* **1**: 217-223.
9. Alexander, W. R. M., and Potter, J. L. (1963). Rhodamine-conjugated papain as a counterstain in fluorescence microscopy. *Immunology* **6**: 450-452.
10. Alkan, W. J., Evenchik, Z., and Eshchar, J. (1965). Q fever and infectious hepatitis. *Am. J. Med.* **38**: 54-61.
11. Allen, J. C., and Cluff, L. E. (1963). Identification of toxinogenic C. *diphtheriae* with fluorescent antitoxin: Demonstration of its non-specificity. *Proc. Soc. Exptl. Biol. Med.* **112**: 194-199.
12. Allen, R., Sims, R. A., and Sulkin, S. E. (1964). Studies with cultured brown adipose tissue. I. Persistence of rabies virus in bat brown fat. *Am. J. Hyg.* **80**: 11-24.
13. Allen, R., Sims, R. A., and Sulkin, S. E. (1964). Studies with cul-

tured brown adipose tissue. II. Influence of low temperature on rabies virus infection in bat brown fat. *Am. J. Hyg.* **80**: 25-52.

14. Ambroise-Thomas, M. P. (1963). L'immuno-fluorescence dans le diagnostic direct et indirect des parasitases: Applications à la toxoplasmose. M.D. thesis. Laboratory of Parasitology, Faculty of Medicine, University of Lyons, France.

15. Ambroise-Thomas, M. P. (1965). Les acquisitions et les perspectives de l'immuno-fluorescence en parasitologie. *J. Med. Lyon,* June 5, 1965: 1055-1068.

16. Anderson, R. I., Sadun, E. H., and Williams, J. S. (1961). A technique for the use of minute amounts of dried blood in the fluorescent antibody test for schistosomiasis. *Exptl. Parasitol.* **11**: 111-116.

17. Anderson, R. I., Sadun, E. H., and Williams, J. S. (1961). Preserved cercariae in the fluorescent antibody (FA) test for schistosomiasis. *Exptl. Parasitol.* **11**: 226-230.

18. Andrade, Z. A., Paronetto, F., and Popper, H. (1961). Immuno-cytochemical studies in schistosomiasis. *Am. J. Pathol.* **39**: 589-598.

19. Angelino, P. F., and Vacca, G. (1964). Immunofluorescence on the human myocardium of rheumatic subjects. (Italian) *Minerva Med.* **55**: 49-54.

20. Anthony, D. W., Madden, P. A., and Gates, D. W. (1964). *Anaplasma marginale* Theiler observed in the gut and excreta of *Dermacentor andersoni* Stiles (*Dermacentor venustus* Marx). *Am. J. Vet. Res.* **25**: 1464-1472.

21. Appel, S. H., and Bornstein, M. B. (1964). The application of tissue culture to the study of experimental allergic encephalo-myelitis. II. Serum factors responsible for demyelination. *J. Exptl. Med.* **119**: 303-312.

22. Apted, F. I. (1964). Rickettsial diseases. *Trop. Diseases Bull.* **61**: 981-988.

23. Arquilla, E. R., and Coblence, C. (1960). The isolation of rabbit insulin antibodies. *Anat. Record* **138**: 203-209.

24. Asherson, G. L. (1964). Experimental production of autoantibody to gut antigens. *Proc. Roy. Soc. Med.* **57**: 813-814.

25. Atanasiu, P., Lepine, P., and Dragonas, P. (1963). Kinetic study of the rabies virus in tissue culture using fluorescent antibodies and ultra-thin sections. (French) *Ann. Inst. Pasteur* **105**: 813-824.

26. Atherton, J. G., Chaparas, S. D., Cremer, M., and Gordon, I. (1965). Mechanism of polykaryocytosis associated with noncytopathic infection by measles virus. *J. Bacteriol.* **90**: 213-219.

27. Ayoub, E. M., and Wannamaker, L. W. (1964). Identification of Group A streptococci. Evaluation of the use of the fluorescent-antibody technique. *J. Am. Med. Assoc.* **187**: 908-913.

28. Balfour, B. M. (1961). Immunological studies on a freeze-substi-tution method of preparing tissue for fluorescent antibody staining. *Immunology* **4**: 206-218.

29. Balfour, B. M., Doniach, D., Roitt, I. M., and Couchman, K. G. (1961). Fluorescent antibody studies in human thyroiditis: Auto-antibodies to an antigen of the thyroid colloid distinct from thyroglobulin. *Brit. J. Exptl. Pathol.* **42**: 307-316.
30. Barile, M. F., Malizia, W. F., and Riggs, D. B. (1962). Incidence and detection of pleuropneumonia-like organisms in cell cultures by fluorescent antibody and cultural procedures. *J. Bacteriol.* **84**: 130-136.
31. Barnes, R., Carmichael, D., and Johnson, G. B. (1962). Comparison between the latex nucleoprotein test and the fluorescent method for the demonstration of antinuclear factor. *Ann. Rheumatic Diseases* **21**: 287-292.
32. Barrow, J. H., Jr., and Taylor, B. C. (1966). Fluorescent-antibody studies of haplosporidian parasites of oysters in Chesapeake and Delaware Bays. *Science* **153**: 1531-1533.
33. Bartfeld, H. (1965). Rheumatoid arthritic and non-rheumatoid synovium in cell culture. Morphological observations, acridine orange, and fluorescent fraction II studies. *Ann. Rheumatic Diseases* **24**: 31-39.
34. Bates, H. A., Pomeroy, B. S., Seal, U. S., and Jay, A. R. (1965). Ornithosis: Experimental immunofluorescent studies. *Avian Diseases* **9**: 24-30.
35. Batty, I., and Walker, P. D. (1963). Differentiation of *Clostridium septicum* and *Clostridium chauvoei* by the use of fluorescent labelled antibodies. *J. Pathol. Bacteriol.* **85**: 517-521.
36. Batty, I., and Walker, P. D. (1964). The identification of *Clostridium novyi* (*Clostridium oedematiens*) and *Clostridium tetani* by the use of fluorescent labelled antibodies. *J. Pathol. Bacteriol.* **88**: 327-328.
37. Baumstark, J. S., Laffin, R. J., and Bardowill, W. A. (1964). A preparative method for the separation of 7S gamma globulin from human serum. *Arch. Biochem. Biophys.* **108**: 514-522.
38. Beale, G. H., and Kacser, H. (1957). Studies on the antigens of *Paramecium aurelia* with the aid of fluorescent antibodies. *J. Gen. Microbiol.* **17**: 68-74.
39. Beale, G. H., and Mott, M. R. (1962). Further studies on the antigens of *Paramecium aurelia* with the aid of fluorescent antibodies. *J. Gen. Microbiol.* **28**: 617-624.
40. Beauregard, M., Magwood, S. E., Bannister, G. L., Robertson, A., Boulanger, P., Ruckerbauer, G. M., and Appel, M. (1965). A study of *Toxoplasma* infection in chickens and cats on a family farm. *Can. J. Comp. Med. Vet. Sci.* **29**: 286-291.
41. Beck, J. S. (1963). Auto-antibodies to cell nuclei. *Scot. Med. J.* **8**: 373-388.
42. Beck, J. S., Anderson, J. R., and Bloch, K. J. (1965). Antinuclear and precipitating auto-antibodies in Sjögren's syndrome. *Ann. Rheumatic Diseases* **24**: 16-22.

43. Beck, J. S., and Walker, P. J. (1964). Antigenicity of trypanosome nuclei: Evidence that DNA is not coupled to histone in these protozoa. *Nature* **204**: 194-195.

44. Belden, E. L., and Robertstad, G. W. (1965). Application of fluorescent antibody technique for serotyping *Vibrio fetus*. *Am. J. Vet. Res.* **26**: 1437-1441.

45. Bellett, A. J., and Mercer, E. H. (1964). The multiplication of sericesthis iridescent virus in cell cultures from *Antheraea eucalypti* Scott. I. Qualitative experiments. *Virology* **24**: 645-653.

46. Bellett, A. J. (1965). The multiplication of sericesthis iridescent virus in cell cultures from *Antheraea eucalypti* Scott. II. An *in vitro* assay for the virus. *Virology* **26**: 127-131.

47. Bellett, A. J. (1965). The multiplication of sericesthis iridescent virus in cell cultures from *Antheraea eucalypti* Scott. III. Quantitative experiments. *Virology* **26**: 132-141.

48. Bellone, A. G., and Leigheb, G. (1964). Observations on the F.T.A. test with particular regard to untreated primary syphilis. (Italian) *Giorn. Ital. Dermatol.* **105**: 175-184.

49. Benda, R. (1965). Demonstration of B virus (herpes virus simiae) in HeLa cells by the fluorescent antibody technique. *Acta Virol.* **9**: 172-179.

50. Bereczky, E., Hughes, R., Bowen, J. M., Munyon, W., and Dmochowski, L. (1965). Study of DNA synthesis and antigen formation in polyoma virus-infected mouse embryo cells by autoradiography and immunofluorescence. *Texas Rept. Biol. Med.* **23**: 3-15.

51. Beregi, E., Perenyi, L., and Simon, J. (1963). Immunofluorescence studies in experimental periarteritis nodosa in rabbits of different ages. *Gerontologia* **8**: 233-241.

52. Bergman, S., Forsgren, A., and Swahn, B. (1966). Effect of normally occurring rabbit antibodies on fluorescent-antibody reactions. *J. Bacteriol.* **91**: 1664-1665.

53. Bernkopf, H., Treu, G., and Maythar, B. (1964). Human infection experiments with three cell-cultured trachoma agents. *Arch. Ophthalmol.* **71**: 693-700.

54. Beutner, E. H. (1961). Immunofluorescent staining: The fluorescent antibody method. *Bacteriol. Rev.* **25**: 49-76.

55. Beutner, E. H., and Witebsky, I. (1962). Studies on organ specificity XIV. Immunofluorescent studies of thyroid reactive autoantibodies in human sera. *J. Immunol.* **88**: 462-475.

56. Beutner, E. H., Witebsky, E., Rose, N. R., and Gerbasi, J. R. (1958). Localization of thyroid and spinal cord autoantibodies by fluorescent antibody technic. *Proc. Soc. Exptl. Biol. Med.* **97**: 712-716.

57. Bhamarapravati, N., Halstead, S. B., Sookavachana, P., and Boonyapaknavik, V. (1964). Studies on dengue virus infection. 1. Immunofluorescent localization of virus in mouse tissue. *Arch. Pathol.* **77**: 538-543.

58. Biagi, F., and Pina, A. (1964). Presence of antigens in calcareous corpuscles of cysticercus. *Rev. Inst. Med. Trop. Sao Paulo* **6**: 114-116.

59. Biberfeld, G., Johnsson, T., and Jonsson, J. (1965). Studies on *Mycoplasma pneumoniae* infection in Sweden. *Acta Pathol. Microbiol. Scand.* **63**: 469-475.

60. Biegeleisen, J. Z., Jr. (1964). . Immunofluorescence techniques in retrospective diagnosis of human listeriosis. *J. Bacteriol.* **87**: 1257-1258.

61. Biegeleisen, J. Z., Jr. (1964). Immunofluorescent staining of *Bacillus anthracis* in dried beef. *J. Bacteriol.* **88**: 260-261.

62. Biegeleisen, J. Z., Jr., Bradshaw, B. R., and Moody, M. D. (1962). Demonstration of *Brucella* antibodies in human serum. A comparison of the fluorescent antibody and agglutination techniques. *J. Immunol.* **88**: 109-112.

63. Biegeleisen, J. Z., Jr., Cherry, W. B., Skaley, P., and Moody, M. D. (1962). The demonstration of *Bacillus anthracis* in environmental specimens by conventional and fluorescent antibody techniques. *Am. J. Hyg.* **75**: 230-239.

64. Biegeleisen, J. Z., Jr., Mitchell, M. S., Marcus, B. B., Rhoden, D. L., and Blumberg, R. W. (1965). Immunofluorescence techniques for demonstrating bacterial pathogens associated with cerebrospinal meningitis. I. Clinical evaluation of conjugates on smears prepared directly from cerebrospinal fluid sediments. *J. Lab. Clin. Med.* **65**: 976-989.

65. Biegeleisen, J. Z., Jr., Mosquera, R., and Cherry, W. B. (1964). A case of human meliodosis: Clinical, epidemiological and laboratory findings. *Am. J. Trop. Med. Hyg.* **13**: 89-99.

66. Biegeleisen, J. Z., Jr., Scott, L. V., and Lewis, V., Jr. (1959). Rapid diagnosis of herpes simplex virus infection with fluorescent antibody. *Science* **129**: 640-641.

67. Billen, J. L., Griffin, J. W., and Waldron, C. A. (1964). Investigations for pyronin bodies and fluorescent antibodies in 5:5 diphenylhydantoin gingival hyperplasia. *Oral. Surg., Oral Med., Oral Pathol.* **18**: 773-782.

68. Bird, A. F. (1964). Serological studies on the plant parasitic nematode, *Meloidogyne javanica. Exptl. Parasitol.* **15**: 350-360.

69. Birge, W. J. (1959). A photometer head assembly for use in microphotometry. *J. Histochem. Cytochem.* **7**: 395-397.

70. Blaskovic, D., Albrecht, P., Lackovic, V., Lesso, J., Rathova, V., and Styk, B. (1963). Rapid diagnosis of influenza by the fluorescent antibody method. *Acta Virol.* **7**: 192.

71. Blaskovic, D., Szanto, J., Albrecht, P., Sadecky, E., and Lackovic, V. (1964). Demonstration of swine influenza virus in pigs by the fluorescent antibody method. *Acta Virol.* **8**: 401-409.

72. Blau, S., Janis, R., Hamerman, D., and Sandson, J. (1965). Cellular origin of hyaluronateprotein in human synovial membrane. *Science* **150**: 353-355.

73. Bloomfield, N., Gordon, M. A., and Elmendorf, D. F., Jr. (1963). Detection of *Cryptococcus neoformans* antigen in body fluids by latex particle agglutination. *Proc. Soc. Exptl. Biol. Med.* **114**: 64-67.

74. Boand, A. V., Jr., Kempf, J. E., and Hanson, R. J. (1957). Phagocytosis of influenza virus. I. *In vitro* observations. *J. Immunol.* **79**: 416-421.

75. Bona, C., Ciplea, A. G., and Ianco, L. (1964). The mechanisms of acquired immunity in infections with *Plasmodium vivax*. Fluorescent antibody technics in the complex of cyto-sero-chemical tests of the blood system during the process of immunogenesis. (French) *Arch. Roumaines Pathol. Exptl. Microbiol.* **23**: 749-762.

76. Boothroyd, M., and Georgala, D. L. (1964). Immunofluorescent identification of *Clostridium botulinum*. *Nature* **202**: 515-516.

77. Borek, F. (1961). The fluorescent antibody method in medical and biological research. *Bull. World Health Organ.* **24**: 249-256.

78. Borek, F., and Silverstein, A. M. (1960). A new fluorescent label for antibody proteins. *Arch. Biochem. Biophys.* **87**: 293-297.

79. Boris, M., Thomason, B. M., Hines, V. D., Montagu, T. S., and Sellers, T. F. (1964). A community epidemic of enteropathogenic *Escherichia coli* 0126:B16:NM gastroenteritis associated with asymptomatic respiratory infection. *Pediatrics* **33**: 18-29.

80. Boss, J. H. (1965). A comparative study of kidney and muscle membrane antigens in the human and rat. *Exptl. Mol. Pathol.* **4**: 416-430.

81. Boss, J. H., and Jones, W. A. (1963). Hepatic localization of infectious agent in murine viral hepatitis. *Arch. Pathol.* **76**: 4-8.

82. Boyer, G. S., Denny, F. W., Jr., and Ginsberg, H. S. (1959). Intracellular localization of type 4 adenovirus. II. Cytological and fluorescein-labelled antibody studies. *J. Exptl. Med.* **109**: 85-96.

83. Boyer, G. S., Denny, F. W., Jr., and Ginsburg, H. S. (1959). Sequential cellular changes produced by types 5 and 7 adenoviruses in HeLa cells and in human amniotic cells. *J. Exptl. Med.* **110**: 827-843.

84. Bozeman, F. M., and Elisberg, B. L. (1963). Serological diagnosis of scrub typhus by indirect immunofluorescence. *Proc. Soc. Exptl. Biol. Med.* **112**: 568-573.

85. Brandsberg, J. W., Tosh, F. E., and Furcolow, M. L. (1964). Concurrent infection with *Histoplasma capsulatum* and *Blastomyces dermatitidis*. *New Engl. J. Med.* **270**: 874-877.

86. Bray, R. S., and Lainson, R. (1965). The immunology and serology of leishmaniasis. I. The fluorescent antibody staining technique. *Trans. Roy. Soc. Trop. Med. Hyg.* **59**: 535-544.

87. Breitenfeld, P. M., and Schafer, W. (1957). The formation of fowl plague virus antigens in infected cells, as studied with fluorescent antibodies. *Virology* **4**: 328-345.

88. Brooks, J. B., Lewis, V. J., and Pittman, B. (1965). Separation of

fluorescent antibody conjugates into 7S and 19S globulin components by gel filtration. *Proc. Soc. Exptl. Biol. Med.* **119**: 748-751.

89. Brown, E. R., and Bittner, J. J. (1961). Fluorescent antibody reactions against the mouse mammary tumor agent. *Proc. Soc. Exptl. Biol. Med.* **106**: 303-306.

90. Brown, G. C. (1963). Fluorescent antibody techniques for the diagnosis of enteric infections. *Arch. Ges. Virusforsch.* **13**: 30-34.

91. Brown, G. C., Maassab, H. F., Veronelli, J. A., and Francis, T. (1964). Rubella antibodies in human serum: Detection by the indirect fluorescent-antibody technique. *Science* **145**: 943-945.

92. Brown, P. C., Glynn, L. E., and Holborow, E. J. (1963). The pathogenesis of experimental allergic orchitis in guinea-pigs. *J. Pathol. Bacteriol.* **86**: 505-520.

93. Brzosko, W. J., and Nowoslawski, A. (1963). Immunohistochemical studies on *Pneumocystis pneumonia*. *Bull. Acad. Polon. Sci. Sér. Sci. Biol.* **11**: 563-564.

94. Brzosko, W. J., Nowoslawski, A., and Madalinski, K. (1964). Identification of immune complexes in lungs from *Pneumocystis carinii* pneumonia cases in infants. *Bull. Acad. Polon. Sci. Sér. Sci. Biol.* **12**: 137-142.

95. Buck, A. A., Sadun, E. H., Anderson, R. I., and Shaffa, E. (1964). Comparative studies of some immunologic screening tests for schistosomiasis in Ethiopia. *Am. J. Hyg.* **80**: 75-84.

96. Buck, A. A., and Spruyt, D. J. (1964). Seroreactivity in the Venereal Disease Research Laboratory slide test and the fluorescent treponemal antibody test. *Am. J. Hyg.* **80**: 91-102.

97. Buckley, S. M. (1956). Visualization of poliomyelitis virus by fluorescent antibody. *Arch. Ges. Virusforsch.* **6**: 388-400.

98. Buckley, S. M. (1957). Cytopathology of poliomyelitis virus in tissue culture. Fluorescent antibody and tinctorial studies. *Am. J. Pathol.* **33**: 691-707.

99. Buckley, S. M. (1965). Junin and tacaribe work in HeLa cells. *Am. J. Trop. Med. Hyg.* **14**: 792-794.

100. Buckley, S. M., Whitney, E., and Rapp, F. (1955). Identification by fluorescent antibody of developmental forms of psittacosis virus in tissue culture. *Proc. Soc. Exptl. Biol. Med.* **90**: 226-230.

101. Burgdorfer, W. (1961). Evaluation of the fluorescent antibody technique for the detection of Rocky Mountain spotted fever rickettsiae in various tissues. *Pathol. Microbiol.* **24**: Suppl., 27-39.

102. Burgdorfer, W., and Lackman, D. (1960). Identification of the virus of Colorado tick fever in mouse tissues by means of fluorescent antibodies. *J. Bacteriol.* **80**: 131-136.

103. Burgdorfer, W., and Lackman, D. (1960). Identification of *Rickettsia rickettsii* in the wood tick, *Dermacentor andersoni,* by means of fluorescent antibodies. *J. Infect. Diseases* **107**: 241-244.

104. Burkholder, P. M., Littell, A. H., and Klein, P. G. (1961). Sectioning at room temperature of unfixed tissue, frozen in a gelatin

matrix, for immunohistologic procedures. *Stain Technol.* **36**: 89-91.

105. Burton, P., and Buffi, D. (1963). Immunofluorescent studies of human plasma cells in γ and B$_2$A myelomas. *Proc. Soc. Exptl. Biol. Med.* **114**: 171-175.

106. Butler, M., and Leach, R. H. (1964). A *Mycoplasma* which induces acidity and cytopathic effect in tissue culture. *J. Gen. Microbiol.* **34**: 285-294.

107. Calabresi, P., Edwards, E. A., and Schilling, R. F. (1959). Fluorescent antiglobulin studies in leukopenic and related disorders. *J. Clin. Invest.* **38**: 2091-2100.

108. Calderon, S. (1964). Immunological studies in onchocerciasis. (Spanish) *Salud Publica Mex.* **6**: 553-559.

109. Camargo, M. E. (1964). Improved technique of indirect immunofluorescence for serological diagnosis of toxoplasmosis. *Rev. Inst. Med. Trop. Sao Paulo* **6**: 117-118.

110. Carmichael, L. E. (1965). An incomplete cycle of adenovirus type 4 multiplication in canine cell cultures and in dogs. *Am. J. Vet. Res.* **26**: 15-23.

111. Caron, G., Martineau, J., and de Repentigny, J. (1964). Quantitative differentiation, using fluorescent antibodies, between strains of staphylococcus isolated from healthy carriers or from clinical cases of different severity. (French) *Rev. Can. Biol.* **23**: 455-459.

112. Carski, T. R. (1960). A fluorescent antibody study of the simian foamy agent. *J. Immunol.* **84**: 426-433.

113. Carski, T. R., Cozad, G. C., and Larsh, H. W. (1962). Detection of *Histoplasma capsulatum* in sputum by means of fluorescent antibody staining. *Am. J. Clin. Pathol.* **37**: 465-469.

114. Carski, T. R., Hoshiwara, I., Yarbrough, W. B., and Robinson, R. Q. (1962). A survey of respiratory illnesses in a population. II. Fluorescent antibody aspects. *Am. J. Hyg.* **75**: 28-32.

115. Carski, T. R., and Shepard, C. C. (1961). Pleuropneumonia-like (*Mycoplasma*) infections of tissue culture. *J. Bacteriol.* **81**: 626-635.

116. Carski, T. R., Wilsnack, R. E., and Sikes, R. K. (1962). Pathogenesis of rabies in wildlife. II. Fluorescent antibody studies. *Am. J. Vet. Res.* **23**: 1048-1051.

117. Carter, C. H. (1959). Staining of coagulase-positive staphylococci with fluorescent antisera. *J. Bacteriol.* **77**: 670-671.

118. Carter, C. H., and Leise, J. M. (1958). Specific staining of various bacteria with a single fluorescent antiglobulin. *J. Bacteriol.* **76**: 152-154.

119. Carter, G. B. (1965). The rapid detection, titration, and differentiation of variola and vaccinia viruses by a fluorescent antibody-coverslip cell monolayer system. *Virology* **25**: 659-662.

120. Carver, R. K., and Goldman, M. (1959). Staining *Toxoplasma gondii* with fluorescein-labelled antibody. III. The reaction in frozen and paraffin sections. *Am. J. Clin. Pathol.* **32**: 159-164.

121. Cebra, J. J., and Goldstein, G. (1965). Chromatographic purification of tetramethylrhodamine-immune globulin conjugates and their use in the cellular localization of rabbit γ-globulin polypeptide chains. *J. Immunol.* **95**: 230-245.

122. Chadwick, C. S., and Fothergill, J. E. (1962). Fluorochromes and their conjugation with proteins. *In* "Fluorescent Protein Tracing" (R. C. Nairn, ed.), pp. 4-30. Williams & Wilkins, Baltimore, Maryland.

123. Chadwick, C. S., McEntegart, M. G., and Nairn, R. C. (1958). Fluorescent protein tracers. A simple alternative to fluorescein. *Lancet,* Feb. 22, 1958: 411-414.

124. Chadwick, C. S., McEntegart, M. G., and Nairn, R. C. (1958). Fluorescent protein tracers; a trial of new fluorochromes and the development of an alternative to fluorescein. *Immunology* **1**: 315-327.

125. Chadwick, C. S., and Nairn, R. C. (1960). Fluorescent protein tracers; the unreacted fluorescent material in fluorescein conjugates and studies of conjugates with other green fluorochromes. *Immunology* **3**: 363-370.

126. Chadwick, P. (1966). The relative sensitivity of fluorescent antibody and cultural methods in detection of small numbers of pathogenic serotypes of *Escherichia coli. Am. J. Epidemiol.* **84**: 150-155.

127. Chadwick, P., and Abbott, L. (1964). Specificity and sensitivity of a microcolony technique for fluorescent antibody identification of pathogenic *Escherichia coli* serotypes. *Can. J. Microbiol.* **10**: 853-859.

128. Chadwick, P., and Slade, J. H. R. (1960). Identification of bacteria by specific antibody conjugated with fluorescein isothiocyanate. *J. Hyg.* **58**: 147-156.

129. Chance, B., and Legaliais, V. (1959). Differential microfluorometer for the localization of reduced pyridine nucleotide in living cells. *Rev. Sci. Instr.* **30**: 732-735.

130. Chanock, R. M., Cook, M. K., Fox, H. H., Parrott, R. H., and Huebner, R. J. (1960). Serologic evidence of infection with Eaton agent in lower respiratory illness in childhood. *New Engl. J. Med.* **262**: 648-654.

131. Chanock, R. M., Mufson, M. A., Somerson, N. L., and Couch, R. B. (1963). Role of *Mycoplasma* (PPLO) in human respiratory disease. *Am. Rev. Respirat. Diseases* **88**: Suppl., 218-239.

132. Chernukha, Y. G., and Korn, M. Y. (1965). Results of use of the fluorescence technique in study of leptospirae. *J. Hyg. Epidemiol., Microbiol., Immunol. (Prague)* **1**: 240-246.

133. Cherry, B. W., and Freeman, E. M. (1959). Staining bacterial smears with fluorescent antibody. V. The rapid identification of *Bacillus anthracis* in culture and in human and murine tissues. *Zentr. Bakteriol., Parasitenk., Abt. I. Orig.* **175**: 582-604.

134. Cherry, W. B., Goldman, M., and Carski, T. R. (1960). Fluorescent antibody techniques in the diagnosis of communicable diseases. *U.S. Public Health Serv. Publ.* **729.**

135. Cherry, W. B., and Moody, M. D. (1965). Fluorescent-antibody techniques in diagnostic bacteriology. *Bacteriol. Rev.* **29:** 222-250.

136. Cherry, W. B., Thomason, B. M., Pomales-Lebron, A., and Ewing, W. H. (1961). Rapid presumptive identification of enteropathogenic *Escherichia coli* in faecal smears by means of fluorescent antibody. III. Field evaluation. *Bull. World Health Organ.* **25:** 159-171.

137. Cheville, N. F., and Olson, C. (1964). Cytology of the canine oral papilloma. *Am. J. Pathol.* **45:** 849-872.

138. Chiappino, G., and Pernis, B. (1964). Demonstration with immunofluorescence of 19S macroglobulins and 7S gamma globulins in different cells of the human spleen. *Pathol. Microbiol.* **27:** 8-15.

139. Chu, T. H., Cheever, F. S., Coons, A. H., and Daniels, J. B. (1951). Distribution of mumps virus in the experimentally infected monkey. *Proc. Soc. Exptl. Biol. Med.* **76:** 571-574.

140. Chung, K. L., Hawirko, R. Z., and Isaac, P. K. (1964). Cell wall replication. I. Cell wall growth of *B. cereus* and *B. megaterium*. *Can. J. Microbiol.* **10:** 43-48.

141. Chung, K. L., Hawirko, R. Z., and Isaac, P. K. (1964). Cell wall replication. II. Cell wall growth and crosswall formation of *Escherichia coli* and *Streptococcus fecalis*. *Can. J. Microbiol.* **10:** 473-482.

142. Chung, K. L., Hawirko, R. Z., and Isaac, P. K. (1965). Cell wall replication in *Saccharomyces cerevisiae*. *Can. J. Microbiol.* **11:** 953-957.

143. Clark, H. F., and Shepard, C. C. (1963). A dialysis technique for preparing fluorescent antibody. *Virology* **20:** 642-644.

144. Clark, H. W., Bailey, J. S., Fowler, R. C., and Brown, T. McP. (1963). Identification of *Mycoplasmataceae* by the fluorescent antibody method. *J. Bacteriol.* **85:** 111-118.

145. Clark, H. W., Fowler, R. C., and Brown, T. McP. (1961). Preparation of pleuropneumonia-like organisms for microscopic study. *J. Bacteriol.* **81:** 500-502.

146. Clayton, R. M. (1954). Localization of embryonic antigens by antisera labelled with fluorescent dyes. *Nature* **174:** 1059.

147. Clayton, R. M. (1960). Labelled antibodies in the study of differentiation. *In* "New Approaches in Cell Biology" (P. M. B. Walker, ed.), pp. 66-88. Academic Press, New York.

148. Clyde, W. A., Jr. (1961). Demonstration of Eaton's agent in tissue culture. *Proc. Soc. Exptl. Biol. Med.* **107:** 715-718.

149. Clyde, W. A., Jr. (1963). Studies on Eaton agent in tissue culture. *Am. Rev. Respirat. Diseases* **88:** Suppl., 212-217.

150. Clyde, W. A., Jr., Denny, F. W., Jr., and Dingle, J. H. (1961). Fluorescent-stainable antibodies to the Eaton agent in human

primary atypical pneumonia transmission studies. *J. Clin. Invest.* **40**: 1638-1647.

151. Cochrane, C. G. (1963). Studies on the localization of circulating antigen-antibody complexes and other macromolecules in vessels. I. Structural studies. *J. Exptl. Med.* **118**: 489-502.

152. Cochrane, C. G., and Weigle, W. O. (1958). The cutaneous reaction to soluble antigen-antibody complexes. A comparison with the Arthus phenomenon. *J. Exptl. Med.* **108**: 591-604.

153. Cochrane, C. G., Weigle, W. O., and Dixon, F. J. (1959). The role of polymorphonuclear leukocytes in the initiation and cessation of the Arthus vasculitis. *J. Exptl. Med.* **110**: 481-494.

154. Coffin, D. L., and Liu, C. (1957). Studies on canine distemper infection by means of fluorescein-labeled antibody. II. The pathology and diagnosis of the naturally occurring disease in dogs and the antigenic nature of the inclusion body. *Virology* **3**: 132-145.

155. Coffin, D. L., and Maestrone, G. (1962). Detection of Leptospires by fluorescent antibody. *Am. J. Vet. Res.* **23**: 159-164.

156. Coghill, N. F., Doniach, D., Roitt, I. M., Mollin, D. L., and Williams, A. W. (1965). Autoantibodies in simple atrophic gastritis. *Gut* **6**: 48-56.

157. Cohen, J. O., Cowart, G. S., and Cherry, W. B. (1961). Antibodies against *Staphylococcus aureus* in nonimmunized rabbits. *J. Bacteriol.* **82**: 110-114.

158. Cohen, J. O., Newton, W. L., Cherry, W. B., and Updyke, E. L. (1963). Normally occurring staphylococcal antibodies in germfree mice. *J. Immunol.* **90**: 358-367.

159. Cohen, J. O., and Oeding, P. (1962). Serological typing of staphylococci by means of fluorescent antibodies. I. Development of specific reagents for seven serological factors. *J. Bacteriol.* **84**: 735-741.

160. Cohen, S., Ohta, G., Singer, E. J., and Popper, H. (1960). Immunocytochemical study of gamma globulin in liver in hepatitis and postnecrotic cirrhosis. *J. Exptl. Med.* **111**: 285-293.

161. Cohen, S. M., Gordon, I., Rapp, F., Macaulay, J. C., and Buckley, S. M. (1955). Fluorescent antibody and complement-fixation tests of agents isolated in tissue culture from measles patients. *Proc. Soc. Exptl. Biol. Med.* **90**: 118-122.

162. Cole, F. E., Jr., and Hetrick, F. M. (1965). Persistent infection of human conjunctiva cell cultures by myxovirus parainfluenza 3. *Can. J. Microbiol.* **11**: 513-521.

163. Cole, R. M. (1964). Cell wall replication in *Salmonella typhosa*. *Science* **143**: 820-822.

164. Cole, R. M. (1965). Symposium on the fine structure and replication of bacteria and their parts. 3. Bacterial cell-wall replication followed by immunofluorescence. *Bacteriol. Rev.* **29**: 326-344.

165. Cole, R. M., and Hahn, J. J. (1962). Cell wall replication in *Streptococcus pyogenes*. *Science* **135**: 722-724.

166. Collins, W. E., Contacos, P. G., Skinner, J. C., Chin, W., and Guinn,

E. (1967). Fluorescent-antibody studies on simian malaria. I. Development of antibodies to *Plasmodium knowlesi*. *Am. J. Trop. Med. Hyg.* **16**: 1-6.

167. Collins, W. E., Jeffery, G. M., and Skinner, J. C. (1964). Fluorescent antibody studies in human malaria. I. Development of antibodies to *Plasmodium malariae*. *Am. J. Trop. Med. Hyg.* **13**: 1-5.

168. Collins, W. E., Jeffery, G. M., and Skinner, J. C. (1964). Fluorescent antibody studies in human malaria. II. Development and persistence of antibodies to *Plasmodium falciparum*. *Am. J. Trop. Med. Hyg.* **13**: 256-260.

169. Collins, W. E., Jeffery, G. M., and Skinner, J. C. (1964). Fluorescent antibody studies in human malaria. III. Development of antibodies to *Plasmodium falciparum* in semi-immune patients. *Am. J. Trop. Med. Hyg.* **13**: 777-782.

170. Collins, W. E., Skinner, J. C., and Guinn, E. G. (1966). Antigenic variations in the plasmodia of lower primates as detected by immunofluorescence. *Am. J. Trop. Med. Hyg.* **15**: 483-485.

171. Collins, W. E., Skinner, J. C., Dobrovolny, C. G., and Jones, F. E. (1965). Fluorescent antibody reactions against six species of simian malaria in monkeys from India and Malaysia. *J. Parasitol.* **5**: 81-84.

172. Convit, J., and Kerdel-Vegas, F. (1965). Disseminated cutaneous leishmaniasis, inoculation to laboratory animals, electron microscopy and fluorescent antibody studies. *Arch. Dermatol.* **91**: 439-447.

173. Cook, M. K., Chanock, R. M., Fox, H. H., Huebner, R. J., Buescher, E. L., and Johnson, R. T. (1960). Role of Eaton agent in disease of lower respiratory tract. Evidence for infection in adults. *Brit. Med. J.* **I**: 905-911.

174. Cookson, L. O. (1963). Some investigations with the fluorescent antibody technique. *Central African J. Med.* **9**: 429-434.

175. Cookson, L. O. (1963) Some investigations with the fluorescent antibody technique. II. Experiments with advanced fluorescent equipment. *Central African J. Med.* **9**: 469-478.

176. Cookson, L. O., Clarke, V., and Pirie, E. (1964). Some investigations with fluorescent antibody technique. III. The threshold fluorescent antibody test in schistosomiasis. *Central African J. Med.* **10**: 12-16.

177. Coons, A. H. (1951). Fluorescent antibodies as histochemical tools. *Federation Proc.* **10**: 558-559.

178. Coons, A. H. (1954). Labelled antigens and antibodies. *Ann. Rev. Microbiol.* **8**: 333-352.

179. Coons, A. H. (1956). Histochemistry with labeled antibody. *Intern. Rev. Cytol.* **5**: 1-23.

180. Coons, A. H. (1958). Fluorescent antibody methods. *In* "General Cytochemical Methods" (J. F. Danielli, ed.), Vol. 1, pp. 399-422. Academic Press, New York.

181. Coons, A. H. (1959). Antibodies and antigens labelled with fluorescein. *Schweiz. Z. Allgem. Pathol. Bakteriol.* **22**: 693-699.
182. Coons, A. H. (1959). The diagnostic application of fluorescent antibodies. *Schweiz. Z. Allgem. Pathol. Bakteriol.* **22**: 700-723.
183. Coons, A. H. (1960). Immunofluorescence. *Public Health Rept.* **75**: 937-943.
184. Coons, A. H. (1961). The beginnings of immunofluorescence. *J. Immunol.* **87**: 499-503.
185. Coons, A. H. (1964). Labeling techniques in the diagnosis of viral diseases. *Bacteriol. Rev.* **28**: 397-399.
186. Coons, A. H., Creech, H. J., and Jones, R. N. (1941). Immunological properties of an antibody containing a fluorescent group. *Proc. Soc. Exptl. Biol. Med.* **47**: 200-202.
187. Coons, A. H., Creech, H. J., Jones, R. N., and Berliner, E. (1942). The demonstration of pneumococcal antigen in tissues by the use of fluorescent antibody. *J. Immunol.* **45**: 159-170.
188. Coons, A. H., and Kaplan, M. H. (1950). Localization of antigen in tissue cells. II. Improvements in a method for the detection of antigen by means of fluorescent antibody. *J. Exptl. Med.* **91**: 1-13.
189. Coons, A. H., Leduc, E. H., and Connolly, J. M. (1955). Studies on antibody production. I. A method for the histochemical demonstration of specific antibody and its application to a study of the hyper-immune rabbit. *J. Exptl. Med.* **102**: 49-60.
190. Coons, A. H., Leduc, E. H., and Kaplan, M. H. (1951). Localization of antigen in tissue cells. VI. The fate of injected foreign proteins in the mouse. *J. Exptl. Med.* **93**: 173-188.
191. Coons, A. H., Snyder, J. C., Cheever, F. S., and Murray, E. S. (1950). Localization of antigen in tissue cells. IV. Antigens of rickettsiae and mumps virus. *J. Exptl. Med.* **91**: 31-38.
192. Corey, H. S., and McKinney, R. M. (1962). Chromatography of nitrofluoresceins, aminofluoresceins, and fluorescein isothiocyanates. *Anal. Biochem.* **4**: 57-68.
193. Cormack, D. H., Easty, G. C., and Ambrose, E. J. (1961). Interaction of enzymes with normal and tumor cells. *Nature* **190**: 1207-1208.
194. Corradetti, A., Verolini, F., Sebastiani, A., Proietti, A. M., and Amati, L. (1964). Fluorescent antibody testing with sporozoites of plasmodia. *Bull. World Health Organ.* **30**: 747-750.
195. Cotran, R. S. (1963). Retrograde *Proteus* pyelonephritis in rats. Localization of antigen and antibody in treated sterile pyelonephritic kidneys. *J. Exptl. Med.* **117**: 813-822.
196. Cotran, R. S., Thrupp, L. D., Hajj, S. N., Zangwill, D. P., Vivaldi, E., and Kass, E. H. (1963). Retrograde *E. coli* pyelonephritis in the rat: A bacteriologic, pathologic, and fluorescent antibody study. *J. Lab. Clin. Med.* **61**: 987-1004.
197. Cotran, R. S., Vivaldi, E., Zangwill, D. P., and Kass, E. H. (1963).

Retrograde *Proteus* pyelonephritis in rats. Bacteriologic, pathologic and fluorescent-antibody studies. *Am. J. Pathol.* **43**: 1-31.

198. Cottenot, F. (1964). Quantitative evaluation on the murine leprosy bacillus of serum antibodies detectable in human leprosy. (French). *Compt. Rend. Soc. Biol.* **158**: 1004-1005.

199. Cowart, G. S., and Thomason, B. M. (1965). Immunofluorescent detection of *Escherichia coli*. *Am. J. Diseases Children* **110**: 131-136.

200. Cox, M. T. (1964). Malignant lymphoma of the thyroid. *J. Clin. Pathol.* **17**: 591-601.

201. Craig, J. M. (1965). Histological distribution of ferritin, especially in the newborn. *Arch. Pathol.* **79**: 435-440.

202. Craig, J. M., and Gitlin, D. (1957). The nature of the hyaline thrombi in thrombotic thrombocytogenic purpura. *Am. J. Pathol.* **33**: 251-265.

203. Cramer, H. (1964). Fluorescence serological demonstration of antibodies against leptospira with a formalin antigen. *Z. Hyg. Infektionskrankh.* **150**: 108-113.

204. Crandall, C. A., Echevarria, R., and Arean, V. M. (1963). Localization of antibody binding sites in the larvae of *Ascaris lumbricoides* var. *suum* by means of fluorescent technics. *Exptl. Parasitol.* **14**: 296-303.

205. Crandall, R. B., Belkin, L. M., and Saadallah, S. (1966). Complement staining with fluorescent antibody for detection of antibody in experimental trichinosis. *J. Parasitol.* **52**: 1219-1220.

206. Crandell, R. A. (1965). Laboratory investigation of arctic strains of rabies virus. *Acta Pathol. Microbiol. Scand.* **63**: 587-596.

207. Crawford, H. J., Wood, R. M., and Lessof, M. H. (1959). Detection of antibodies by fluorescent-spot technique. *Lancet* Dec. 26, 1959: 1173-1174.

208. Creech, H. J., and Jones, R. N. (1941). The conjugation of horse serum albumin with isocyanates of certain polynuclear aromatic hydrocarbons. *J. Am. Chem. Soc.* **63**: 1661-1669.

209. Cremer, N., and Watson, D. W. (1957). Influence of stress on distribution of endotoxin in RES determined by fluorescent antibody technic. *Proc. Soc. Exptl. Biol. Med.* **95**: 510-513.

210. Cruickshank, B., and Currie, A. R. (1958). Localization of tissue antigens with the fluorescent antibody technique; application to human anterior pituitary hormones. *Immunology* **1**: 13-26.

211. Cruickshank, B., and Hill, A. G. S. (1953). The histochemical identification of a connective-tissue antigen in the rat. *J. Pathol. Bacteriol.* **66**: 283-289.

212. Curtain, C. C. (1958). Electrophoresis of fluorescent antibody. *Nature* **182**: 1305-1306.

213. Curtain, C. C. (1961). Localization of 18S gamma-macroglobulin in plasmacytoid cells of the bone marrow of a case of macroglobulinaemia. *Australian J. Exptl. Biol. Med. Sci.* **39**: 391-396.

214. Curtain, C. C. (1961). The chromatographic purification of fluorescein-antibody. *J. Histochem. Cytochem.* **9**: 484-486.
215. Curtain, C. C. (1964). Immuno-cytochemical localization of two abnormal serum globulins in the one bone-marrow smear. *Australasian Ann. Med.* **13**: 136-138.
216. Curtain, C. C., Kidson, C., Champness, D. L., and Gorman, J. G. (1964). Malaria antibody content of gamma 2-7S globulin in tropical populations. *Nature* **203**: 1366-1367.
217. Curtain, C. C., and O'Dea, J. F. (1959). Possible sites of macroglobulin synthesis. A study made with fluorescent antibody. *Australasian Ann. Med.* **8**: 143-150.
218. Dacres, W. G. (1961). Fluorescein-labeled antibody technique for identification of leptospiral serotypes. *Am. J. Vet. Res.* **22**: 570-572.
219. Dacres, W. G. (1963). Fluorescein-labeled antibody technique for identification of leptospiral serotypes–refixation of formalin-fixed organisms with osmic acid vapor. *Am. J. Vet. Res.* **24**: 1321-1323.
220. Dajani, A. S., Clyde, W. A., Jr. and Denny, F. W. (1965). Experimental infection with *Mycoplasma pneumoniae* (Eaton's agent). *J. Exptl. Med.* **121**: 1071-1086.
221. Dales, S., Gomatos, P. J., and Hsu, K. C. (1965). The uptake and development of reovirus in strain L cells followed with labeled viral ribonucleic acid and ferritin-antibody conjugates. *Virology* **25**: 193-211.
222. Dallenbach, F., and Piekarski, G. (1960). Uber den Nachweis von *Toxoplasma gondii* in Gewebe mit Hilfe markierter fluorescienender Antikorper (Methode nach Coons). *Arch. Pathol. Anat. Physiol.* **333**: 607-618.
223. Danielsson, D. (1963). The demonstration of *N. gonorrhoeae* with the aid of fluorescent antibodies. I. Immunological studies of antigonococcal sera and their fluorescein-labelled globulins, with particular regard to specificity. *Acta Dermato-Venerol.* **43**: 451-464.
224. Danielsson, D. (1963). The demonstration of *N. gonorrhoeae* with the aid of fluorescent antibodies. II. A comparison between the fluorescent antibody technique and conventional methods of detecting *N. gonorrhoeae* in men and women. *Acta Dermato-Venereol.* **43**: 511-521.
225. Danielsson, D. (1965). The demonstration of *N. gonorrhoeae* with the aid of fluorescent antibodies. III. Studies by immunofluorescence and double diffusion-in-gel technique on the antigenic relationship between strains of *N. gonorrhoeae. Acta Pathol. Microbiol. Scand.* **64**: 243-266.
226. Danielsson, D. (1965). The demonstration of *N. gonorrhoeae* with the aid of fluorescent antibodies. IV. Studies by immunofluorescence and double diffusion-in-gel technique on the antigenic relationship between *N. gonorrhoeae* and other *Neisseria* strains. *Acta Pathol. Microbiol. Scand.* **64**: 267-276.
227. Danielsson, D. (1965). The demonstration of *N. gonorrhoeae* with

the aid of fluorescent antibodies. V. A comparison of different techniques—absorption, one-step inhibition, and counterstaining—for elimination of cross reactions. *Acta Dermato-Venereol.* **45**: 61-73.

228. Danielsson, D. (1965). The demonstration of *N. gonorrhoeae* with the aid of fluorescent antibodies. VI. A comparison of conventional methods and fluorescent antibody (FA) techniques with counterstaining for the demonstration of *N. gonorrhoeae*. *Acta Dermato-Venereol.* **45**: 74-80.

229. Danielsson, D., and Laurell, G. (1964). Detection of enteropathogenic *Escherichia coli* in a Swedish watercourse (the river Fyris) by means of fluorescent antibodies and by conventional methods. *Acta Paediat.* **53**: 49-54.

230. Danielsson, D., and Laurell, G. (1965). A membrane filter method for the demonstration of bacteria by the fluorescent antibody technique. II. The application of the method for detection of small numbers of bacteria in water. *Acta Pathol. Microbiol. Scand.* **63**: 604-608.

231. D'Antona, D. (1964). Anaerobic and aerobic tetanus bacillus studies with the immuno-fluorescence reaction (contribution to the study of the genesis of tetanus toxin). *Nuovi Ann. Igiene Microbiol.* **15**: 254-262.

232. D'Antona, D., and Mannucci, E. (1961). Fluorescent antibodies in laboratory diagnosis (principles of the techniques). (Italian) *Ann. Sclavo* **3**: 37-48.

233. Darken, M. A. (1961). Natural and induced fluorescence in microscopic organisms. *Appl. Microbiol.* **9**: 354-360.

234. Davies, M. E. (1965). Cellulolytic bacteria in some ruminants and herbivores as shown by fluorescent antibody. *J. Gen. Microbiol.* **39**: 139-141.

235. Dayan, A. D., Morgan, H. G., Hope-Stone, H. F., and Boucher, B. J. (1964). Disseminated herpes zoster in the reticuloses. *Am. J. Roentgenol., Radium Therapy Nucl. Med.* **92**: 116-123.

236. Deacon, W. E., Falcone, V. H., and Harris, A. (1957). A fluorescent test for treponemal antibodies. *Proc. Soc. Exptl. Biol. Med.* **96**: 477-480.

237. Deacon, W. E., and Freeman, E. M. (1960). Fluorescent treponemal antibody studies. *J. Invest. Dermatol.* **34**: 249-253.

238. Deacon, W. E., Freeman, E. M., and Harris, A. (1960). Fluorescent treponemal antibody test. Modification based on quantitation (FTA-200). *Proc. Soc. Exptl. Biol. Med.* **103**: 827-829.

239. Deacon, W. E., and Hunter, E. F. (1962). Treponemal antigens as related to identification and syphilis serology. *Proc. Soc. Exptl. Biol. Med.* **110**: 352-356.

240. Deacon, W. E., Peacock, W. L., Jr., Freeman, E. M., and Harris, A. (1959). Identification of *Neisseria gonorrhoeae* by means of fluorescent antibody. *Proc. Soc. Exptl. Biol. Med.* **101**: 322-325.

241. Deacon, W. E., Peacock, W. L. Jr., Freeman, E. M., Harris, A., and Bunch, W. L., Jr. (1960). Fluorescent antibody tests for detection of the gonococcus in women. *Public Health Rept.* **75**: 125-129.

242. Dean, D. J., Evans, W. M., and McClure, R. C. (1963). Pathogenesis of rabies. *Bull. World Health Organ.* **29**: 803-811.

243. deBarbieri, A., and Scevola, M. E. (1958). Sulla preparazione di alcuni enzimi fluorescenti e loro attivita biochimica. *Boll. Soc. Ital. Biol. Sper.* **34**: 1189-1192.

244. Dedmon, R. E., Holmes, A. W., and Deinhardt, F. (1965). Preparation of fluorescein isothiocyanate-labeled γ-globulin by dialysis, gel filtration, and ion-exchange chromatography in combination. *J. Bacteriol.* **89**: 734-739.

245. Deibel, R., and Hotchin, J. E. (1959). Quantitative applications of fluorescent antibody technique to influenza-virus-infected cell cultures. *Virology* **8**: 367-380.

246. de La Vaissiere, C., and Goiffon, B. (1963). Immunofluorescence diagnosis of toxic gastroenteritis caused by colibacillary pathogens in infants. (French) *Concours Med.* **85**: 185-188.

247. Denny, F. W., Jr., and Ginsberg, H. S. (1959). Intracellular localization of type 4 adenovirus. I. Cellular fractionation studies. *J. Exptl. Med.* **109**: 69-83.

248. de Repentigny, J., and Frappier, A. (1956). Studies on *H. pertussis* liquid cultures. III. Localization of surface antigens by means of fluorescent antibody. *Can. J. Microbiol.* **2**: 677-683.

249. de Repentigny, J., Sonea, S., and Frappier, A. (1961). Étude microfluorometrique des micro-organismes. I. La fluorescence première (autofluorescence). *Ann. Inst. Pasteur* **101**: 353-366.

250. de Repentigny, J., Sonea, S., and Frappier, A. (1963). Comparison of quantitative immunofluorescence and immunodiffusion for the evaluation of antigenic materials from *Staphylococcus aureus*. *J. Bacteriol.* **86**: 1348-1349.

251. de Repentigny, J., Sonea, S., and Frappier, A. (1964). Differentiation by immunodiffusion and by quantitative immunofluorescence between 5-fluorouracil-treated and normal cells from a toxinogenic *Staphylococcus aureus* strain. *J. Bacteriol.* **88**: 444-448.

252. de Sala, A. R., Menendez-Corrada, R., and Rodriguez-Molina, R. (1962). Detection of circumoval precipitins by the fluorescent antibody technic. *Proc. Soc. Exptl. Biol. Med.* **111**: 212-215.

253. Deutsch, H. F. (1952). Separation of antibody-active proteins from various animal sera by ethanol fractionation techniques. *Methods Med. Res.* **5**: 284-300.

254. Diamond, L., and Crawford, L. V. (1964). Some characteristics of large-plaque and small-plaque lines of polyoma virus. *Virology* **22**: 235-244.

255. Diderholm, H. (1963). A fluorescent antibody study on the forma-

tion of simian virus 40 in monkey kidney cells. *Acta Pathol. Microbiol. Scand.* **57**: 348-352.

256. Diggs, C. L., and Sadun, E. H. (1965). Serological cross reactivity between *Plasmodium vivax* and *Plasmodium falciparum* as determined by a modified fluorescent antibody test. *Exptl. Parasitol.* **16**: 217-223.

257. Dineen, J. K., and Ada, G. L. (1957). Rapid extraction with ethyl acetate of free fluorescein derivatives from fluorescein isocyanate-globulin conjugate. *Nature* **180**: 1284.

258. Dinter, Z., Hermodsson, S., and Hermodsson, L. (1964). Studies on myxovirus yucaipa; its classification as a member of the paramyxovirus group. *Virology* **22**: 297-304.

259. Dixon, F. J., Feldman, J. D., and Vasquez, J. J. (1961). Experimental glomerulonephritis. The pathogenesis of a laboratory model resembling the spectrum of human glomerulonephritis. *J. Exptl. Med.* **113**: 899-920.

260. Dixon, F. J., and McConahey, P. J. (1963). Enchancement of antibody formation by whole body x-irradiation. *J. Exptl. Med.* **117**: 833-848.

261. Djanian, A. Y., Beutner, E. H., and Witebsky, E. (1964). Tanned-cell hemagglutination test for detection of antibodies in sera of patients with myasthenia gravis. *J. Lab. Clin. Med.* **63**: 60-70.

262. Domingue, G. J., and Pierce, W. A., Jr. (1965). Effect of partially purified streptococcal M protein in the *in vitro* phagocytosis of *Streptococcus pyogenes. J. Bacteriol.* **89**: 583-588.

263. Donaldhare, J., and Morgan, H. R. (1964). Polyoma virus and L cell relationship. II. A curable carrier system not dependent on interferon. *J. Natl. Cancer Inst.* **33**: 765-775.

264. Doniach, D., and Roitt, I. M. (1962). Auto-antibodies in disease. *Ann. Rev. Med.* **13**: 213-240.

265. Douglas, W. (1965). The digital artery lesion of rheumatoid arthritis: an immunofluorescent study. *Ann. Rheumatic Diseases* **24**: 40-45.

266. Dowdle, W. R., and Hansen, P. A. (1959). Labeling of antibodies with fluorescent azo dyes. *J. Bacteriol.* **77**: 669-670.

267. Dowdle, W. R., and Hansen, P. A. (1961). A phage-fluorescent antiphage staining system for *Bacillus anthracis. J. Infect. Diseases* **108**: 125-135.

268. Duncan, D. A., Drummond, K. N., Michael, A. F., and Vernier, R. L. (1965). Pulmonary hemorrhage and glomerulonephritis. Report of six cases and study of the renal lesion by the fluorescent antibody technique and electron microscopy. *Ann. Internal Med.* [N.S.] **62**: 920-938.

269. Dutcher, T. F., and Fahey, J. L. (1960). Immunocytochemical demonstration of intranuclear localization of 18S gamma macroglobulin in macroglobulinemia of Waldenstrom. *Proc. Soc. Exptl. Biol. Med.* **103**: 452-455.

270. Duxbury, R. E., and Sadun, E. H. (1964). Fluorescent antibody test for the serodiagnosis of visceral leishmaniasis. *Am. J. Trop. Med. Hyg.* **13**: 525-529.

271. Dvorak, H. F., and Cohen, R. B. (1965). Localization of skeletal muscle phosphorylase using a fluorescent antibody technique and its correlation with histochemical observations. *J. Histochem. Cytochem.* **13**: 454-460.

272. Dzagurov, S. G., Chumakov, M. P., Karmysheva, V. Y., Kolyaskina, G. I., Graevskaya, N. A., Kuroshkina, N. P., and Panosyan, L. B. (1964). Use of fluorescent antibody method to study intracellular locale of simian virus 40 and for its rapid detection in vaccines. *Federation Proc.* **23**: Transl. Suppl., 548-550.

273. Eagle, H., Smith, D., and Vickers, P. (1936). The effect of combination with diazo compounds on the immunological reactivity of antibodies. *J. Exptl. Med.* **63**: 617-643.

274. Easterbrook, K. B., and Davern, C. I. (1963). The effect of 5-bromodeoxyuridine on the multiplication of vaccinia virus. *Virology* **19**: 509-520.

275. Easterday, B. C., and Jaeger, R. F. (1963). The detection of Rift Valley Fever virus by a tissue culture fluorescein-labeled antibody method. *J. Infect. Diseases* **112**: 1-6.

276. Eaton, M. D., Farnham, A. E., Levinthal, J. D., and Scala, A. R. (1962). Cytopathic effect of the atypical pneumonia organism in culture of human tissue. *J. Bacteriol.* **84**: 1331-1337.

277. Edwards, E. A. (1962). Detecting *Treponema pallidum* in primary lesions by the fluorescent antibody technique. *Public Health Rept.* **77**: 427-430.

278. Ehrlich, R., and Ehrmantraut, H. C. (1955). Instrumental estimation of bacterial population by fluorescence microscopy. *Appl. Microbiol.* **3**: 231-234.

279. Ellinger, P. (1940). Fluorescence microscopy in biology. *Biol. Rev.* **15**: 323-350.

280. Ellison, D. W., and Baker, H. J. (1964). The indirect fluorescent antibody technique in scrub typhus studies. *Med. J. Malaya* **19**: 65-66.

281. Elves, M. W., Roath, S., Taylor, G., and Israels, M. C. G. (1963). *In vitro* production of antibody lymphocytes. *Lancet,* **7294**: 1292-1293.

282. Emmart, E. W. (1958). Observations on the absorption spectra of fluorescein, fluorescein derivatives and conjugates. *Arch. Biochem.* **73**: 1-8.

283. Emmart, E. W., Bates, R. W., and Turner, W. A. (1965). Localization of prolactin in rat pituitary and in transplantable mammotropic pituitary tumor using fluorescent antibody. *J. Histochem. Cytochem.* **13**: 182-190.

284. Emmart, E. W., and Cole, R. M. (1955). Studies on streptococcal hyaluronidase and antihyaluronidase. I. The development *in vitro* of

streptococcal (Group C) hyaluronidase, its isolation and use as an antigen in rabbits. *J. Bacteriol.* **70**: 596-607.

285. Emmart, E. W., Cole, R. M., May, E. L., and Longley, J. B. (1958). Studies on streptococcal hyaluronidase and antihyaluronidase. II. The localization of sites of absorption of streptococcal hyaluronidase (Group C) with fluorescent antibody. *J. Histochem. Cytochem.* **6**: 161-173.

286. Emmart, E. W., and Crisp, L. R. (1956). Improved freeze-drying and embedding apparatus for frozen tissue. *Rev. Sci. Instr.* **27**: 315-318.

287. Emmart, E. W., and Helander, E. (1960). Distribution of muscle protein in the fibers of the conduction system of the beef heart. *Arch. Pathol.* **70**: 730-739.

288. Emmart, E. W., Kominz, D. R., and Miguel, J. (1963). The localization and distribution of glyceraldehyde-3-phosphate dehydrogenase in myoblasts and developing muscle fibers growing in cultures. *J. Histochem. Cytochem.* **11**: 207-217.

289. Emmart, E. W., Schimke, R. T., Spicer, S. S., and Turner, W. A. (1963). The localization of glyceraldehyde-3-phosphate dehydrogenase in kidney tissue by means of fluorescent antibody. *Exptl. Cell Res.* **30**: 460-475.

290. Emmart, E. W., Spicer, S. S., and Bates, R. W. (1963). Localization of prolactin within the pituitary by specific fluorescent antiprolactin globulin. *J. Histochem. Cytochem.* **11**: 365-373.

291. Emmart, E. W., Spicer, S. S., Turner, W. A., and Henson, J. G. (1962). The localization of glyceraldehyde-3-phosphate dehydrogenase within the muscle of the roach, *Periplaneta americana*, by means of fluorescent antibody. *Exptl. Cell Res.* **26**: 78-97.

292. Emmart, E. W., and Turner, W. A. (1960). Studies on streptococcal hyaluronidase and antihyaluronidase. III. The production and cellular localization of hyaluronidase following streptococcal infection. *J. Histochem. Cytochem.* **8**: 273-283.

293. Emmons, R. W., and Lennette, E. H. (1966). Immunofluorescent staining in the laboratory diagnosis of Colorado tick fever. *J. Lab. Clin. Med.* **68**: 923-929.

294. Eng, J., Nielsen, H. A., and Wereide, K. (1963). A comparative study of fluorescent treponemal antibody (FTA) and *Treponema pallidum* immobilization (TPI) testing in 50 untreated syphilitic patients. *Bull. World Health Organ.* **28**: 533-535.

295. Essenfeld, E., and Fennell, R. H., Jr. (1964). Immunofluorescent study of experimental *Trypanosoma cruzi* infection. *Proc. Soc. Exptl. Biol. Med.* **116**: 728-730.

296. Estela, L. A., and Shuey, H. E. (1963). Comparison of fluorescent antibody, precipitin, and bacitracin disk methods in the identification of group A streptococci. *Am. J. Clin. Pathol.* **40**: 591-597.

297. Eveland, W. C. (1963). Demonstration of *Listeria monocytogenes*

in direct examination of spinal fluid by fluorescent-antibody technique. *J. Bacteriol.* **85**: 1448-1450.

298. Eveland, W. C. (1964). Use of a fluorescein-labeled sonically disrupted bacterial antigen to demonstrate antibody-producing cells. *J. Bacteriol.* **88**: 1476-1481.

299. Fahey, J. L., and Horbett, A. P. (1959). Human gamma globulin fractionation on anion exchange cellulose columns. *J. Biol. Chem.* **234**: 2645-2651.

300. Feder, N., and Sidman, R. L. (1958). Methods and principles of fixation by freeze-substitution. *J. Biophys. Biochem. Cytol.* **4**: 593-601.

301. Fedova, D., and Zelenkova, L. (1965). The use of the fluorescent antibody method for the rapid identification of the A2 influenza virus. I. The identification of influenza virus in the epithelial cell sediment of allantoic or amniotic fluid of infected chick embryos. *J. Hyg., Epidemiol., Microbiol., Immunol. (Prague)* **9**: 127-134.

302. Fedova, D., and Zelenkova, L. (1965). The use of the fluorescent antibody method for the rapid identification of the A2 influenza virus. II. The identification of influenza virus in nasal smears by the fluorescent antibody technique. *J. Hyg., Epidemiol., Microbiol., Immunol. (Prague)* **9**: 135-166.

303. Felton, L. C., and McMillion, C. R. (1961). Chromatographically pure fluorescein and tetramethylrhodamine isothiocyanates. *Anal. Biochem.* **2**: 178-187.

304. Fernandes, M. V., and Moorehead, P. S. (1965). Transformation of African green monkey kidney cultures infected with simian vacuolating virus (SV40). *Texas Rept. Biol. Med.* **23**: Suppl. 1, 242-258.

305. Fernandes, M. V., Wiktor, T. J., and Koprowski, H. (1964). Endosymbiotic relationship between animal viruses and host cells. *J. Exptl. Med.* **120**: 1099-1116.

306. Fife, E. H., Jr., Bryan, B. M., Saunders, R. W., and Muschel, L. H. (1961). Evaluation of the fluorescent treponemal antibody (FTA) test for syphilis. *Am. J. Clin. Pathol.* **36**: 105-113.

307. Fife, E. H., Jr., and Muschel, L. H. (1959). Fluorescent-antibody technic for serodiagnosis of *Trypanosoma cruzi* infection. *Proc. Soc. Exptl. Biol. Med.* **101**: 540-543.

308. Filho, A. M., Krupp, I. M., and Malek, E. A. (1965). Localization of antigen and presence of antibody in tissues of mice infected with *Schistosoma mansoni,* as indicated by fluorescent antibody technics. *Am. J. Trop. Med. Hyg.* **14**: 84-99.

309. Finck, H., Holtzer, H., and Marshall, J. M., Jr. (1956). An immunochemical study of the distribution of myosin in glycerol extracted muscle. *J. Biophys. Biochem. Cytol.* **2**: 175-178.

310. Fink, M. A., Karon, M., Rauscher, F. J., Malmgren, R. A., and Orr, H. C. (1966). Further observations on the immunofluorescence of cells in human leukemia. *Cancer* **18**: 1317-1321.

311. Fink, M. A., and Malmgren, R. A. (1963). Fluorescent antibody studies of the viral antigen in a murine leukemia (Rauscher). *J. Natl. Cancer Inst.* **31**: 1111-1118.

312. Fink, M. A., Malmgren, R. A., Rauscher, F. J., Orr, H. C., and Karon, M. (1964). Application of immunofluorescence to the study of human leukemia. *J. Natl. Cancer Inst.* **33**: 581-588.

313. Fink, M. A., Manaker, R. A., Dalton, A. J., and Cranford, V. L. (1966). Immunofluorescence of tissue cultured cells derived from human lymphoid diseases. *Proc. Intern. Wenner-Gren Symp., Stockholm, 1965,* pp. 145-155. Pergamon Press, Oxford.

314. Fitch, F. W. (1962). Immunohistochemical study of Ehrlich ascites tumor. *Arch. Pathol.* **73**: 144-160.

315. Fleck, J., Minck, R., and Kirn, A. (1962). Etude de l'action inhibitrice spécifique des antiserums sur les cultures L des bactéries. III. Localization de l'antigen H par la technique de l'immunofluorescence. *Ann. Inst. Pasteur* **102**: 243-246.

316. Fletcher, S. (1965). Indirect fluorescent antibody technique in the serology of *Toxoplasma gondii. J. Clin. Pathol.* **18**: 193-199.

317. Fogel, M., and Sachs, L. (1964). The induction of Forssmanantigen synthesis in hamster and mouse cells in tissue culture, as detected by the fluorescent-antibody technic. *Exptl. Cell Res.* **34**: 448-462.

318. Formal, S. B., Labrec, E. H., Kent, T. H., and Falkow, S. (1965). Abortive intestinal infection with an *Escherichia coli-Shigella flexneri* hybrid strain. *J. Bacteriol.* **89**: 1374-1382.

319. Formal, S. B., Labrec, E. H., and Schneider, H. (1965). Pathogenesis of bacillary dysentery in laboratory animals. *Federation Proc.* **24**: 29-34.

320. Forman, J. (1964). A current bibliography on allergy and applied immunology. *Rev. Allergy Appl. Immunol.* **18**: 80-116.

321. Fothergill, J. E. (1962). Properties of conjugated serum proteins. *In* "Fluorescent Protein Tracing" (R. E. Nairn, ed.), pp. 31-55. Williams & Wilkins, Baltimore, Maryland.

322. Fothergill, J. E., and Nairn, R. C. (1961). Purification of fluorescent protein conjugates: comparison of charcoal and Sephadex. *Nature* **192**: 1073-1074.

323. Fox, E. A. (1962). Measurement of streptococcal antigen synthesis with fluorescent antibody. *Proc. Soc. Exptl. Biol. Med.* **109**: 577-579.

324. Franek, J. (1964). Application of fluorescent antibodies for demonstrating *B. anthracis* in the organs of infected animals. *J. Hyg., Epidemiol., Microbiol., Immunol. (Prague)* **8**: 111-119.

325. Franek, J., and Prochazka, O. (1965). Fluorescent antibody demonstration of *Pasteurella tularensis. Folia Microbiol. (Prague)* **10**: 77-84.

326. Franek, J., and Wolfova, J. (1965). Use of the immunofluorescence

method in an epidemic focus of tularaemia. *Folia Microbiol. (Prague)* **10**: 85-92.

327. Fraser, K. B., and Crawford, E. M. (1965). Immunofluorescent and electron-microscopic studies of polyoma virus in transformation reactions with BHK21 cells. *Exptl. Mol. Pathol.* **4**: 51-65.

328. Fraser, K. B., Nairn, R. C., McEntegart, M. G., and Chadwick, C. S. (1959). Neurotropic and non-neurotropic influenza-A infection of mouse brain studied with fluorescent antibody. *J. Pathol. Bacteriol.* **78**: 423-433.

329. Fredrickson, L. E. (1963). Rabies in an endemic area and the value of the fluorescent antibody technique. *J. Tenn. State Med. Assoc.* **56**: 311-313.

330. Freed, J. J. (1955). Freeze-drying technics in cytology and cytochemistry. *Lab. Invest.* **4**: 106-122.

331. Frezzotti, R., and Berengo, A. (1963). Identification of *Toxoplasma gondii* with fluorescein-labelled antibodies in the cerebrospinal fluid of patients with neuro-ophthalmic toxoplasmosis. *Ophthalmologia* **145**: 72-76.

332. Friedman, M. E., and White, J. D. (1965). Immunofluorescent demonstration of cell-associated staphylococcal enterotoxin B. *J. Bacteriol.* **89**: 1155.

333. Friou, G. J. (1964). Immunofluorescence and antinuclear antibodies. *Arthritis Rheumat.* **7**: 161-166.

334. Friou, G. J., Finck, S. C., and Detre, K. D. (1958). Interaction of nuclei and globulin from lupus erythematosis serum demonstrated with fluorescent antibody. *J. Immunol.* **80**: 324-329.

335. Frommhagen, L. H. (1965). The solubility and other physicochemical properties of human γ-globulin labeled with fluoresceinisothiocyanate. *J. Immunol.* **95**: 442-445.

336. Frommhagen, L. H., and Martins, M. J. (1963). A comparison of fluorescein-labeled γ-globulins purified by Rivanol and DEAE chromatography. *J. Immunol.* **90**: 116-120.

337. Frommhagen, L. H., and Spendlove, R. S. (1962). The staining properties of human serum proteins conjugated with purified fluorescein isothiocyanate. *J. Immunol.* **89**: 124-131.

338. Fry, C. S., and Wilkinson, A. E. (1964). Immunofluorescence techniques as an aid to the diagnosis of gonorrhoea. *Brit. J. Venereal Diseases* **40**: 125-128.

339. Frye, F. L., and Enright, J. B. (1964). Observations on erythrocytic inclusion bodies from mice infected with rabies virus. *Proc. Soc. Exptl. Biol. Med.* **115**: 689-691.

340. Gadeke, R. (1959). Lokalisation eines ECHO-9-Virus in geweben infizierter Sauglingmause mittels fluoreszierender Antikorper. *Schweiz. Z. Allgem. Pathol. Bakteriol.* **22**: 751-758.

341. Gane, N. F. G., Hunt, A. L. C., and Booth, R. L. (1964). Some aspects of the fluorescent antibody test for bilharziasis. *Central African J. Med.* **10**: 407-410.

342. Garbin, S., and Piacentini, I. (1965). Contribution to the study of passage of antitreponemal antibodies from the mother to the fetus. (Italian) *Boll. Ist. Sieroterap. Milan.* **44**: 102-103.

343. Garin, J. P., and Ambroise-Thomas, P. (1963). The serological diagnosis of toxoplasmosis by the fluorescent antibody method (indirect technic). (French) *Presse Med.* **71**: 2485-2488.

344. Garnham, P. C. C., and Voller, A. (1965). Experimental studies on *Babesia divergens* in rhesus monkeys with special reference to its diagnosis by serological methods. *Acta Protozool.* **3**: 183-187.

345. Gebbie, D. A. M., Hamilton, P. J. S., Hutt, M. S. R., Marsden, P. D., Voller, A., and Wilks, N. E. (1964). Malarial antibodies in idiopathic splenomegaly in Uganda. *Lancet* **II**: 392-393.

346. Geck, P., Dan, P., and Nasz, I. (1964). Examination of the cytopathic effect of adenoviruses by immunofluorescence. *Acta Microbiol. Acad. Sci. Hung.* **11**: 19-22.

347. Geck, P., Osvath, P., Voltay, B., Backhausz, R., Losonezy, G., Vigh, G., and Bognar, S. (1963). Immunofluorescence and passive haemagglutination in infantile enterocolitis. *Acta Microbiol. Acad. Sci. Hung.* **10**: 1-6.

348. Geck, P., and Szanto, R. (1964-1965). Comparative examination of chronic typhoid carriers with immunofluorescent and cultural methods. *Acta Microbiol. Acad. Sci. Hung.* **11**: 211-214.

349. Geder, L., Koller, M., Gonczol, E., Jeney, E., and Gonczol, I. (1963). Isolation of herpes zoster virus strains. *Acta Microbiol. Acad. Sci. Hung.* **10**: 155-161.

350. Gelfand, M. (1964). Criteria for making a diagnosis of schistosomiasis. *J. Trop. Med. Hyg.* **67**: 114-116.

351. Gelfand, M., Clarke, V. de V., and Turnbull, C. (1964). The detection of antibodies to *Schistosoma spp.* in newly born infants of mothers having the same antibodies. *J. Trop. Med. Hyg.* **67**: 254.

352. Georgala, D. L., and Boothroyd, M. (1964). A rapid immunofluorescence technique for detecting salmonellae in raw meat. *J. Hyg.* **62**: 319-327.

353. Georgala, D. L., and Boothroyd, M. (1965). Preparation of fluorescent polyvalent salmonella antisera. *Nature* **205**: 521-522.

354. George, W., and Walton, K. W. (1961). Purification and concentration of dye-protein conjugates by gel filtration. *Nature* **192**: 1188-1189.

355. Ghose, T., and Tso, S. C. (1964). Uptake of protein by regenerating liver cells. *Nature* **204**: 1210-1211.

356. Gilden, R. V., Carp, R. I., Taguchi, F., and Defendi, V. (1965). The nature and localization of the SV 40-induced complement-fixing antigen. *Proc. Natl. Acad. Sci. U.S.* **53**: 684-692.

357. Gill, B. S. (1965). Studies on the serological diagnosis of *Trypanosoma evansi*. *J. Comp. Pathol. Therap.* **75**: 175-183.

358. Gill, F. A., and Cole, R. M. (1965). The fate of a bacterial antigen

(streptococcal M protein) after phagocytosis by macrophages. *J. Immunol.* **94**: 898-915.

359. Gitlin, D., and Craig, J. M. (1957). Variations in the staining characteristics of human fibrin. *Am. J. Pathol.* **33**: 267-283.

360. Gitlin, D., Landing, B. H., and Whipple, A. (1953). The localization of homologous plasma proteins in the tissues of young human beings as demonstrated with fluorescent antibodies. *J. Exptl. Med.* **97**: 163-176.

361. Glynn, L. E., Holborow, E. H., and Johnson, G. D. (1957). The distribution of blood-group substances in human gastric and duodenal mucosa. *Lancet* **II**: 1083-1088.

362. Goldin, R. B., and Krasnik, F. I. (1963). Specific staining of ornithosis virus by fluorescein-labelled incomplete antibodies. *Acta Virol.* **7**: 561.

363. Goldman, M. (1953). Cytochemical differentiation of *Endamoeba histolytica* and *Endamoeba coli* by means of fluorescent antibody. *Am. J. Hyg.* **58**: 319-328.

364. Goldman, M. (1954). Use of fluorescein-tagged antibody to identify cultures of *Endamoeba histolytica* and *Endamoeba coli. Am. J. Hyg.* **59**: 318-325.

365. Goldman, M. (1957). Staining *Toxoplasma gondii* with fluorescein-labelled antibody. I. The reaction in smears of peritoneal exudate. *J. Exptl. Med.* **105**: 549-556.

366. Goldman, M. (1957). Staining *Toxoplasma gondii* with fluorescein-labeled antibody. II. A new serologic test for antibodies to *Toxoplasma* based upon inhibition of specific staining. *J. Exptl. Med.* **105**: 557-573.

367. Goldman, M. (1960). Antigenic analysis of *Entamoeba histolytica* by means of fluorescent antibody. I. Instrumentation for microfluorimetry of stained amebae. *Exptl. Parasitol.* **9**: 25-36.

368. Goldman, M. (1961). Immunochemical staining with fluorescent antibody. *In* "International Review of Tropical Medicine" (D. R. Lincicome, ed.), Vol. 1, pp. 215-245. Academic Press, New York.

369. Goldman, M. (1963). Fluorescence techniques in microbiology. *J. Am. Med. Technologists* **25**: 453-461.

370. Goldman, M. (1964). Fluorescent antibody methods in the diagnosis of amebiasis. *Proc. 7th Intern. Congr. Trop. Med. Malaria, Rio de Janeiro*, 1963, Vol. 2, pp. 278-279.

371. Goldman, M. (1966). Evaluation of a fluorescent antibody test for amebiasis using two widely differing ameba strains as antigen. *Am. J. Trop. Med. Hyg.* **15**: 694-700.

372. Goldman, M. (1967). An improved microfluorimeter for measuring brightness of fluorescent antibody reactions. *J. Histochem. Cytochem.* **15**: 38-45.

373. Goldman, M., and Cannon, L. T. (1967). Antigenic analysis of *Entamoeba histolytica* by means of fluorescent antibody. V. Com-

parison of 15 strains of *Entamoeba* with information on their pathogenicity to guinea pigs. *Am. J. Trop. Med. Hyg.* **16**: 245-254.

374. Goldman, M., and Carver, R. K. (1957). Preserving fluorescein isocyanate for simplified preparation of fluorescent antibody. *Science* **126**: 839-840.

375. Goldman, M., and Carver, R. K. (1961). Microfluorimetry of cells stained with fluorescent antibody. *Exptl. Cell. Res.* **23**: 265-280.

376. Goldman, M., and Carver, R. K. (1962). Fluorescence inhibition test for toxoplasmosis. *Public Health Lab.* **20**: 80-87.

377. Goldman, M., Carver, R. K., and Gleason, N. N. (1960). Antigenic analysis of *Entamoeba histolytica* by means of fluorescent antibody. II. *E. histolytica* and *E. hartmanni*. *Exptl. Parasitol.* **10**: 366-388.

378. Goldman, M., and Gleason, N. N. (1962). Antigenic analysis of *Entamoeba histolytica* by means of fluorescent antibody. IV. Relationships of two strains of *E. histolytica* and one of *E. hartmanni* demonstrated by cross-absorption techniques. *J. Parasitol.* **48**: 778-783.

379. Goldman, M., Gleason, N. N., and Carver, R. K. (1962). Antigenic analysis of *Entamoeba histolytica* by means of fluorescent antibody. III. Reactions of the Laredo strain with five anti-*histolytica* sera. *Am. J. Trop. Med. Hyg.* **11**: 341-346.

380. Goldman, M., Gordon, M. A., and Carver, R. K. (1962). Comparison of titers of dye and fluorescence-inhibition tests in the serologic diagnosis of toxoplasmosis. *Am. J. Clin. Pathol.* **37**: 541-550.

381. Goldstein, G., Slizys, I. S., and Chase, M. W. (1961). Studies on fluorescent antibody staining. I. Non-specific fluorescence with fluorescein-coupled sheep anti-rabbit globulins. *J. Exptl. Med.* **114**: 89-110.

382. Goldstein, G., Spalding, B. H., and Hunt, W. B., Jr. (1962). Studies on fluorescent antibody staining. II. Inhibition by sub-optimally conjugated antibody globulins. *Proc. Soc. Exptl. Biol. Med.* **111**: 416-421.

383. Goldstein, M., Hiramoto, R., and Pressman, D. (1959). Comparative fluorescein labeling and cytotoxicity studies with human cell strains, HeLa, Raos, and 407 Liver and with fresh surgical specimens of cervical carcinoma, osteogenic sarcoma and normal adult liver. *J. Natl. Cancer Inst.* **22**: 697-705.

384. Goldwasser, R. A., and Kissling, R. E. (1958). Fluorescent antibody staining of street and fixed rabies virus antigens. *Proc. Soc. Exptl. Biol. Med.* **98**: 219-223.

385. Goldwasser, R. A., Kissling, R. E., Carski, T. R., and Nosty, T. S. (1959). Fluorescent antibody staining of rabies virus antigens in the salivary glands of rabid animals. *Bull. World Health Organ.* **20**: 579-588.

386. Goldwasser, R. A., and Shepard, C. C. (1958). Staining of comple-

ment and modification of fluorescent antibody procedures. *J. Immunol.* **80**: 122-131.

387. Goldwasser, R. A., and Shepard, C. C. (1959). Fluorescent antibody methods in the differentiation of murine and epidemic typhus; specificity changes resulting from previous immunization. *J. Immunol.* **82**: 373-380.

388. Gordon, M. A. (1958). Differentiation of yeasts by means of fluorescent antibody. *Proc. Soc. Exptl. Biol. Med.* **97**: 694-698.

389. Gordon, M. A. (1959). Fluorescent staining of *Histoplasma capsulatum. J. Bacteriol.* **77**: 678-681.

390. Gordon, M. A. (1962). Differentiation and classification of yeasts by the Coons fluorescent antibody technic. *In* "Fungi and Fungous Diseases" (G. Dalldorf, ed.), pp. 207-219. Thomas, Springfield, Illinois.

391. Gordon, M. A., and Al-Doory, Y. (1965). Application of fluorescent antibody procedures to the study of pathogenic dematiaceous fungi. II. Serological relationships of the genus *Fonsecaea. J. Bacteriol.* **89**: 551-556.

392. Gordon, M. A., Edwards, M. R., and Tompkins, J. N. (1962). Refinement of fluorescent antibody by gel filtration. *Proc. Soc. Exptl. Biol. Med.* **109**: 96-99.

393. Gornall, A. G., Bardawill, C. J., and David, M. M. (1949). Determination of serum proteins by means of the Biuret reaction. *J. Biol. Chem.* **177**: 751-766.

394. Gotoff, S. P., Fellers, F. X., Vawter, G. F., Janeway, C. A., and Rosen, F. S. (1965). The beta-1C globulin in childhood nephrotic syndrome: Laboratory diagnosis of progressive glomerulonephritis. *New Engl. J. Med.* **273**: 524-529.

395. Goudie, R. B., and McCallum, H. M. (1963). Loss of tissue-specific autoantigen in thyroid tumours: A demonstration by immunofluorescence. *Lancet* **II**: 1035-1038.

396. Green, G. M., and Kass, E. H. (1964). The role of the alveolar macrophage in the clearance of bacteria from the lung. *J. Exptl. Med.* **119**: 167-176.

397. Griffin, C. W., Carski, T. R., and Warner, G. S. (1961). Labeling procedures employing crystalline fluorescein isothiocyanate. *J. Bacteriol.* **82**: 534-537.

398. Griffin, J. W. (1963). Fluorescent antibody study of herpes simplex virus lesions and recurrent aphthae. *Oral Surg., Oral Med., Oral Pathol.* **16**: 945-952.

399. Griffin, J. W. (1965). Recurrent intraoral herpes simplex virus infection. *Oral Surg., Oral Med., Oral Pathol.* **19**: 209-213.

400. Grogan, C. H., and Roboz, E. (1955). Simple apparatus for concentrating biologic fluids of low protein content. *J. Lab. Clin. Med.* **45**: 495-498.

401. Gross, W. M., and Ball, M. R. (1964). Use of fluorescein-labeled

antibody to study *Borrelia anserina* infection (avian spirochetosis) in the chicken. *Am. J. Vet. Res.* **25**: 1734-1739.

402. Grossman, M., Sussman, S., Gottfried, D., Quock, C., and Ticknor, W. (1964). Immunofluorescent techniques in bacterial meningitis, identification of *Neisseria meningitidis* and *Hemophilus influenzae*. *Am. J. Diseases Children* **107**: 356-362.

403. Grunberg, E., and Cleeland, R. (1966). Fluorescence and visibility of *Proteus mirabilis* stained directly with fluorescein isothiocyanate. *J. Bacteriol.* **92**: 23-27.

404. Guarguaglini, M. (1964). Evaluation of the treponema agglutination (TPA) test as compared with the Nelson-Mayer (TPI) test and immunofluorescence (FTA) test in serodiagnosis of syphilis. (Italian) *Boll. Ist. Sieroterop. Milan.* **43**: 221-233.

405. Gurvich, E. B., and Roihel, V. M. (1965). Use of the fluorescent antibody technique in the detection and differential diagnosis of smallpox. *Acta Virol.* **9**: 165-171.

406. Guthe, T., Vaisman, A., and Paris-Hamelin, A. (1964). Fluorescent antibody technic using dried and eluated blood. Study of the preservation and shipment of samples at high temperatures. (French) *Bull. World Health Organ.* **31**: 87-94.

407. Haglund, J. R., Ayres, J. C., Paton, A. M., Kraft, A. A., and Quinn, L. Y. (1964). Detection of salmonella in eggs and egg products with fluorescent antibody. *Appl. Microbiol.* **12**: 447-450.

408. Hahn, J. J., and Cole, R. M. (1963). Studies on the mechanism of the long chain phenomenon of group A streptococci. *J. Exptl. Med.* **117**: 583-594.

409. Hahn, J. J., and Cole, R. M. (1963). Streptococcal M antigen location and synthesis, studied by immunofluorescence. *J. Exptl. Med.* **118**: 659-666.

410. Hahon, N., and Nakamura, R. M. (1964). Quantitative assay of psittacosis virus by the fluorescent cell-counting technique. *Virology* **23**: 203-208.

411. Halikis, D. N., and Arquilla, E. R. (1961). Studies on the physical, immunological and biological properties of insulin conjugated with fluorescein isothiocyanate. *Diabetes* **10**: 142-147.

412. Hall, C. T., and Hansen, P. A. (1962). Chelated azo dyes used as counterstains in the fluorescent antibody technic. *Zentr. Bakteriol., Parasitenk., Abt. I. Orig.* **184**: 548-554.

413. Halparen, S., Donaldson, P., and Sulkin, S. E. (1958). Identification of streptococci in bacterial mixtures and clinical specimens with fluorescent antibody. *J. Bacteriol.* **76**: 223-224.

414. Hamard, M., Cannat, A., and Seligmann, M. (1964). Detection of antinuclear antibodies by immunofluorescence. (French) *Rev. Franc. Etudes Clin. Biol.* **9**: 716-728.

415. Hamperl, H. (1947). Die Methoden der Fluoreszenzmikroskopie. *Mikroskopie* **2**: 152-155.

416. Hampton, E. G. (1964). Viral antigen in rat embryo in culture

infected with the H-1 virus isolated from transplantable human tumors: Cytochemical studies. *Cancer Res.* **24**: 1534-1543.

417. Han, S. S., Johnson, A. G., and Han, I. H. (1965). The antibody response in the rat. I. A histometric study of the spleen following a single injection of bovine gamma globulin with and without endotoxin *J. Infect. Diseases* **115**: 149-158.

418. Hanna, L., and Bernkopf, H. (1964). Trachoma viruses isolated in the United States. 8. Separation of TRIC viruses from related agents by immunofluorescence. *Proc. Soc. Exptl. Biol. Med.* **116**: 827-831.

419. Hansen, P. A. (1964). Fluorescent compounds used in protein tracing. Absorption and emission data. Publication from University of Maryland, College Park, Maryland.

420. Hanson, L. A., and Tan, E. M. (1965). Characterization of antibodies in human urine. *J. Clin. Invest.* **44**: 703-715.

421. Hanson, R. J., Kempf, J. E., and Board, A. V., Jr. (1957). Phagocytosis of influenza virus. II. Its occurrence in normal and immune mice. *J. Immunol.* **79**: 422-427.

422. Harris, T. N., Dray, S., Ellsworth, B., and Harris S. (1963). Rabbit gamma-globulin allotypes as genetic markers for the source of antibody produced in recipients of *Shigella* incubated lymph node cells. *Immunology* **6**: 169-178.

423. Hartley, B. S., and Massey, V. (1956). The active centre of chymotrypsin. 1. Labelling with a fluorescent dye. *Biochim. Biophys. Acta* **21**: 58-70.

424. Hartroft, P. M., Sutherland, L. E., and Hartroft, W. S. (1964). Juxtaglomerular cells as the source of renin: further studies with the fluorescent antibody technique and the effect of passive transfer of antirenin. *Can. Med. Assoc. J.* **90**: 163-166.

425. Hassan, S. A., Rabin, E. R., and Melnick, J. L. (1965). Reovirus myocarditis in mice: an electron microscopic, immunofluorescent, and virus assay study. *Exptl. Mol. Pathol.* **4**: 66-80.

426. Hatch, M. H. (1963). Identification of coxsackie and ECHO virus isolates with fluorescent antibody. *Proc. Soc. Exptl. Biol. Med.* **114**: 161-165.

427. Head, W. E. (1962). Immunochemical study of the diptheria toxin-fluorescent antitoxin system. *J. Pharm. Sci.* **51**: 662-665.

428. Hebert, G. A., and Pittman, B. (1965). Factors affecting removal of $(NH_4)_2SO_4$ from salt fractionated serum globulins employing a spectrophotometric procedure for determination of sulfate. *Health Lab. Sci.* **2**: 48-53.

429. Helander, E., and Emmart, E. W. (1959). Localization of myosin in the conduction bundle of beef heart. *Proc. Soc. Exptl. Biol. Med.* **101**: 838-842.

430. Henle, G., and Henle, W. (1965). Evidence for a persistent viral infection in a cell line derived from Burkitt's lymphoma. *J. Bacteriol.* **89**: 252-258.

431. Henle, G., and Henle, W. (1965). Cross-reactions among γ-globulins of various species in indirect immunoflourescence. *J. Immunol.* **95**: 118-124.

432. Henle, G., and Henle, W. (1966). Immunofluorescence in cells derived from Burkitt's lymphoma. *J. Bacteriol.* **91**: 1248-1256.

433. Herbeuval, R., Duheille, J., and Goedert-Herbeuval, C. (1965). Diagnosis of unusual blood cells by immunofluorescence. *Acta Cytol.* **9**: 73-82.

434. Herman, R. (1965). Fluorescent antibody studies on the intracellular form of *Leishmania donovani* grown in cell culture. *Exptl. Parasitol.* **17**: 218-228.

435. Hers, J. F. (1963). Fluorescent antibody technique in respiratory viral diseases. *Am. Rev. Respirat. Diseases.* **88**: Suppl., 316-333.

436. Hess, E. V., Fink, C. W., Taranta, A., and Ziff, M. (1964). Heart muscle antibodies in rheumatic fever and other diseases. *J. Clin. Invest.* **43**: 886-893.

437. Hess, E. V., Hunter, D. K., and Ziff, M. (1965). Gonococcal antibodies in acute arthritis. *J. Am. Med. Assoc.* **191**: 531-534.

438. Hess, R., and Pearse, A. G. E. (1959). Labelling of proteins with cellulose-reactive dyes. *Nature* **183**: 260-261.

439. Hicks, J. D., and Matthaei, E. (1955). Fluorescence in histology. *J. Pathol. Bacteriol.* **70**: 1-12.

440. Hill, A. G. S., and Cruickshank, B. (1953). A study of antigenic components of kidney tissue. *Brit. J. Exptl. Pathol.* **34**: 27-34.

441. Hill, A. G. S., Deane, H. W., and Coons, A. H. (1950). Localization of antigen in tissue cells. V. Capsular polysaccharide of Friedlander bacillus, Type B, in the mouse. *J. Exptl. Med.* **92**: 35-44.

442. Hinton, W. E., Evers, C. G., and Brunson, J. G. (1964). The influence of adrenal medullary hormones on nephrotoxic nephritis in rabbits. *Lab. Invest.* **13**: 1374-1380.

443. Hinuma, Y., and Hummeler, K. (1961). Studies on the complement-fixing antigens of poliomyelitis. III. Intracellular development of antigen. *J. Immunol.* **87**: 367-375.

444. Hinuma, Y., Ohta, R., Miyamoto, T., and Ishida, N. (1962). Evaluation of the complement method of fluorescent antibody technique with myxoviruses. *J. Immunol.* **89**: 19-26.

445. Hirai, T., and Hirai, A. (1964). Tobacco mosaic virus: cytological evidence of the synthesis in the nucleus. *Science* **145**: 589-591.

446. Hiramoto, R., Bernecky, J., Jurand, J., and Hamlin, M. (1964). The effect of hydrogen ion concentration on fluorescent labeled antibodies. *J. Histochem. Cytochem.* **12**: 271-274.

447. Hiramoto, R., Engel, K., and Pressman, D. (1958). Tetramethylrhodamine as immunochemical fluorescent label in the study of chronic thyroiditis. *Proc. Soc. Exptl. Biol. Med.* **97**: 611-614.

448. Hiramoto, R., Goldstein, M., and Pressman, D. (1958). Reactions of antisera prepared against HeLa cells and normal fetal liver cells with adult human tissues. *Cancer Res.* **18**: 668-669.

449. Hiramoto, R., and Hamlin, M. (1965). Detection of two anti-bodies in single plasma cells by the paired fluorescence technique. *J. Immunol.* **95**: 214-224.

450. Hiramoto, R., Jurand, J., Bernecky, J., and Pressman, D. (1962). Lack of staining of testicular tumors by anti-sperm and anti-testis antibodies. *Proc. Soc. Exptl. Biol. Med.* **111**: 505-507.

451. Hiramoto, R., Jurandowski, J., Bernecky, J., and Pressman, D. (1959). Precise zone of localization of anti-kidney antibody in various organs. *Proc. Soc. Exptl. Biol. Med.* **101**: 583-586.

452. Hiramoto, R., Jurandowski, J., Bernecky, J., and Pressman, D. (1961). Immunochemical differentiation of rhabdomyosarcomas. *Cancer Res.* **21**: 383-386.

453. Hiramoto, R., Jurandowski, J., Bernecky, J., and Pressman, D. (1961). Immunohistochemical identification of tissue culture cells. *Proc. Soc. Exptl. Biol. Med.* **108**: 347-353.

454. Hiramoto, R., and Pressman, D. (1957). Immunohistochemical staining properties of human skin and some related tumors. *Cancer Res.* **17**: 1135-1137.

455. Hiramoto, R., Yagi, Y., and Pressman, D. (1958). *In vivo* fixation of antibodies in the adrenal. *Proc. Soc. Exptl. Biol. Med.* **98**: 870-874.

456. Hiramoto, R., Yagi, Y., and Pressman, D. (1959). Immunohisto-chemical studies in anti-Murphy-lymphosarcoma sera. *Cancer Res.* **19**: 874-879.

457. Hobbs, T. R., and Mascoli, C. C. (1965). Studies on experimental infection of weanling mice with reoviruses. *Proc. Soc. Exptl. Biol. Med.* **118**: 847-853.

458. Hobson, P.N., and Mann, S. O. (1957). Some studies on the identi-fication of rumen bacteria with fluorescent antibodies. *J. Gen. Microbiol.* **16**: 463-471.

459. Hochberg, M., Cooper, J. K., Redys, J. J., and Caceres, C. A. (1966). Identification of fluorescent-antibody labeled group A streptococci by fluorometry. *Appl. Microbiol.* **14**: 386-390.

460. Holborow, E. J., Brown, P. C., Roitt, I. M., and Doniach, D. (1959). Cytoplasmic localization of "complement-fixing" auto-antigen in human thyroid epithelium. *Brit. J. Exptl. Pathol.* **40**: 583-588.

461. Holborow, E. J., Weir, D. M., and Johnson, G. D. (1957). A serum factor in lupus erythematosus with affinity for tissue nuclei. *Brit. Med. J.* **II**: 732-734.

462. Holman, M. S., Koornhof, H. J., and Hayden-Smith, S. (1964). The laboratory diagnosis of gonorrhoea in the female, *S. African J. Lab. Clin. Med.* **10**: 95-98.

463. Holmes, A. W., Caldwell, R. G., Dedmon, R. E., and Deinhardt, F. (1964). Isolation and characterization of a new herpes virus. *J. Immunol.* **92**: 602-610.

464. Holter, H., and Marshall, J. M., Jr. (1954). Studies on pinocytosis

in the amoeba *Chaos chaos*. *Compt. Rend. Trav. Lab. Carlsberg* **29**: 7-26.

465. Holwerda, J., and Eldering, G. (1963). Culture and fluorescent-antibody methods in diagnosis of whooping cough. *J. Bacteriol.* **86**: 449-451.

466. Hopkins, S. J., and Wormall, A. (1933). Phenyl isocyanate protein compounds and their immunological reactions. *Biochem. J.* **27**: 740-753.

467. Horesji, J., and Smetana, R. (1956). The isolation of gamma globulin from blood serum by rivanol. *Acta Med. Scand.* **155**: 65-70.

468. Hornung, J. E. (1965). Immunofluorescent studies of *Shigella* in infants and young children. *Am. J. Med. Technol.* **31**: 239-255.

469. Horowitz, R. E., Burrow, L., Paronetto, F., Dreiling, D., and Karp, A. E. (1965). Immunologic observations of homografts. II. The canine kidney. *Transplantation* **3**: 318-325.

470. Horowitz, R. E., Stuyvesant, V. W., Wigmore, W., and Tatter, D. (1965). Fibrinogen as a component of amyloid. *Arch. Pathol.* **79**: 238-244.

471. Hsu, K. C., Rifkind, R. A., and Zabriskie, J. B. (1963). Fluorescent, electron microscopic and immunoelectrophoretic studies of labeled antibodies. *Science* **142**: 1471-1473.

472. Hudson, B. W. (1961). Column adsorption of fluorescein isothiocyanate-labeled antibodies. *Bull. World Health Organ.* **24**: 291-292.

473. Hudson, B. W., and Quan, S. F. (1960). Use of fluorescent antibody technique for detection of *Pasteurella pestis* in rodents. *Trans. Roy. Soc. Trop. Med. Hyg.* **54**: 599-600.

474. Huebner, R. J., Chanock, R. M., Rubin, B. A., and Casey, M. J. (1964). Induction by adenovirus type 7 of tumors in hamsters having the antigenic characteristics of SV40 virus. *Proc. Natl. Acad. Sci. U.S.* **52**: 1333-1340.

475. Hughes, P. E. (1958). The significance of staining reaction of preneoplastic rat liver with fluorescein-globulin complexes. *Cancer Res.* **18**: 426-432.

476. Hughes, P. E., and Louis, C. J. (1959). Differential staining of normal and neoplastic tissue with fluorescein-egg albumen. *Arch. Pathol.* **68**: 508-512.

477. Hunter, E. F., Deacon, W. E., and Meyer, P. E. (1964). Improved FTA test for syphilis, absorption procedure (FTA-ABS). *Public Health Rept.* **79**: 410-412.

478. Husain, M. H., and Sommerville, R. G. (1964). Presence of herpes-simplex virus on eczematous skin. *Lancet* **II**: 391-392.

479. Imamura, S., and Ashizawa, Y. (1965). Studies on the serological reactions of leptospira, especially on the sensitized-erythrocyte lysis test and the fluorescent antibody test. *Japan. J. Hyg.* **19**: 365-368.

480. Imre, G., Korchmaros, I., Geck, P., Nasz, I., and Dan, P. (1964). Antigenic specificity of inclusion bodies in epidemic keratoconjunctivitis. *Ophthalmologia* **148**: 7-12.

481. Ingram, R. L., and Carver, R. K. (1963). Malaria parasites: Fluorescent antibody technique for tissue stage study. *Science* **139**: 405-406.

482. Ingram, R. L., Otken, L. B., Jr., and Jumper, J. R. (1961). Staining of malarial parasites by the fluorescent antibody technic. *Proc. Soc. Exptl. Biol. Med.* **106**: 52-54.

483. Ishida, N., Hinuma, Y., Sekino, K., Shiratori, T., and Kudo, H. (1963). Experimental human influenza infections studied by means of immunofluorescent staining of nasal smears. *Tohoku J. Exptl. Med.* **78**: 390-397.

484. Ishizaki, R., and Shimizu, T. (1964). Sequential development of antigens of equine rhinopneumonitis virus in infected hamster liver cells as studied with fluorescent antibodies. *Natl. Inst. Animal Health Quart.* **4**: 194-204.

485. Ito, M., Ikegami, M., Shiroki, K., and Tagaya, I. (1964). Studies on the multiplication of simian virus 40 (vacuolating virus) by means of fluorescent antibody technique. *Japan. J. Med. Sci. Biol.* **17**: 179-193.

486. Ito, M., and Nishioka, K. (1959). Two reagents for fluorescent antibody technique and the visualization of the viral antigen synthesized in Ehrlich ascites tumor cells infected with ED virus. *Japan. J. Microbiol.* **3**: 71-83.

487. Jachowski, L. A., Jr., Anderson, R. I., and Sadun, E. H. (1963). Serologic reactions to *Schistosoma mansoni*. I. Quantitative studies on experimentally infected monkeys (*Macaca mulatta*). *Am. J. Hyg.* **77**: 137-145.

488. Jackson, G. J. (1959). Fluorescent antibody studies of *Trichinella spiralis* infections. *J. Infect. Diseases* **105**: 97-117.

489. Jackson, G. J. (1960). Fluorescent antibody studies of *Nippostrongylus muris* infections. *J. Infect. Diseases* **106**: 20-36.

490. Jaeger, R. F., Spertzel, R. O. and Kuehne, R. W. (1961). Detection of air-borne *Pasteurella tularensis* using the fluorescent antibody technique. *Appl. Microbiol.* **9**: 585-587.

491. Jamison, R. M., Mayor, H. D., and Melnick, J. L. (1963). Studies on ECHO 4 virus (picornavirus group) and its intracellular development. *Exptl. Mol. Pathol.* **2**: 188-202.

492. Jankovic, B. D. (1959). Histochemical identification of antigen in red cells. *Exptl. Cell Res.* **17**: 183-184.

493. Jawetz, E., Rose, L., Hanna, L., and Thygeson, P. (1965). Experimental inclusion conjunctivitis in man: measurements of infectivity and resistance. *J. Am. Med. Assoc.* **194**: 620-632.

494. Jeanes, A. L. (1964). The application of immunoflourescence techniques to the diagnosis of infection. *Guy's Hosp. Rept.* **113**: 136-142.

495. Jeanes, A. L. (1964). Immunofluorescent diagnosis of amoebiasis. *Brit. Med. J.* Dec. 12, 1964: 1531.

496. Jeanes, A. L. (1966). Indirect fluorescent antibody test in diagnosis of hepatic amoebiasis. *Brit. Med. J.* June 11, 1966: 1464.
497. Jensen, K. E. (1963). Measurement of growth-inhibiting antibody for *Mycoplasma pneumoniae. J. Bacteriol.* **86:** 1349-1350.
498. Jeon, K. W., and Bell, I. G. (1964). Behavior of cell membrane in relation to locomotion in *Amoeba proteus. Exptl. Cell Res.* **33:** 531-539.
499. Jerushalmy, Z., Kaminsky, E., Kohn, A., and DeVries, A. (1963). Interaction of Newcastle disease virus with megakaryocytes in cell cultures of guinea pig bone marrow. *Proc. Soc. Exptl. Biol. Med.* **114:** 687-690.
500. Jobbagy, A., and Kiraly, K. (1966). Chemical characterization of fluorescein isothiocyanate-protein conjugates. *Biochim. Biophys. Acta* **124:** 166-175.
501. Johnson, C. F., and Scott, A. D. (1964). Cytological studies of Newcastle disease virus (NDV) in HEP-2 cells. *Proc. Soc. Exptl. Biol. Med.* **115:** 281-286.
502. Johnson, G. D. (1961). Simplified procedure for removing non-specific staining components from fluorescein-labeled conjugates. *Nature* **191:** 70-71.
503. Johnson, G. D., and Holborow, E. J. (1963). Immunofluorescent test for infectious mononucleosis. *Nature* **198:** 1316-1317.
504. Johnson, R. T. (1964). The pathogenesis of herpes virus encephalitis. I. Virus pathways to the nervous system of suckling mice demonstrated by fluorescent antibody staining. *J. Exptl. Med.* **119:** 343-356.
505. Johnson, R. T. (1965). Experimental rabies. Studies of cellular vulnerability and pathogenesis using fluorescent antibody staining. *J. Neuropathol. Exptl. Neurol.* **24:** 662-674.
506. Johnson, R. T. (1965). Virus invasion of the central nervous system: A study of Sindbis virus infection in the mouse using fluorescent antibody. *Am. J. Pathol.* **6:** 929-943.
507. Johnson, R. T., and Mercer, E. H. (1964). The development of fixed rabies virus in mouse brain. *Australian J. Exptl. Biol. Med. Sci.* **42:** 449-456.
508. Joncas, J. (1964). The direct fluorescent antibody technique studied with reovirus type 1. *Rev. Can. Biol.* **23:** 333-338.
509. Jones, W. D., Jr., Saito, H., and Kubica, G. P. (1965). Fluorescent antibody techniques with mycobacteria. *Am. Rev. Respirat. Diseases* **92:** 255-260.
510. Jones, W. L., and Foster, J. W. (1966). Papain-treated globulins in specific and cross-reacting immunofluorescent staining. *J. Bacteriol.* **91:** 984-986.
511. Kagan, I. G., Sulzer, A. J., and Carver, R. K. (1965). An evaluation of the fluorescent antibody test for the diagnosis of schistosomiasis. *Am. J. Epidemiol.* **81:** 63-70.

512. Kantor, F. S. (1964). Fate of streptococcal M protein after exposure to plasmin and human leukocytes. *Yale J. Biol. Med.* **36**: 259-267.
513. Kantor, F. S. (1965). Fibrinogen precipitation by streptococcal M protein. II. Renal lesions induced by intravenous injection of M protein into mice and rats. *J. Exptl. Med.* **121**: 861-872.
514. Kaplan, M. H. (1958). Localization of streptococcal antigen in tissues. I. Histologic distribution and persistence of M protein, types 1, 5, 12 and 19 in the tissue of the mouse. *J. Exptl. Med.* **107**: 341-352.
515. Kaplan, M. H. (1958). Immunologic studies of heart tissue. I Production in rabbits of antibodies reactive with an autologous myocardial antigen following immunization with heterologous heart tissue. *J. Immunol.* **80**: 254-267.
516. Kaplan, M. H. (1958). Immunologic studies of heart tissue. II. Differentiation of a myocardial sarcoplasmic antigen and cardiolipin. *J. Immunol.* **80**: 268-277.
517. Kaplan, M. H. (1959). The fluorescent antibody technic as a research tool in the study of connective tissue diseases. *Arthritis Rheumat.* **2**: 568-573.
518. Kaplan, M. H. (1963). Immunologic relation of streptococcal and tissue antigens. I. Properties of an antigen in certain strains of Group A streptococci exhibiting an immunologic cross-reaction with human heart tissue. *J. Immunol.* **90**: 595-606.
519. Kaplan, M. H., Coons, A. H., and Deane, H. W. (1950). Localization of antigen in tissue cells. III. Cellular distribution of pneumococcal polysaccharides types II and III in the mouse. *J. Exptl. Med.* **91**: 15-30.
520. Kaplan, M. H., and Dallenbach, F. D. (1961). Immunologic studies of heart tissue. III. Occurrence of bound gamma globulin in auricular appendages from rheumatic hearts. Relationship to certain histopathologic features of rheumatic heart disease. *J. Exptl. Med.* **113**: 1-15.
521. Kaplan, M. H., and Meyeserian, M. (1962). Immunologic studies of heart tissue. V. Antigens related to heart tissue revealed by cross-reactions of rabbit antisera to heterologous heart. *J. Immunol.* **88**: 450-461.
522. Kaplan, M. H., Meyeserian, M., and Kushner, L. (1961). Immunologic studies of heart tissue. IV. Serologic reactions with human heart tissue as revealed by immunofluorescent methods: Isoimmune, Wasserman and auto-immune reactions. *J. Exptl. Med.* **113**: 17-35.
523. Kaplan, W., and Clifford, M. K. (1964). Production of fluorescent antibody reagents specific for the tissue form of *Coccidioides immitis. Am. Rev. Respirat. Diseases* **89**: 651-658.
524. Kaplan, W., and Gonzalez-Ochoa, A. (1963). Application of the fluorescent antibody technique to the rapid diagnosis of sporotrichosis. *J. Lab. Clin. Med.* **62**: 835-841.

525. Kaplan, W., and Ivens, M. S. (1960). Fluorescent antibody staining of *Sporotrichum schenckii* in cultures and clinical materials. *J. Invest. Dermatol.* **35**: 151-159.

526. Kaplan, W., and Kaufman, L. (1963). Specific fluorescent antiglobulins for the detection and identification of *Blastomyces dermatitidis* yeast-phase cells. *Mycopathol. Mycol. Appl.* **19**: 173-180.

527. Karakawa, W. W., Borman, E. K., and McFarland, C. R. (1964). Typing of group A streptococci by immunofluorescence. I. Preparation and properties of type I fluorescein-labeled antibody. *J. Bacteriol.* **87**: 1377-1382.

528. Karakawa, W. W., Krause, R. M., and Borman, E. K. (1965). Immunochemical aspects of the cross-reactivity between groups A and C streptococci as detected by the fluorescent antibody technique. *J. Immunol.* **94**: 282-288.

529. Karakawa, W. W., Rotta, J., and Krause, R. M. (1965). Detection of M protein in colonies of streptococcal L forms by immunofluorescence. *Proc. Soc. Exptl. Biol. Med.* **118**: 198-201.

530. Karakawa, W. W., Sedgwick, A. K., and Borman, E. K. (1964). Typing of *Haemophilus influenzae* with fluorescent antibody reagent. *Health Lab. Sci.* **1**: 114-118.

531. Karasszon, D., and Bodon, L. (1963). Demonstration of the swine-fever virus in tissue culture by immunofluorescence. *Acta Microbiol. Acad. Sci. Hung.* **10**: 287-291.

532. Kartman, L. (1960). The role of rabbits in sylvatic plague epidemiology, with special attention to human cases in New Mexico and use of the fluorescent antibody technique for detection of *Pasteurella pestis* in field specimens. *Zoonoses Res.* **1**: 1-27.

533. Kase, A., and Marshall, J. D. (1960). A study of *Cryptococcus neoformans* by means of the fluorescent antibody technic. *Am. J. Clin. Pathol.* **34**: 52-56.

534. Kato, S., Miyamoto, H., Takahashi, M., and Kamahora, J. (1963). Shope fibroma and rabbit myxoma viruses. II. Pathogenesis of fibromas in domestic rabbits. *Biken's J.* **6**: 135-143.

535. Kato, S., Takahashi, M., Miyamoto, H., and Kamahora, J. (1963). Shope fibroma and rabbit myxoma viruses. I. Autoradiographic and cytoimmunological studies on "B" type inclusions. *Biken's J.* **6**: 127-134.

536. Katzenelson, E., and Bernkopf, H. (1965). Serologic differentiation of trachoma strains and other agents of the psittacosis-lymphogranuloma venereum-trachoma group with the aid of the direct fluorescent antibody method. *J. Immunol.* **94**: 467-474.

537. Kaufman, L., and Blumer, S. (1966). Occurrence of serotypes among *Histoplasma capsulatum* strains. *J. Bacteriol.* **91**: 1434-1439.

538. Kaufman, L., and Brandt, B. (1964). Fluorescent-antibody studies of the mycelial form of *Histoplasma capsulatum* and morphologically similar fungi. *J. Bacteriol.* **87**: 120-126.

539. Kaufman, L., Brandt, B., and McLaughlin, D. (1964). Evaluation

of the fluorescent antibody and agar gel precipitin tests for detecting *Histoplasma* antibodies in anticomplementary sera. *Am. J. Hyg.* **79**: 181-185.

540. Kaufman, L., and Cherry, W. B. (1961). Technical factors affecting the preparation of fluorescent antibody reagents. *J. Immunol.* **87**: 72-79.

541. Kaufman, L., and Kaplan, W. (1961). Preparation of a fluorescent antibody specific for the yeast phase of *Histoplasma capsulatum*. *J. Bacteriol.* **82**: 729-735.

542. Kaufman, L., and Kaplan, W. (1963). Serological characterization of pathogenic fungi by means of fluorescent antibodies. I. Antigenic relationships between yeast and mycelial forms of *Histoplasma capsulatum* and *Blastomyces dermatitidis*. *J. Bacteriol.* **85**: 986-991.

543. Kaufman, L., Schubert, J., and Kaplan, W. (1962). Fluorescent antibody inhibition test for histoplasmosis. *J. Lab. Clin. Med.* **59**: 1033-1038.

544. Kelen, A. E., Ayllon-Leindl, L., and Labzoffsky, N. A. (1962). Indirect fluorescent antibody method in serodiagnosis of toxoplasmosis. *Can. J. Microbiol.* **8**: 545-554.

545. Kellogg, D. S., Jr., and Deacon, W. E. (1964). A new rapid immunofluorescent staining technique for identification of *Treponema pallidum* and *Neisseria gonorrhoeae*. *Proc. Soc. Exptl. Biol. Med.* **115**: 963-965.

546. Kendall, F. E. (1937). Studies on serum proteins. I. Identification of a single serum globulin by immunological means. Its distribution in the sera of normal individuals and of patients with cirrhosis of the liver and with chronic glomerulonephritis. *J. Clin. Invest.* **16**: 921-931.

547. Kent, S. P. (1961). A study of mucins in tissue sections using the fluorescent antibody technique. I. The preparation and specificity of bovine submaxillary gland mucin antibody. *J. Histochem. Cytochem.* **9**: 491-497.

548. Kent, S. P. (1963). Study of tissue mucins using the fluorescent antibody technique. II. The preparation and specificity of human submaxillary gland mucin antibody. *J. Histochem. Cytochem.* **11**: 273-282.

549. Kent, S. P. (1964). The demonstration and distribution of water soluble blood group O (H) antigen in tissue sections using a fluorescein labelled extract of *Ulex europeus* seed. *J. Histochem. Cytochem.* **12**: 591-599.

550. Keutel, H. J. (1965). Localization of uromucoid in human kidney and in sections of human kidney stone with the fluorescent antibody technique. *J. Histochem. Cytochem.* **13**: 155-160.

551. Killander, J., Ponten, J., and Roden, L. (1961). Rapid preparation of fluorescent antibodies using gel-filtration. *Nature* **192**: 182-183.

552. King, D. A., and Croghan, D. L. (1965). Immunofluorescence of

feline panleucopenia virus in cell culture: Determination of immunological status of felines by serum neutralization. *Can. J. Comp. Med.* **29**: 85-89.

553. King, E. S., Jr., Hughes, P. E., and Louis, C. S. (1958). The species non-specificity of globulins in the globulin-fluorescein staining of tissues. *Brit. J. Cancer* **12**: 5-13.

554. King, E. S., Jr., Hughes, P. E., and Louis, C. J. (1959). Differential fluorescence staining of normal and neoplastic tissues: use of various serum proteins. *Cancer* **12**: 741-752.

555. Kirsh, D., and Kissling, R. (1963). The use of immunofluorescence in the rapid presumptive diagnosis of variola. *Bull. World Health Organ.* **29**: 126-128.

556. Kirsner, J. B. (1965). The immunologic response of the colon. *J. Am. Med. Assoc.* **191**: 809-814.

557. Kisch, A. L., and Fraser, K. B. (1964). The effect of pH on transformation of BMK21 cells by polyoma virus. I. Relationship between transformation rate and synthesis of viral antigen. *Virology* **24**: 186-192.

558. Kisch, A. L., Johnson, K. M., and Chanock, R. M. (1962). Immunofluorescence with respiratory syncytial virus. *Virology* **16**: 177-189.

559. Kitahara, T., Butel, J. S., Rapp, F., and Melnick, J. L. (1965). Correlation between complement-fixing cell antibody and immunofluorescent nuclear antibody in hamsters bearing 'SV40'-induced tumors. *Nature* **205**: 717.

560. Klainer, A. S., Madoff, M. A., Cooper, L. Z., and Weinstein, L. (1964). Staphylococcal alphahemolysin: Detection on the erythrocyte membrane by immunofluorescence. *Science* **145**: 714-715.

561. Klatzo, I., Howath, B., and Emmart, E. W. (1958). Demonstration of myosin in human striated muscle by fluorescent antibody. *Proc. Soc. Exptl. Biol. Med.* **97**: 135-140.

562. Klein, E., and Klein, G. (1964). Antigenic properties of lymphomas induced by the Moloney agent. *J. Natl. Cancer Inst.* **32**: 547-568.

563. Klein, E., and Klein, G. (1964). Mouse antibody production test for the assay of the Moloney virus. *Nature* **204**: 339-342.

564. Klein, E., and Klein, G. (1965). Antibody response and leukemia development in mice inoculated neonatally with the Moloney virus. *Cancer Res.* **25**: 851-854.

565. Klein, G., Clifford, P., Klein, E., and Stjernsward, J. (1966). Search for tumor specific immune reactions in Burkitt lymphoma patients by the membrane immunofluorescence reaction. *Proc. Natl. Acad. Sci. U.S.* **55**: 1628-1635.

566. Klingenberg, H. G., Lipp, W., and Miller, F. (1961). The effect of protamine and acridine orange on the muscular activity of the guinea pig uterus. *Exptl. Cell Res.* **23**: 1-8.

567. Klotz, A. W. (1965). Application of FA techniques to detection of *Clostridium perfringens*. *Public Health Reports* **80**: 305-311.

568. Klugerman, M. R. (1966). Chemical and physical variables affecting the properties of fluorescein isothiocyanate and its protein conjugates. *J. Immunol.* **95**: 1165-1173.
569. Kniker, W. T., and Cochrane, C. T. (1965). Pathogenic factors in vascular lesions of experimental serum sickness. *J. Exptl. Med.* **122**: 83-98.
570. Koffler, D. (1964). Giant cell pneumonia, fluorescent antibody and histochemical studies on alveolar giant cells. *Arch. Pathol.* **78**: 267-273.
571. Koffler, D., and Friedman, A. H. (1964). Localization of immunoglobulins in chronic thyroiditis. *Lab. Invest.* **13**: 239-245.
572. Koffler, D., Garlock, J., and Rothman, W. (1962). Immunocytochemical reactions from ulcerative colitis patients. *Proc. Soc. Exptl. Biol. Med.* **109**: 358-360.
573. Koffler, D., and Paronetto, F. (1965). Serologic and immunofluorescent studies of humoral antibody and gamma-globulin localization in experimental autoimmune thyroiditis. *J. Immunol.* **94**: 329-336.
574. Kohn, J. (1959). A simple method for the concentration of fluids containing proteins. *Nature* **183**: 1055.
575. Kolker, I. I. (1965). Immunopathological data on pathogenesis of burn disease and glomerulonephritis. *Federation Proc.* **24**: Transl. Suppl., 507-511.
576. Koller, M., Gonczol, E., and Vaczi, L. (1963). Study of the multiplication of varicella-zoster virus by the fluorescent antibody test. *Acta. Microbiol. Acad. Sci. Hung.* **10**: 183-188.
577. Komminos, G. N., and Tompkins, V. N. (1963). A simple method of eliminating the cross-reaction of staphylococcus in the fluorescent antibody technic. *Am. J. Clin. Pathol.* **40**: 319-324.
578. Kopf, A. W., Morrill, S. D., and Silberberg, I. (1965). Broad spectrum of leukoderma acquisitum centrifugum. *Arch. Dermatol.* **92**: 14-35.
579. Kornfeld, P., Siegal, S., Weiner, L. B., and Osserman, K. E. (1965). Studies in myasthenia gravis. Immunologic response in thymectomized and nonthymectomized patients. *Ann. Internal Med.* [N.S.] **63**: 416-428.
580. Kovacs, E., Baratawidjaja, R. K., and Labzoffsky, N. A. (1963). Visualization of poliovirus type III in paraffin sections of monkey spinal cord by indirect immuno-fluorescence. *Nature* **200**: 497-498.
581. Kraft, S. C., Fitch, F. W., and Kirsner, J. B. (1963). Histologic and immunohistochemical features of the Auer "colitis" in rabbits. *Am. J. Pathol.* **43**: 913-927.
582. Kramar, J. (1963). Versuch der verwendung markierter fluorescierender antikorper in der serologischen diagnose der toxoplasmose. In "Progress in Protozoology" (J. Ludvik *et al.* eds.), pp. 381-383. Academic Press, New York.

583. Krasnik, F. I. (1963). Demonstration of *Rickettsia prowazeki* in cell cultures by the fluorescent antibody method. *Acta Virol.* **7**: 190.

584. Kratchko, A., Natler, R., and Thivolet, J. (1964). Méthode rapide de recherche du virus vaccinal par mise en culture sur cellules et identification par immunofluorescence direct (note preliminaire). *Ann. Inst. Pasteur* **107**: 184-189.

585. Krier, J. P., and Ristic, M. (1963). Morphologic, antigenic, and pathogenic characteristics of *Eperythrozoon ovis and Eperythrozoon wenyoni. Am. J. Vet. Res.* **24**: 488-500.

586. Kreier, J. P., and Ristic, M. (1963). Anaplasmosis. XI. Immuno-serologic characteristics of the parasites present in the blood of calves infected with the Oregon strain of *Anaplasma marginale. Am. J. Vet. Res.* **24**: 688-696.

587. Kreier, J. P., and Ristic, M. (1964). Detection of a *Plasmodium berghei*-antibody complex formed *in vivo. Am. J. Trop. Med. Hyg.* **13**: 6-10.

588. Krigman, M. R., and Manuelidis, E. E. (1965). Morphological and permeability changes in the cerebral parenchyma adjacent to heterologous intracerebral tumors. *J. Neuropathol. Exptl. Neurol.* **24**: 49-62.

589. Krooth, R. S., Tobie, J. E., Tjio, J. H., and Goodman, H. C. (1961). Reaction of human sera with mammalian chromosomes shown by fluorescent antibody technique. *Science* **134**: 284-286.

590. Kundin, W. D. (1963). Studies on West Nile virus infection by means of fluorescent antibodies. II. Pathogenesis of West Nile virus infection in experimentally inoculated chicks. *Arch. Ges. Virusforsch.* **12**: 529-536.

591. Kundin, W. D., and Liu, C. (1963). Effects of acetone, ultraviolet irradiation and formalin on West Nile virus infectivity and immunofluorescent antigenicity. *Proc. Soc. Exptl. Biol. Med.* **114**: 359-360.

592. Kundin, W. D., Liu, C., Harmon, P., and Rodina, P. (1964). Pathogenesis of scrub typhus infection (*Rickettsia tsutsugamushi*) as studied by immunofluorescence. *J. Immunol.* **93**: 772-781.

593. Kundin, W. D., Liu, C., Hysell, P., and Hamachige, S. (1963). Studies on West Nile virus infection by means of fluorescent antibodies. I. Pathogenesis of West Nile virus infection in experimentally inoculated suckling mice. *Arch. Ges. Virusforsch.* **12**: 514-528.

594. Kunz, C. (1958). Fluorescent-serological examination for demonstration of *Candida albicans* antigen in pneumonia of premature infants. (German). *Zentr. Bakteriol., Parasitenk., Abt. I. Orig.* **172**: 446-448.

595. Kunz, C. (1958). Untersuchungen mit fluorescein-markierten antikorpern an Hefen. *Schweiz. Z. Allgem. Pathol. Bakteriol.* **21**: 892-899.

596. Kunz, C. (1959). Fluoreszenz-serologische Untersuchungen an einem pathogenen Pilzstamm (*Sporotrichum schenckii*). *Arch. Klin. Exptl. Dermatol.* **209**: 200-205.

597. Kunz, C. (1959). Weitere fluoreszenz-serologioche Untersuchungen on Pilzen. *Schweiz. Z. Allgem. Pathol. Bakteriol.* **22**: 742-746.

598. Kunz, C. (1964). The use of the immunofluorescent method and microphotometry for the differentiation of arboviruses. *Virology* **24**: 672-674.

599. Kuvin, S. F., Tobie, J. E., Evans, C. B., Coatney, G. R., and Contacos, P. G. (1962). Antibody production in human malaria as determined by the fluorescent antibody technique. *Science* **135**: 1130-1131.

600. Kuvin, S. F., Tobie, J. E., Evans, C. B., Coatney, G. R., and Contacos, P. G. (1962). Fluorescent antibody studies on the course of antibody production and serum gamma globulin levels in normal volunteers infected with human and simian malaria. *Am. J. Trop. Med. Hyg.* **11**: 429-436.

601. Kuvin, S. F., and Voller, A. (1963). Malarial antibody titres of West Africans in Britain. *Brit. Med. J.* **5355**: 477-479.

602. LaBrec, E. H., Formal, S. B., and Schneider, H. (1959). Serological identification of *Shigella flexneri* by means of fluorescent antibody technique. *J. Bacteriol.* **78**: 384-391.

603. Labzoffsky, N. A., Baratawidjaja, R. K., Kuitunen, E., Lewis, F. N., Kavelman, D. A., and Morrissey, L. P. (1964). Immunofluorescence as an aid in the early diagnosis of trichinosis. *Can. Med. Assoc. J.* **90**: 920-921.

604. Lacy, P. E. (1959). Electron microscopic and fluorescent antibody studies on islets of Langerhans. *Exptl. Cell Res.* Suppl. 7: 296-308.

605. Lacy, P. E., and Davies, J. (1957). Preliminary studies on the demonstration of insulin in the islets by the fluorescent antibody technic. *Diabetes* **6**: 354-357.

606. Lacy, P. E., and Davies, J. (1959). Demonstration of insulin in mammalian pancreas by the fluorescent antibody method. *Stain Technol.* **34**: 85-89.

607. Laffin, R. L., Bardawil, W. A., Pachas, W. N., and McCarthy, J. S. (1964). Immunofluorescent studies on the occurrence of antinuclear factor in normal human serum. *Am. J. Pathol.* **45**: 465-480.

608. Laurence, D. J. R. (1957). Fluorescence techniques for the enzymologist. *In* "Methods in Enzymology" (S. P. Colowick and N. O. Kaplan, eds.), Vol. 4, pp. 174-212. Academic Press, New York.

609. Lazarus, J. M., Sellers, D. P., and Marine, W. M. (1965). Meningitis due to the group B beta-hemolytic streptococcus. *New Engl. J. Med.* **272**: 146-147.

610. Lebrun, J. (1956). Cellular localization of herpes simplex virus by means of fluorescent antibody. *Virology* **2**: 496-510.

611. Lebrun, J. (1957). L'antigene poliomyelitique au cour du development intracellulaire des virus. *Ann. Inst. Pasteur* **93**: 225-229.

612. Leduc, E. H., Coons, A. H., and Connally, J. M. (1955). Studies on antibody production. II. The primary and secondary responses in the popliteal lymph node of the rabbit. *J. Exptl. Med.* **102**: 61-72.

613. Lee, L., and McCluskey, R. T. (1962). Immunohistochemical demonstration of the reticuloendothelial clearance of circulating fibrin aggregates. *J. Exptl. Med.* **116**: 611-618.

614. Leibovitz, A., Oberhofer, T. R., Meacham, J. T., Jr., and Diestelhorst, T. N. (1963). Enhancement of specificity of the fluorescent treponemal antibody test as compared with the TPI test. *Am. J. Clin. Pathol.* **40**: 480-486.

615. Lennette, E. H., Woodie, J. D., Nakamura, K., and Magoffin, R. L. (1965). The diagnosis of rabies by fluorescent antibody method (FRA) employing immune hamster serum. *Health Lab. Sci.* **2**: 24-34.

616. Leone, R. (1964). Cutaneous candidiasis. I. Immunofluorescence, agglutination and fungistasis reactions. (Italian) *Minerva Dermatol.* **39**: 231-235.

617. Lesso, J., Szanto, J., and Albrecht, P. (1963). Mumps virus infection of HeLa cells studied by the fluorescent antibody method. *Acta Virol.* **7**: 37-41.

618. Lessof, M. H., Crawford, H. J., and Wood, R. M. (1959). Antibody to thyroglobulin in patients with thyroid disease. *Lancet* Dec. 26, 1959: 1172-1173.

619. Leuchtenberger, C. (1958). Quantitative determination of DNA in cells by Feulgen microspectrophotometry. *In* "General Cytochemical Methods" (J. F. Danielli, ed.) Vol. 1, pp. 219-278. Academic Press, New York.

620. Levenson, H., and Cochrane, C. G. (1964). Nonprecipitating antibody and the Arthus vasculitis. *J. Immunol.* **92**: 118-127.

621. Levine, S. I., Goulet, N. R., and Liu, O. C. (1965). Beta-propiolactone decontamination of simian virus-40 as determined by a rapid fluorescent-antibody assay. *Appl. Microbiol.* **13**: 70-72.

622. Levine, S., Zimmerman, H. M., Wenk, E. J., and Gonatas, N. K. (1963). Experimental leukoencephalophathies due to implantation of foreign substances. *Am. J. Pathol.* **42**: 97-117.

623. Levinthal, J. D., Takacs, B., and Eaton, M. D. (1963). The distribution of polyoma viral antigen as detected by immunofluorescence in the tissues of infected mice. *Acta Unio Intern. Contra Cancrum* **19**: 318-321.

624. Levinthal, J. M., and Shein, H. M. (1964). Propagation of a simian tumor agent (Yaba virus) in cultures of human and simian renal cells as detected by immunofluorescence. *Virology* **23**: 268-270.

625. Levy, H. B., and Sober, H. A. (1960). A simple chromatographic method for preparation of gamma globulin. *Proc. Soc. Exptl. Biol. Med.* **103**: 250-252.

626. Levy, J. A., and Henle, G. (1966). Indirect immunofluorescence

tests with sera from African children and cultured Burkitt lymphoma cells. *J. Bacteriol.* **92**: 275-276.

627. Lewis, V. J., and Brooks, J. B. (1964). Comparison of fluorochromes for the preparation of fluorescent-antibody reagents. *J. Bacteriol.* **88**: 1520-1521.

628. Lewis, V. J., Jones, W. L., and Brooks, J. B. (1964). Technical considerations in the preparation of fluorescent-antibody conjugates. *Appl. Microbiol.* **12**: 343-348.

629. Leznoff, A., Fishman, J., Goodfriend, L., McGarry, E., Beck, J., and Rose, B. (1960). Localization of fluorescent antibodies to human growth hormone in human anterior pituitary gland. *Proc. Soc. Exptl. Biol. Med.* **104**: 232-235.

630. Lichtenberg, F. von (1964). Studies on granuloma formation. III. Antigen sequestration and destruction in the schistosome pseudotubercle. *Am. J. Pathol.* **45**: 75-94.

631. Leiss, B. (1963). Fluorescence serologic studies on cell cultures after infection with rinderpest virus, with a contribution to the problem of a group specific seroreaction between measles virus and rinderpest antibody. (German) *Zentr. Bakteriol. Parasitenk., Abt. I. Orig.* **190**: 424-443.

632. Leiss, B., and Plowright, W. (1963). The propagation and growth characteristics of rinderpest virus in HeLa cells. *Arch. Ges. Virusforsch.* **14**: 27-38.

633. Lind, K. (1965). Role of fresh human or guinea-pig serum in the indirect fluorescent antibody test for *Mycoplasma pneumoniae* antibodies in human sera. *Acta Pathol. Microbiol. Scand.* **63**: 639-640.

634. Linz, R., and LeJour, M. (1964). Diagnosis by immunofluorescence of *Escherichia coli* gastroenteritis. (French) *Acta Clin. Belg.* **19**: 237-247.

635. Lipp, W. (1961). Use of gel filtration and polyethylene glycol in the preparation of fluorochrome-labelled proteins. *J. Histochem. Cytochem.* **9**: 458-459.

636. Liu, C. (1955). Studies on influenza infection in ferrets by means of fluorescein-labelled antibody. I. The pathogenesis and diagnosis of the disease. *J. Exptl. Med.* **101**: 665-676.

637. Liu, C. (1955). Studies on influenza infection in ferrets by means of fluorescein-labelled antibody. II. The role of "soluble antigen" in nuclear fluorescence and cross-reactions. *J. Exptl. Med.* **101**: 677-685.

638. Liu, C. (1956). Rapid diagnosis of human influenza infection from nasal smears by means of fluorescein-labelled antibody. *Proc. Soc. Exptl. Biol. Med.* **92**: 883-887.

639. Liu, C. (1957). Studies on primary atypical pneumonia. I. Localization, isolation, and cultivation of a virus in chick embryos. *J. Exptl. Med.* **106**: 455-466.

640. Liu, C. (1961). Diagnosis of influenzal infection by means of

fluorescent antibody staining. *Am. Rev. Respirat. Diseases* **88**: 130-133.

641. Liu, C. (1961). Studies on primary atypical pneumonia. III. A factor in normal serum which enhances the reaction between PAP virus and convalescent serum. *J. Exptl. Med.* **113**: 111-123.

642. Liu, C. (1963). Immunofluorescent technic: Application in the study and diagnosis of infectious diseases. *Clin. Pediat.* (*Philadelphia*) **2**: 490-497.

643. Liu, C. (1964). Fluorescent-antibody techniques. In "Diagnostic Procedures for Viral and Rickettsial Diseases" (E. H. Lennette and N.J. Schmidt, eds.), 3rd ed., pp. 177-193. Public Health Assoc., New York.

644. Liu, C., and Coffin, D. L. (1957). Studies on canine distemper infection by means of fluorescein-labeled antibody. I. The pathogenesis, pathology and diagnosis of the disease in experimentally infected ferrets. *Virology* **3**: 115-131.

645. Liu, C., Eaton, M. D., and Heyl, J. T. (1959). Studies on primary atypical pneumonia. II. Observations concerning the development and immunological characteristics of antibody in patients. *J. Exptl. Med.* **109**: 545-556.

646. Llanes-Rodas, R., and Liu, C. (1965). A study of measles virus infection in tissue culture cells with particular reference to the development of intranuclear inclusion bodies. *J. Immunol.* **95**: 840-845.

647. Llanes-Rodas, R., and Liu, C. (1956). Rapid diagnosis of measles from urinary sediments stained with fluorescent antibody. *New Engl. J. Med.* **275**: 516-523.

648. Loffler, H. (1964). Immunofluorescence of oncogenic viruses. (German) *Bull. Schweiz. Akad. Med. Wiss.* **20**: 48-53.

649. Loh, P. C., and Payne, F. E. (1965). Effect of p-fluorophenylalanine on the synthesis of vaccinia virus. *Virology* **25**: 560-574.

650. Loh, P. C., and Payne, F. E. (1965). Effect of 5-fluoro-2'-deoxyuridine on the synthesis of vaccinia virus. *Virology* **25**: 575-584.

651. Loh, P. C., and Riggs, J. L. (1961). Demonstration of the sequential development of vaccinial antigens and virus in infected cells: Observations with cytochemical and differential fluorescent procedures. *J. Exptl. Med.* **114**: 149-160.

652. Longhi, A., Caleffi, M. L., and Toniutti, M. (1964). Data on the value and significance of the immunofluorescence test (fluorescent treponemal antibody test) in the serological study of syphilis. (Italian) *Arch. Ital. Dermatol., Sifilog. Venereol.* **32**: 256-300.

653. Louis, C. J. (1958). The significance of the cell type in the fluorescein-globulin staining of tissues. *Brit. J. Cancer* **12**: 537-546.

654. Louis, C. J. (1961). Fluorescein-globulin staining of tumor transplants. *Arch. Pathol.* **72**: 593-598.

655. Louis, C. J., and White, J. (1960). Fluorescein-globulin staining of cells in tissue cultures. *Lab. Invest.* **9**: 273-282.

656. Lowry, O. H., Rosebrough, N. J., Farr, A. L., and Randall, R. J. (1951). Protein measurement with the Folin phenol reagent. *J. Biol. Chem.* **193**: 265-275.

657. Lucasse, C. (1962). Fluorescent antibody test for onchocerciasis. *Z. Tropenmed. Parasitol.* **13**: 404-408.

658. Lucasse, C. (1964). Fluorescent antibody test as applied to cerebro-spinal fluid in human sleeping sickness. *Bull. Soc. Pathol. Exotique* **57**: 283-292.

659. Lucasse, C., and Hoeppli, R. (1963). Immunofluorescence in onchocerciasis. *Z. Tropenmed. Parasitol.* **14**: 262-269.

660. Lunzenauer, K., Henze, K., and Seidler, E. (1965). On the problem of type specificity and duration of usability of fluorescein-labeled antibodies of *Shigella flexneri* type 4A (German) *Deut. Gesundheitsw.* **20**: 277-280.

661. Luporini, G., Del Giacco, G. S., and Novi, C. (1964). Latest research on experimental kidney disease due to antigen-antibody complexes. *Boll. Ist. Sieroterap. Milan.* **43**: 253-265.

662. Luscher, E. F., and Kaser-Glanzmann, R. (1961). A new method for the quantitative determination of fibrinolytic activities, based on the use of fluorescent fibrin as a substrate. *Vox Sanguinis* **6**: 116-119.

663. Maassab, H. F., and Loh, P. C. (1962). Fluorescent antibody studies in tissue culture of parainfluenza 3 infection. *Proc. Soc. Exptl. Biol. Med.* **109**: 897-900.

664. Maestrone, G. (1963). Demonstration of leptospiral and viral antigens in formalin-fixed tissues. *Nature* **197**: 409-410.

665. Maestrone, G. (1963). The use of an improved fluorescent antibody procedure in the demonstration of *Leptospira* in animal tissues. *Can. J. Comp. Med. Vet. Sci.* **27**: 108-112.

666. Maestrone, G., and Benjamin, M. A. (1962). Leptospira infection in the gold fish (*Carassium auratus*). *Nature* **195**: 719-720.

667. Maestrone, G., and Coffin, D. L. (1961). Studio della Leptospirosi sperimentale nell'uova embrionato di pollo. *Arch. Vet. Ital.* **12**: 23-36.

668. Maestrone, G., and Coffin, D. L. (1961). Studio della mallattia di Newcastle a mezzo della tecnica degli anticorpi fluorescenti. I. Osservazioni sulla infezione sperimentale dell'uovo embrionato di pollo. *Arch. Vet. Ital.* **12**: 97-106.

669. Maestrone, G., and Coffin, D. L. (1961). Studio della malattia di Newcastle a mezzo della tecnica degli anticorpi fluorescenti. II. Osservazione sulla infezione sperimentale nel pulcino. *Arch. Vet. Ital.* **12**: 193-199.

670. Maestrone, G., and Coffin, D. L. (1964). Study of Newcastle disease by means of fluorescent antibody technique. *Am. J. Vet. Res.* **25**: 217-223.

671. Magureanu, E., Musetescu, M., and Grobnicu, M. (1965). Histo-

logical study of adenovirus type 14 development in cell cultures. *J. Hyg.* **63**: 99-104.

672. Maiztegui, J. L., Biegeleisen, J. Z., Jr., Cherry, W. B., and Kass, E. H. (1965). Bacteremia due to gram-negative rods. *New Engl. J. Med.* **272**: 222-229.

673. Malizia, W. F., Barile, M. F., and Riggs, D. B. (1961). Immuno-fluorescence of pleuropneumonia-like organisms isolated from tissue cell cultures. *Nature* **191**: 190-191.

674. Mallucci, L. (1965). Observations on the growth of mouse hepatitis virus (MHV-3) in mouse macrophages. *Virology* **25**: 30-37.

675. Malmgren, R. A., Fink, M. A., and Mills, W. (1960). Demonstration of the intracellular location of Rous sarcoma virus antigen by fluorescein-labeled antiserums. *J. Natl. Cancer Inst.* **24**: 995-1001.

676. Maloney, E. D., and Kaufman, H. E. (1965). Dissemination of corneal herpes simplex. *Invest. Ophthalmol.* **4**: 872-875.

677. Mancini, R. E., Andrada, J. A., Saraceni, D., Bachmann, A. E., Lavier, J. C., and Nemirovsky, M. (1965). Immunological and testicular response in man sensitized with human testicular homogenate. *J. Clin. Endocrinol.* **25**: 859-875.

678. Mancini, E. E., Davidson, O. W., Vilar, O., Nemirovsky, M., and Bueno, D. C. (1962). Localization of achrosomal antigenicity in guinea pig testes. *Proc. Soc. Exptl. Biol. Med.* **111**: 435-438.

679. Mancini, E. E., Vilar, O., Dellacha, J. M., Davidson, O. W., and Castro, A. A. (1961). Histological localization in rat tissues of intra-venously injected thyrotrophin labelled with a fluorescent dye. *J. Histochem. Cytochem.* **9**: 271-277.

680. Mancini, E. E., Vilar, O., Gomez, C., Dellacha, J. M., Davidson, O. W., and Castro, A. (1961). Histological study of distribution of fluorescent serum proteins in connective tissue. *J. Histochem. Cytochem.* **9**: 356-362.

681. Mandras, A., Vanini, G. C., and Ciarlini, E. (1962). Immuno-fluorescence reaction for the demonstration of antibodies against *Toxoplasma gondii*. (*Italian*) *Igiene Mod.* (*Parma*) **56**: 636-644.

682. Mansberg, H. P., and Kusnetz, J. (1966). Quantitative fluorescence microscopy: fluorescent antibody automatic scanning techniques. *J. Histochem. Cytochem.* **14**: 260-273.

683. Marie, J., Herzog, F., Badillet, M., and Gaiffe, M. (1964). Diagnosis of whooping cough by the immuno-fluorescence technic. (French) *Pediatrie* **19**: 53-59.

684. Marie, J., Herzog, F., and Gaiffe, M. (1963). The rapid diagnosis of whooping cough with the fluorescent antibody technic. (French) *Ann. Pediat., Semaine Hop.* **10**: 53-56.

685. Markowitz, A. S., and Lange, C. F., Jr. (1964). Streptococcal related glomerulo-nephritis. I. Isolation, immunochemistry and comparative chemistry of soluble fractions from type 12 nephrito-genic streptococci and human glomeruli. *J. Immunol.* **92**: 565-575.

686. Marmion, B. P., Perceval, A., and Ennis, G. C. (1965). Respiratory illness and *Mycoplasma pneumoniae* (Eaton agent). *Med. J. Australia* **2**: 233-235.

687. Marrack, J. (1934). Nature of antibodies. *Nature* **133**: 292-293.

688. Marsden, H. B., Hyde, W. A., and Bracegirdle, E. (1965). Immuno-fluorescence in the diagnosis of enteropathogenic *Escherichia coli* infections. *Lancet* **I**: 189-191.

689. Marshall, J. D., Jr., Eveland, W. C., and Smith, C. W. (1958). Superiority of fluorescein isothiocyanate (Riggs) for fluorescent antibody technic with a modification of its application. *Proc. Soc. Exptl. Biol. Med.* **98**: 898-900.

690. Marshall, J. D., Jr., Hansen, P. A., and Eveland, W. C. (1961). Histobacteriology of the genus *Pasteurella*. I. *Pasteurella anatipestifer. Cornell Vet.* **51**: 24-34.

691. Marshall, J. M., Jr. (1951). Localization of adrenocorticotropic hormone by histochemical and immunochemical methods. *J. Exptl. Med.* **94**: 21-30.

692. Marshall, J. M., Jr. (1954). Distribution of chymotrypsinogen, procarboxypeptidase, desoxyribonuclease and ribonuclease in bovine pancreas. *Exptl. Cell Res.* **6**: 240-242.

693. Martin, A. J., and O'Brien, M. (1965). Detection of enteropathogenic *Escherichia coli* in fecal cultures by use of a modified fluorescent-antibody technique. *J. Bacteriol.* **89**: 570-573.

694. Martin, J. E., Jr., Peacock, W. L., Jr., and Thayer, J. D. (1965). Further studies with a selective medium for cultivating *Neisseria gonorrhoeae. Brit. J. Venereal Diseases* **41**: 199-201.

695. Matumoto, M., Saburi, Y., Aoyama, Y., and Mutai, M. (1964). A neurotropic variant of measles virus in suckling mice. *Arch. Ges. Virusforsch.* **14**: 683-696.

696. May, J. W. (1962). Sites of cell-wall extension demonstrated by the use of fluorescent antibody. *Exptl. Cell Res.* **27**: 170-172.

697. Mayersbach, H. (1958). Immunohistological methods. II. Another tagging stain: 1-dimethylaminonaphthalene-5-sulfonic acid. (German) *Acta Histochem.* **5**: 351-368.

698. Mayersbach, H. (1959). Die Anwendung der Gefriertrocknung fur die Immunohistologie. *Acta Histochem.* **8**: 524-534.

699. Mayersbach, H. (1969). Unspecific interactions between serum and tissue sections in the fluorescent-antibody technique for tracing antigens in tissues. *J. Histochem. Cytochem.* **7**: 427.

700. Mayersbach, H., and Pearse, A.G.E. (1965). The metabolism of fluorescein-labelled and unlabelled egg-white in the renal tubules of the mouse. *Brit. J. Exptl. Pathol.* **37**: 81-89.

701. Mayersbach, H., and Schubert, G. (1960). Immunohistological methods. III. The nonspecific reactions between tagged sera and tissues in the immuno-histological technic. (German) *Acta Histochem.* **10**: 44-82.

702. Mayor, H. D. (1961). Cytochemical and fluorescent antibody studies

on the growth of polio virus in tissue culture. *Texas Rept. Biol. Med.* **19**: 106-122.

703. McCluskey, R. T., Vasalli, P., Gallo, G., and Baldwin, D. S. (1966). An immunofluorescent study of pathogenic mechanisms in glomerular diseases. *New Eng. J. Med.* **274**: 695-701.

704. McCormick, J. N. (1962). Use of fluorescein-labelled rheumatoid factor for locating sites of antibody fixation in tissues. *Nature* **193**: 302-303.

705. McCurdy, L. E., and Burstone, M. S. (1966). Water soluble plastic mounting media. *J. Histochem. Cytochem.* **14**: 427-428.

706. McDevitt, H. O., Peters, J. H., Pollard, L. W., Harter, J. G., and Coons, A. H. (1963). Purification and analysis of fluorescein-labeled antisera by column chromatography. *J. Immunol.* **90**: 634-642.

707. McEntegart, M. G., Chadwick, C. S., and Nairn, R. C. (1958). Fluorescent antisera in the detection of serological varieties of *Trichomonas vaginale. Brit. J. Venereal Diseases* **34**: 1-3.

708. McGavran, M. H., and White, J. D. (1964). Electron microscopic and immunofluorescent observations on monkey liver and tissue culture cells infected with the Asibi strain of yellow fever virus. *Am. J. Pathol.* **45**: 501-517.

709. McGavran, M. H., White, J. D., Eigelsbach, H. T., and Kerpsack, R. W. (1962). Morphologic and immunohistochemical studies of the pathogenesis of infection and antibody formation subsequent to vaccination of *Macaca irus* with an attenuated strain of *Pasteurella tularensis.* I. Intracutaneous vaccination. *Am. J. Pathol.* **41**: 259-271.

710. McKay, D. G., Gitlin, D., and Craig, J. M. (1959). Immunochemical demonstration of fibrin in the generalized Schwartzman reaction. *Arch. Pathol.* **67**: 270-273.

711. McKinney, R. M., Spillane, J. T., and Pearce, G. W. (1964). Factors affecting the rate of reaction of fluorescein isothiocyanate with serum proteins. *J. Immunol.* **93**: 232-242.

712. McKinney, R. M., Spillane, J. T., and Pearce, G. W. (1964). Storage stability of fluorescein isothiocyanate. *Anal. Biochem.* **8**: 525-526.

713. McQueen, J. L., Lewis, A. L., and Schneider, N. J. (1960). Rabies diagnosis by fluorescent antibody. I. Its evaluation in a public health laboratory. *Am. J. Public Health* **50**: 1743-1752.

714. Mellick, P. W., Winter, A. J., and McEntee, K. (1965). Diagnosis of vibriosis in the bull by use of the fluorescent antibody technic. *Cornell Vet.* **55**: 280-294.

715. Mellors, R. C. (1965). Autoimmune disease in NZB/BL mice. I. Pathology and pathogenesis of a model system of spontaneous glomerulonephritis. *J. Exptl. Med.* **122**: 25-40.

716. Mellors, R. C., Arias-Stella, J., Siegel, M., and Pressman, D. (1955). Analytical pathology. II. Histopathologic demonstration of

glomerular-localizing antibodies in experimental glomerulonephritis. *Am. J. Path.* **31**: 687-716.

717. Mellors, R. C., Heimer, R., Corcos, J., and Korngold, L. (1959). Cellular origin of rheumatoid factor. *J. Exptl. Med.* **110**: 875-886.

718. Mellors, R. C., and Korngold, L. (1963). The cellular origin of human immunoglobulins (γ_2, γ_{1M}, γ_{1A}). *J. Exptl. Med.* **118**: 387-396.

719. Mellors, R. C., and Munroe, J. S. (1960). Cellular localization of Rous sarcoma virus as studied with fluorescent antibody. *J. Exptl. Med.* **112**: 963-974.

720. Mellors, R. C., Nowoslawski, A., and Korngold, L. (1961). Rheumatoid arthritis and the cellular origin of rheumatoid factors. *Am. J. Pathol.* **39**: 533-546.

721. Mellors, R. C., Nowoslawski, A., Korngold, L., and Sengson, B. L. (1961). Rheumatoid factor and the pathogenesis of rheumatoid arthritis. *J. Exptl. Med.* **113**: 475-484.

722. Mellors, R. C., and Ortega, L. G. (1956). Analytic pathology. III. New observations on the pathogenesis of glomerulonephritis, lipid nephrosis, periarteritis nodosa, and secondary amyloidosis in man. *Am. J. Pathol.* **32**: 455-499.

723. Mellors, R. C., Ortega, L. G., and Holman, H. R. (1957). Role of gamma globulin in pathogenesis of renal lesions in systemic lupus erythematosus and chronic membranous glomerulonephritis, with an observation on the lupus erythematosus cell reaction. *J. Exptl. Med.* **106**: 191-202.

724. Mellors, R. C., Siegel, M., and Pressman, D. (1955). Analytic pathology. I. Histochemical demonstration of antibody localization in tissues, with special reference to the antigenic components of kidney and lung. *Lab. Invest.* **4**: 69-89.

725. Mellors, R. C., and Silver, R. (1951). A microfluorometric scanner for the differential detection of cells: Application to exfoliative cytology. *Science* **114**: 356-360.

726. Melnick, J. L., Stinebaugh, S. E., and Rapp. F. (1964). Incomplete simian papovavirus SV40. Formation of non-infectious viral antigen in the presence of fluorouracil. *J. Exptl. Med.* **119**: 313-326.

727. Merklen, F. P., Cottenot, F., and Galistin, P. (1963). Antibodies demonstrated by immunofluorescence in human leprosy serums. (French). *Compt. Rend. Acad. Sci.* **257**: 2212-2213.

728. Metzger, J. F., Banks, I. S., Smith, C. W., and Hoggan, M. D. (1961). Demonstration of Venezuelan equine encephalomyelitis in tissue culture by immunofluorescence. *Proc. Soc. Exptl. Biol. Med.* **106**: 212-215.

729. Metzger, M., and Ruczkowska, J. (1964). Influence of lysozyme upon the reactivity of *Treponema pallidum* in the fluorescent antibody reaction. *Arch. Immunol. Therap. Exptl.* **12**: 702-708.

730. Metzger, J. F., and Smith, C. W. (1960). Rapid identification of

Neisseria meningitidis by fluorescent antibody technic. *U.S. Armed Forces Med. J.* **11**: 1185-1189.

731. Michael, A. F., Jr., Drummond, K. N., Good, R. A., and Vernier, R. L. (1966). Acute post-streptococcal glomerulonephritis: immune deposit disease. *J. Clin. Invest.* **45**: 237-248.

732. Midgley, A. R., and Pierce, G. B. (1962). Immunohistochemical localization of human chorionic gonadotropin, *J. Exptl. Med.* **115**: 289-294.

733. Miller, J. N., Boak, R. A., Carpenter, C. M., and Fazzan, F. (1963). Immuno-fluorescent methods in the diagnosis of infectious diseases. *Am. J. Med. Technol.* **29**: 25-32.

734. Mims, C. A. (1964). Aspects of the pathogenesis of virus diseases. *Bacteriol. Rev.* **28**: 30-71.

735. Minowada, J. (1964). Deoxyribonucleic acid and protein syntheses in polyoma virus-infected mouse kidney cells in culture as studied by autoradiography and immunofluorescence. *Gann* **55**: 267-276.

736. Mirachamsy, H., and Taslimi, H. (1964). Visualization of horse sickness virus by the fluorescent antibody technique. *Immunology* **7**: 213-216.

737. Mitchell, J. R. (1964). Detection of *Toxacara canis* antibodies with fluorescent antibody technique. *Proc. Soc. Exptl. Biol. Med.* **117**: 267-270.

738. Mitchell, M. S., and Biegeleisen, J. Z., Jr. (1965). The effect of penicillin on immunofluorescent staining of *Diplococcus pneumoniae, Neisseria meningitidis,* and *Hemophilus influenzae* in cerebrospinal fluid *in vitro. J. Lab. Clin. Med.* **66**: 53-63.

739. Mitchell, M. S., Marcus, B. B., and Biegeleisen, J. Z., Jr. (1965). Immunofluorescence techniques for demonstrating bacterial pathogens associated with cerebrospinal meningitis. II. Growth, visibility, and immunofluorescent staining of *Hemophilus influenzae, Neisseria meningitidis,* and *Diplococcus pneumoniae* in cerebrospinal fluid. *J. Lab. Clin. Med.* **65**: 990-1003.

740. Mitchell, M. S., Rhoden, D. L., and King, E. O. (1965). Lactose-fermenting organisms resembling *Neisseria meningitidis. J. Bacteriol.* **90**: 560.

741. Miura, T., and Kasai, T. (1964). Autofluorescence of pathogenic fungi. *Tohoku J. Exptl. Med.* **82**: 158-163.

742. Miura, T., and Kasai, T. (1964). Difference in result of the fluorescent antibody staining of dermatophytes due to the difference of fixing procedure. *Tohoku J. Exptl. Med.* **84**: 72-80.

743. Miyamoto, T., Hinuma, Y., and Ishida, N. (1965). Intracellular transfer of hemadsorption type 2 virus antigen during persistent infection of HeLa cell cultures. *Virology* **27**: 28-36.

744. Moggi, P., Pratesi, V., and Mori, S. (1963). Some immunological problems in infants. II. Demonstration, by means of fluorescent antitoxin, of specific antibodies in sensitized lymphocytes. (Italian) *Riv. Clin. Pediat.* **72**: 203-208.

745. Möller, G. (1961). Demonstration of mouse isoantigens at the cellular level by the fluorescent antibody technique. *J. Exptl. Med.* **114**: 415-434.

746. Moody, M. D., Ellis, E. C., and Updyke, E. L. (1958). Staining bacterial smears with fluorescent antibody. IV. Grouping streptococci with fluorescent antibody. *J. Bacteriol.* **75**: 553-560.

747. Moody, M. D., Goldman, M., and Thomason, B. M. (1956). Staining bacterial smears with fluorescent antibody. I. General methods for *Malleomyces pseudomallei*. *J. Bacteriol.* **72**: 357-361.

748. Moody, M. D., and Jones, W. L. (1963). Identification of *Corynebacterium diphtheriae* with fluorescent antibacterial reagents. *J. Bacteriol.* **86**: 285-293.

749. Moody, M. D., Siegel, A. C., Pittman, B., and Winter, C. C. (1963). Fluorescent-antibody identification of group A streptococci from throat swabs. *Am. J. Public Health* **53**: 1083-1092.

750. Moody, M. D., and Winter, C. C. (1959). Rapid identification of *Pasteurella pestis* with fluorescent antibody. III. Staining *Pasteurella pestis* in tissue impression smears. *J. Infect. Diseases* **104**: 288-294.

751. Moon, H. D., and McIvor, B. C. (1960). Elastase in the exocrine pancreas; localization with fluorescent antibody. *J. Immunol.* **85**: 78-80.

752. Moore, M. B., Jr., VanderStoep, E. M., Wende, R. D., and Knox, J. M. (1963). Fluorescent gonococcal antibody technique in gonorrhea in the male. *Public Health Rept.* **78**: 90-92.

753. Mordhorst, C. H. (1965). Trachoma agents isolated in the United States. IX. Complement-fixing and immunofluorescent antibodies in parenterally injected monkeys. *Am. J. Ophthalmol.* **59**: 769-773.

754. Mori, S., Moggi, P., and Pratesi, V. (1963). Some immunological problems in infants. III. Different antibody responses in sensitized lymphocytes of newborn infants and children demonstrated by means of fluorescence (Italian). *Riv. Clin. Pediat.* **72**: 209-213.

755. Morris, R. H., Vassali, P., Beller, F. K., and McLusky, R. T. (1964). Immunofluorescent studies of renal biopsies in the diagnosis of toxemia of pregnancy. *Obstet. Gynecol.* **24**: 32-46.

756. Moulton, J. E. (1956). Fluorescent antibody studies of demyelination in canine distemper. *Proc. Soc. Exptl. Biol. Med.* **91**: 460-464.

757. Moulton, J. E., and Brown, C. H. (1954). Antigenicity of canine distemper inclusion bodies as demonstrated by fluorescent antibody technic. *Proc. Soc. Exptl. Biol. Med.* **86**: 99-102.

758. Moulton, J. E., and Frazier, L. M. (1965). Early nuclear changes in cells infected with canine hepatitis virus. *Am. J. Vet. Res.* **26**: 723-726.

759. Moulton, J. E., and Howarth, J. A. (1957). The demonstration of *Leptospira canicola* in hamster kidneys by means of fluorescent antibody. *Cornell Vet.* **47**: 524-532.

760. Mufson, M. A., Ludwig, W. M., Purcell, R. H., Cate, T. R., Taylor-

Robinson, D., and Chanock, R. M. (1965). Exudative pharyngitis following experimental *Mycoplasma hominis:* Type 1 infection. *J. Am. Med. Assoc.* **192**: 1146-1152.

761. Mukherjea, A. K., Ray, H. N., and Sen, A. K. (1962). Use of rhodamine-tagged antibody for staining *Entamoeba histolytica* from culture. *Bull. Calcutta School Trop. Med.* **10**: 107-108.

762. Muller, F., and Klein, P. (1959). Fluoreszenz-serologische Darstellung der Komplement bindung an Virus-Antikorper Komplexe in der Gewebekultur. *Deut. Med. Wochschr.* **84**: 2195-2198.

763. Muller-Ruchholtz, W., Kraus, E., and Federlin, K. (1965). Studies on "transmission" of Masugi nephritis in rats. VII. Further fluorescence microscopic studies on parabionts and nephritic single animals (German). *Z. Immunol. Allergieforsch.* **128**: 137-160.

764. Munyon, W., Hughes, R., Angermann, J., Bereczky, E., and Dmochowski, L. (1964). Studies on the effect of 5-iododeoxyuridine and p-fluorophenylalanine on polyoma virus formation *in vitro. Cancer Res.* **24**: 1880-1886.

765. Murray, E. S. (1964). Guinea pig inclusion conjunctivitis virus. I. Isolation and identification as a member of the psittacosis-lymphogranuloma-trachoma group. *J. Infect. Diseases* **114**: 1-12.

766. Murray, H. G. (1963). The diagnosis of smallpox by immunofluorescence. Lancet **I**: 847-848.

767. Mussgay, M. (1963). Structure and mode of multiplication of animal virus types. 5. Experimental part: Studies on the multiplication of the Venezuelan equine encephalitis virus, of the vesticular stomatitis virus and the foot-and-mouth disease virus. (German). *Arch. Hyg. Bakteriol.* **147**: 616-644.

768. Myerburg, R. J., Jablon, J. M., Mazzerella, J. A., and Saslaw, M. S. (1964). Evaluation of FA and conventional techniques for identifying group A beta hemolytic streptococci. *Public Health Rept.* **79**: 510-514.

769. Myhre, B. A. (1965). Blood group differentiation using fluorescent antibodies. *Proc. Soc. Exptl. Biol. Med.* **120**: 712-714.

770. Nadel, M. K., and Orsi, E. V. (1964). Immunofluorescence of noncytopathic tissue culture adapted fixed rabies. *Am. J. Med. Technol.* **30**: 173-176.

711. Nagaraj. A. N. (1962). Fluorescent antibody staining of viral antigen in dissociated plant cells. *Virology* **18**: 329-331.

772. Nagaraj. A. N. (1965). Immunofluorescence studies on synthesis and distribution of tobacco mosaic virus antigen in tobacco. *Virology* **25**: 133-142.

773. Nagaraj. A. N., and Black, L. M. (1961). Localization of wound-tumor virus antigen in plant tumors by the use of fluorescent antibodies. *Virology* **15**: 289-294.

774. Nagaraj. A. N., Sinha, R. C., and Black, L. M. (1961). A smear technique for detecting virus antigen in individual vectors by the use of fluorescent antibodes. *Virology* **15**: 205-208.

775. Nairn, R. C. (1962). Direct protein-tracing in experimental physiology and pathology. *In "Fluorescent Protein Tracing"* (R. C. Nairn, ed.), pp. 83-96. Williams & Wilkins, Baltimore, Maryland.

776. Nairn, R. C., Chadwick, C. S., and McEntegart, M. G. (1958). Fluorescent protein tracers in the study of experimental liver damage. *J. Pathol. Bacteriol.* **76**: 143-153.

777. Nairn, R. C., Fraser, K. B., and Chadwick, C. S. (1959). The histological localization of renin with fluorescent antibody. *Brit. J. Exptl. Pathol.* **40**: 155-163.

778. Nairn, R. C., Ghose, T., Fothergill, J. E., and McEntegart, M. G., (1962). Kidney specific antigen and its species distribution. *Nature* **196**: 385-387.

779. Nairn, R. C., Richmond, H. G., and Fothergill, J. E. (1960). Differences in staining of normal and malignant cells by non-immune fluorescent protein conjugates. *Brit. Med. J.* **II**: 1341-1343.

780. Nairn, R. C., Richmond, H. G., McEntegart, M. G., and Fothergill, J. E. (1960). Immunological differences between normal and malignant cells. *Brit. Med. J.* **II**: 1335-1340.

781. Naumann, G. (1964). Fluorescence serological investigations for the demonstration of treponema-specific antibodies. (German) *Z. Ges. Hyg.* **10**: 518-523.

782. Navarette-Reyna, A., Rosenstein, D. L., and Sonnenwirth, A. C. (1965). Bacterial aortic aneurysm due to *Listeria monocytogenes*: first report of an aneurysm caused by *Listeria. Am. J. Clin. Pathol.* **43**: 438-444.

783. Nayak, D. P., Kelley, G. W., Young, G. A., and Underdahl, D. R. (1964). Progressive descending influenza infection in mice determined by immunofluorescence. *Proc. Soc. Exptl. Biol. Med.* **116**: 200-206.

784. Neil, A. L., and Dixon, F. J. (1959). Immunohistochemical detection of antibody in cell-transfer studies. *Arch. Pathol.* **67**: 643-649.

785. Nelson, J. D., Hempstead, B., Tanaka, R., and Pauls, F. P. (1964). Fluorescent antibody diagnosis of infections. *J. Am. Med. Assoc.* **188**: 1121-1124.

786. Nelson, J. D., and Shelton, S. (1963). Immunofluorescent studies of *Listeria monocytogenes* and *Erysipelothrix insidiosa*. Application to clinical diagnosis. *J. Lab. Clin. Med.* **62**: 935-942.

787. Nelson, J. D., and Whitaker, J. A. (1960). Diagnosis of enteropathogenic *E. coli* diarrhea by fluorescein-labeled antibodies. *J. Pediat.* **57**: 684-688.

788. Neurath, A. R. (1965). Fluorometric estimation of antigens (antibodies). *Z. Naturforsch.* **20b**: 974-976.

789. Neurath, A. R., Rubin, B. A., and Vernon, S. K. (1966). Quantitative determination of adenovirus antigens by means of a fluorescent precipitin test. *Experientia* **22**: 653-657.

790. Newton, B. A. (1955). A fluorescent derivative of polymixin: Its

preparation and use in studying the site of action of the antibiotic. *J. Gen. Microbiol.* **12**: 226-236.

791. Nichol, J. C., and Deutsch, H. F. (1948). Biophysical studies of blood plasma proteins. VII. Separation of gamma-globulin from sera of various animals. *J. Am. Chem. Soc.* **70**: 80-83.

792. Nichols, R. L. and McComb, D. E. (1962). Immunofluorescent studies with trachoma and related antigens. *J. Immunol.* **89**: 545-554.

793. Nichols, R. L. and McComb, D. E. (1964). Serologic strain differentiation in trachoma. *J. Exptl. Med.* **120**: 639-654.

794. Nichols, R. L., McComb, D. E., Haddad, N., and Murray, E. S. (1963). Studies on trachoma. II. Comparison of fluorescent antibody, Giemsa and egg isolation methods for detection of trachoma virus in human conjunctival scrapings. *Am. J. Trop. Med. Hyg.* **12**: 223-229.

795. Niel, G., and Fribourg-Blanc, A. (1962). Technique actuelle du test d'immunofluorescence appliqué au diagnostic de la syphilis. *Ann. Inst. Pasteur* **102**: 616-628.

796. Niel, G., and Fribourg-Blanc, A. (1963). Immuno-fluorescence et serologie de la syphilis. *Bull. World Health Organ.* **29**: 429-442.

797. Nielsen, H. A., and Idsoe, O. (1963). Evaluation of the fluorescent treponemal antibody test (FTA). *Acta Pathol. Microbiol. Scand.* **57**: 331-347.

798. Nii, S., and Kamahora, J. (1963). Location of herpetic viral antigen in interphase cells. *Biken's J.* **6**: 145-154.

799. Nii, S., and Kamahora, J., (1964). Detection of measles viral antigen in the lymph nodes of cynomolgus monkeys infected with measles. *Biken's J.* **7**: 71-73.

800. Nir, Y., Beemer, A., and Goldwasser, R. A. (1965). West Nile virus infection in mice following exposure to a viral aerosol. *Brit. J. Exptl. Pathol* **46**: 443-449.

801. Nordén, G. (1953). The rate of appearance, metabolism and disappearance of 3,4-benzpyrene in the epithelium of mouse skin after a single application in a volatile solvent. *Acta Pathol. Microbiol. Scand.* Suppl. 96.

802. Nowoslawski, A., and Brzosko, W. J. (1964). Indirect immunofluorescent test for serodiagnosis of *Pneumocystis carinii* infection. *Bull. Acad. Polon. Sci.* **12**: 143-147.

803. Noyes, W. F., (1955). Visualization of Egypt 101 virus in the mouse's brain and in cultured human carcinoma cells by means of fluorescent antibody. *J. Exptl. Med.* **102**: 243-247.

804. Noyes, W. F. (1959). Studies on the Shope rabbit papilloma virus. II. The location of infective virus in papillomas of the cottontail rabbit. *J. Exptl. Med.* **109**: 423-428.

805. Noyes, W. F., and Mellors, R. C. (1957). Fluorescent antibody detection of the antigens of the Shope papilloma virus in papillomas of the wild and domestic rabbit. *J. Exptl. Med.* **106**: 555-562.

806. Noyes, N. F., and Watson, B. K. (1955). Studies on the increase of vaccine virus in cultured human cells by means of the fluorescent antibody technique. *J. Exptl. Med.* **102**: 237-241.

807. Nuzzolo, L., Ravetta, M., and Vellucci, A. (1963). Immunological relations between some types of adenovirus studied with the immunofluorescence method (Italian). *Nuovi Ann. Igiene Microbiol.* **14**: 44-55.

808. O'Berry, P. A. (1964). A comparison of 3 methods of serum fractionation in the preparation of *Vibrio fetus* fluorescent antibody conjugates. *Am. J. Vet. Res.* **25**: 1669-1672.

809. Ocklitz, H. W., and Weppe, C. M. (1964). The bacteriological diagnosis of pertussis, fluorescence serology and cultivation in comparison. 2. Antibody fluorescent staining of *Bordetella pertussis*. (German) *Zentr. Bakteriol. Parasitenk., Abt. I. Orig.* **194**: 103-114.

810. O'Connor, G. T., Rabson, A. S., Malmgren, R. A., Berezesky, I. K., and Paul, F. J. (1965). Morphologic observations of green monkey kidney cells after single and double infection with adenovirus 12 and simian virus 40. *J. Natl. Cancer Inst.* **34**: 679-693.

811. Oddo, F. G., and Cascio, G. (1963). The immuno-fluorescence test in visceral and cutaneous leishmaniasis. (Italian) *Riv. Ist. Sieroterap. Ital.* **38**: 139-145.

812. O'Dea, J. F., and Dineen, J. K. (1957). Fluorescent antibody studies with herpes simplex virus in unfixed preparations of trypsinized tissue cultures. *J. Gen. Microbiol.* **17**: 19-24.

813. Ogawa, H., Takahashi, R., Honjo, S., Takaska, M., Fujiwara, T., Ando, K., Nakagawa, M., Muto, T., and Imaizumi, K. (1964). Shigellosis in cynomolgus monkeys (*Macaca irus*). III. Histopathological studies on natural and experimental shigellosis. *Japan. J. Med. Sci. Biol.* **17**: 321-332.

814. Ohta, G., Cohen, S., Singer, E. J., Rosenfield, R., and Strauss, L. (1959). Demonstration of gamma globulin in vascular lesions of experimental necrotizing arteritis in the rat. *Proc. Soc. Exptl. Biol. Med.* **102**: 187-189.

815. Okuda, R., Kaplan, M. H., Cuppage, F. E., and Heymann, W. (1965). Deposition of autologous gamma globulin in kidneys of rats with nephrotic renal disease of various etiologies. *J. Lab. Clin. Med.* **66**: 204-215.

816. Olson, R. A. (1960). Rapid scanning microspectrofluorimeter. *Rev. Sci. Instr.* **31**: 844-849.

817. Onodera, T., Hinuma, Y., and Ishida, N. (1964). Ineffectiveness of antibody on the intracellular development of influenza virus WS strain in Ehrlich ascites cells in mice. *J. Immunol.* **92**: 648-656.

818. Opferkuch, W., and Huth, E. (1963). Diagnosis of strains of enteropathogenic colibacilli by fluorescent antibodies. (French). *Pediatrie* **18**: 703-707.

819. Ornstein, L., Mantner, W., Baruch, J. D., and Tamura, R. (1957). New horizons in fluorescence microscopy. *J. Mt. Sinai Hosp., N.Y.* **24**: 1066-1078.
820. Ortega, L. G., and Mellors, R. C. (1956). Analytical pathology. IV. The role of localized antibodies in the pathogenesis of nephrotoxic nephritis in the rat. *J. Exptl. Med.* **104**: 151-170.
821. Osato, T., Mirand, E. A., and Grace, J. T., Jr. (1964). Propagation and immunofluorescent investigations of Friend virus in tissue culture. *Nature* **201**: 52-54.
822. Osato, T,. Mirand, E. A., and Grace, J. T., Jr. (1965). Hemadsorption and immunofluorescence of Friend virus in cell culture. *Proc. Soc. Exptl. Biol. Med.* **119**: 1187-1191.
823. Ovcinnikov, N. M. (1963). An appraisal of the fluorescent antibody method in gonorrhoea. *Bull. World Health Organ.* **29**: 781-788.
824. Page, R. H., Caldroney, G. L., and Stulberg, C. S. (1961). Immunofluorescence in diagnostic bacteriology. I. Direct identification of *Hemophilus influenzae* in smears of cerebrospinal fluid sediments. *Am. J. Diseases Children* **101**: 155-159.
825. Palacios, O. (1965). Cytochemical and fluorescent antibody studies on the growth of measles virus in tissue culture. *Arch. Ges. Virusforsch.* **16**: 83-88.
826. Pappenhagen, A. R., Koppel, J. L., and Olwin, J. H. (1962). Use of fluorescein-labeled fibrin for the determination of fibrinolytic activity. *J. Lab. Clin. Med.* **59**: 1039-1046.
827. Paronetto, F. (1963). The fluorescent antibody technique applied to titration and identification of antigens in solutions or antisera. *Proc. Soc. Exptl. Biol. Med.* **113**: 354-397.
828. Paronetto, F. (1965). Immunocytochemical observations on the vascular necrosis and renal glomerular lesions of malignant nephrosclerosis. *Am. J. Pathol.* **6**: 901-915.
829. Paronetto, F., Horowitz, R. E., Sicular, A., Burrows, L., Kark, A. E., and Popper, H. (1965). Immunologic observations on homografts. I. The canine liver. *Transplantation* **3**: 303-317.
830. Paronetto, F., Schaffner, F., and Popper, H. (1961). Immunocytochemical reaction of serum of patients with hepatic diseases with hepatic structures. *Proc. Soc. Exptl. Biol. Med.* **106**: 216-219.
831. Paronetto, F., Schaffner, F., and Popper, H. (1964). Immunocytochemical and serologic observations in primary biliary cirrhosis. *New Engl. J. Med.* **271**: 1123-1128.
832. Paronetto, F., and Strauss, L. (1962). Immunocytochemical observations in periarteritis nodosa. *Ann. Internal Med.* [N.S.] **56**: 289-295.
833. Pasternak, G. (1965). Serologic studies on cells of Graffi virus-induced myeloid leukemia in mice. *J. Natl. Cancer Inst.* **34**: 71-84.
834. Paton, A. M. (1964). The adaptation of the immunofluorescence technique for use in bacteriological investigations of plant tissue. *J. Appl. Bacteriol.* **27**: 237-243.

835. Patten, S. F., Jr., and Brown, K. A. (1958). Freeze-solvent substitution technic. A review with an application to fluorescence microscopy. *Lab. Invest.* **7**: 209-223.

836. Patterson, R., and Suszko, I. M. (1963). *In vitro* production of antibody by chicken spleen cells. II. Immunofluorescent studies of tissue culture preparations. *J. Immunol.* **90**: 836-842.

837. Patterson, R., Suszko, I. M., and Pruzansky, J. J. (1962). *In vitro* uptake of antigen-antibody complexes by phagocytic cells. *J. Immunol.* **89**: 471-482.

838. Peacock, W. L., and Thayer, J. D. (1964). Direct FA technique using flazo orange counterstain in identification of *Neisseria gonorrhoeae*. *Public Health Rept.* **79**: 1119-1122.

839. Pellegrino, J., and Biocca, E. (1960). Serological diagnosis of schistosomiasis mansoni. II. The immunofluorescence reaction with cercaria of *Schistosoma bovis* and *Cercaria caratinguensis*. (Portuguese) *Rev. Inst. Med. Trop. Sao Paulo* **5**: 257-260.

840. Pepe, F. A. (1961). The use of specific antibody in electron microscopy. I. Preparation of mercury-labeled antibody. *J. Biophys. Biochem. Cytol.* **11**: 515-520.

841. Pepe, F. A., and Finck, H. (1961). The use of specific antibody in electron microscopy. II. The visualization of mercury-labeled antibody in the electron microscope. *J. Biophys. Biochem. Cytol.* **11**: 521-531.

842. Petran, E. I. (1964). Comparison of the fluorescent antibody and the bacitracin disk methods for the identification of group A streptococci. *Tech. Bull. Registry Med. Technologists* **34**: 8-10.

843. Pettit, T. H., Kimura, S. J., and Peters, H. (1964). The fluorescent antibody technique in diagnosis of herpes simplex keratitis. *Arch. Ophthalmol.* **72**: 86-98.

844. Pettit, T. H., Kimura, S. J., Uchida, Y., and Peters, H. (1965). Herpes simplex uveitis: An experimental study with fluorescein-labeled antibody technique. *Invest. Ophthalmol.* **4**: 349-357.

845. Petty, C. S. (1965). Botulism: The disease and the toxin. *Am. J. Med. Sci.* **249**: 345-359.

846. Philipson, L. (1961). Adenovirus assay by the fluorescent cell-counting procedure. *Virology* **15**: 263-268.

847. Pier, A. C., Richard, J. L., and Farrell, E. F. (1964). Fluorescent antibody and cultural techniques in cutaneous streptothricosis. *Am. J. Vet. Res.* **25**: 1014-1020.

848. Pillot, J., and D'Azambuja, S. (1963). Indirect immunfluorescence and the complement fixation reaction realized with *Leptospira icterohaemorrhagiae*. (French) *Ann. Inst. Pasteur* **104**: 137-141.

849. Pine, L., Kaufman, L., and Boone, C. J. (1964). Comparative fluorescent antibody staining of *Histoplasma capsulatum* and *Histoplasma duboisii* with a specific anti-yeast phase *H. capsulatum* conjugate. *Mycopatholo. Mycol. Appl.* **24**: 315-326.

850. Piomelli, S., Stefanini, M., and Mele, H. (1959). Antigenicity of

human vascular endothelium: Lack of relationship to the pathogenesis of vasculitis. *J. Lab. Clin. Med.* **54**: 241-256.

851. Pital, A., and Janowitz, S. L. (1963). Enhancement of staining intensity in the fluorescent antibody reaction. *J. Bacteriol.* **86**: 888-889.

852. Pittman, B., Hebert, G. A., Cherry, W. B., and Taylor, G. C. (1967). The quantitation of non-specific staining as a guide for improvement of fluorescent antibody conjugates. *J. Immunol.* **98**: 1196-1203.

853. Pittman, F. E., and Holub, D. A. (1965). Sjogren's syndrome and adult celiac disease. *Gastroenterology* **48**: 869-876.

854. Poetschke, G., and Killisch, L. (1959). Untersuchungen mit fluoreszenz-markierten Antikorpern. VI. Fluoreszenz-serologische Untersuchungen an Spirochaten (*T. pallidum*, Reiter-Spirochaten) *Bor. recurrens* und Schleimhautspirochaten. *Schweiz. Z. Allgem. Pathol. Bakteriol.* **22**: 765-770.

855. Poetschke, G., Ueleke, H., and Killisch, L. (1957). Untersuchungen mit fluorescein-markierten Antikorpen. I. Allgemeines und Methodisches. *Z. Immunitaetsforsch.* **114**: 393-405.

856. Poetschke, G., Ueleke, H., and Killisch, L. (1957). Untersuchungen mit fluorescein-markierten Antikorpen. II. Das serologische Verhalten der L-phase von *Proteus*. *Z. Immunitaetsforsch.* **114**: 406-415.

857. Pollister, A. W. (1952). Photomultiplier apparatus for microspectrophotometry of cells. *Lab. Invest.* **1**: 106-114.

858. Pollister, A. W., and Ornstein, L. (1959). The photometric chemical analysis of cells. *In* "Analytical Cytology" (R. C. Mellors, ed.), 2nd ed., pp. 431-518.

859. Pope, J. H., and Rowe, W. P. (1964). Detection of specific antigen in SV40-transformed cells by immunofluorescence. *J. Exptl. Med.* **120**: 121-128.

860. Pope, J. H., and Rowe, W. P. (1964). Immunofluorescent studies of adenovirus 12 tumors and of cells transformed or infected by adenoviruses. *J. Exptl. Med.* **120**: 577-588.

861. Porath, J., and Flodin, P. (1959). Gel filtration: A method for desalting and group separation. *Nature* **183**: 1657-1659.

862. Porter, B. M., Comfort, B. K., Menges, R. W., Habermann, T. R., and Smith, C. D. (1965). Correlation of fluorescent antibody, histopathology, and culture on tissues from 372 animals examined for histoplasmosis and blastomycosis. *J. Bacteriol.* **89**: 748-751.

863. Porter, D. D., Dixon, F. J., and Larsen, A. E. (1965). Metabolism and function of gamma globulin in Aleutian disease of mink. *J. Exptl. Med.* **121**: 889-900.

864. Pressman, D., Yagi, Y., and Hiramoto, R. (1958). A comparison of fluorescein and I[131] as labels for determining the *in vivo* localization of anti-tissue antibodies. *Intern. Arch. Allergy Appl. Immunol.* **12**: 125-136.

865. Preston, J. A. (1964). The rapid identification of group A streptococci in throat swabs. A comparative study of two methods. *Mich. Med.* **63**: 704-706.

866. Price, G. R., and Schwartz, S. (1956). Fluorescence microscopy. *In* "Physical Techniques in Biological Research" (G. Oster and A. W. Pollister, eds.), Vol. 3, pp. 91-148. Academic Press, New York.

867. Price, G. R., and Christenson, L. (1957). Combined phase and fluorescence microscopy. *Mikroskopie* **12**: 147-151.

868. Prince, A. M., Fuji, H., and Gershon, R. K. (1964). Immunohistochemical studies on the etiology of anicteric hepatitis in Korea. *Am. J. Hyg.* **79**: 365-381.

869. Prince, A. M., and Ginsberg, H. S. (1967). Immunohistochemical studies on the interaction between Ehrlich ascites tumor cells and Newcastle disease virus. *J. Exptl. Med.* **105**: 177-191.

870. Procknow, J. J., Connelly, A. P., and Ray, C. G. (1962). Fluorescent antibody technique in histoplasmosis. *Arch. Pathol.* **73**: 313-324.

871. Puhvel, S. M., Barafatani, M., Warnick, M., and Sternberg, T. H. (1964). Study of antibody levels to *Corynebacterium acnes*. *Arch. Dermatol.* **90**: 421-427.

872. Quan, S. F., Knapp, W., Goldenberg, M. I., Hudson, B. W., Lawton, W. D., Chen, T. H., and Kartman, L. (1965). Isolation of a strain of *Pasteurella pseudotuberculosis* from Alaska identified as *Pasteurella pestis:* An immunofluorescent false positive. *Am. J. Trop. Med. Hyg.* **14**: 424-432.

873. Rabin, E. R., Hassan, S. A., Jenson, A. B., and Melnick, J. L. (1964). Coxsackie virus B_3 myocarditis in mice. An electron microscopic, immunofluorescent and virus-assay study. *Am. J. Pathol.* **44**: 775-797.

874. Radke, M. G., and Sadun, E. H. (1963). Resistance produced in mice by exposure to irradiated *Schistosoma mansoni* cercariae. *Exptl. Parasitol.* **13**: 134-142.

875. Rado, J. P., Tako, J., Geder, L., and Jeney, E. (1965). Herpes zoster house epidemic in steroid-treated patients. A clinical and viral study. *Arch. Internal Med.* **116**: 329-335.

876. Rahman, A. N., and Luttrell, C. N. (1962). Albumin embedding method for frozen sectioning of fresh tissues for fluorescent antibody and histochemical studies. *Bull. Johns Hopkins Hosp.* **110**: 66-72.

877. Rapp, F., Butel, J. S., Feldman, L. A., Kitahara, T., and Melnick, J. L. (1965). Differential effects of inhibitors on the steps leading to the formation of SV40 tumor and virus antigens. *J. Exptl. Med.* **121**: 935-944.

878. Rapp, F., Butel, J. S., and Melnick, J. L. (1964). Virus-induced intra-nuclear antigen in cells transformed by papovavirus SV40. *Proc. Soc. Exptl. Biol. Med.* **116**: 1131-1135.

879. Rapp, F., and Friend, C. (1963). Early detection and localization

of Swiss mouse leukemia virus. *Acta Unio Intern. Contra Cancrum* **19**: 348-350.

880. Rapp, F., Gordon, I., and Baker, R. F. (1960). Observations of measles virus infection of cultured human cells. I. A study of development and spread of virus antigen by means of immuno-fluorescence. *J. Biophys. Biochem. Cytol.* **7**: 43-48.

881. Rapp, F., Melnick, J. L., Butel, J. S., and Kitahara, T. (1964). The incorporation of SV40 material into adenovirus 7 as measured by intranuclear synthesis of SV40 tumor antigen. *Proc. Natl. Acad. Sci. U.S.* **52**: 1348-1352.

882. Rapp, F., Melnick, J. L., Kitahara, T., and Sheppard, R. (1965). Search for virus-induced antigens in human tumors using the SV40-hamster system as a model. *Proc. Soc. Exptl. Biol. Med.* **118**: 573-576.

883. Rapp, F., Rasmussen, L. E., and Benyesh-Melnich, M. (1963). The immunofluorescent focus technique in studying the replication of cytomegalovirus. *J. Immunol.* **91**: 709-719.

884. Rapp, F., Seligman, S. J., Jarosse, L. B., and Gordon, I. (1959). Quantitative determination of infectious units of measles virus by counts of immunofluorescent foci. *Proc. Soc. Exptl. Biol. Med.* **101**: 289-294.

885. Rapp, F., and Vanderslice, D. (1964). Spread of zoster virus in human embryonic lung cells and the inhibitory effect of iododeoxy-uridine. *Virology* **22**: 321-330.

886. Rappaport, B. Z. (1960). Antigen-antibody reactions in allergic human tissues. I. Preparation and use of fluorescein conjugated reagins for staining the reaction sites. *J. Exptl. Med.* **112**: 55-64.

887. Rappaport, B. Z. (1960). Antigen-antibody reactions in allergic human tissues. II. Study by fluorescence technique of the localization of reagins in human skin and their relation to globulins. *J. Exptl. Med.* **112**: 725-734.

888. Rappaport, B. Z. (1964). Antigen-antibody reactions in allergic human tissues. III. Immunofluorescent study of allergic nasal mucosa. *J. Immunol.* **93**: 792-797.

889. Raskin, J. (1961). Antigen-antibody reaction site in contact dermatitis. *Arch. Dermatol.* **86**: 459-465.

890. Raskin, J. (1963). Molluscum contagiosum. Tissue culture and serologic study. *Arch. Dermatol.* **87**: 552-559.

891. Rauch, H. C., and Raffel, S. (1964). Immunofluorescent localization of encephalitogenic protein in myelin. *J. Immunol.* **92**: 452-455.

892. Rauch, H. C., and Rontz, L. A. (1963). Immunofluorescent identification of group A streptococci in direct throat smears. *J. Lab. Clin. Med.* **61**: 529-536.

893. Rawson, A. J., Abelson, N. M., and Hollander, J. L. (1965). Studies on the pathogenesis of rheumatoid joint inflammation. II. Intra-cytoplasmic particulate complexes in rheumatoid synovial fluids. *Ann. Internal Med.* [N.S.] **62**: 281-284.

894. Reda, I. M., Rott, F., and Schafer, W. (1964). Fluorescent antibody studies with NDV-infected cell systems. *Virology* **22**: 422-425.
895. Redetzki, H. M. (1958). Labelling of antibodies by 5-dimethyl-amino-1-napthalene sulfonyl chloride, its effect on antigen-antibody reaction. *Proc. Soc. Exptl. Biol. Med.* **98**: 120-122.
896. Redmond, D. L., and Kotcher, E. (1963). Comparison of cultural and immunofluorescent procedures in the identification of *Haemophilus vaginalis. J. Gen. Microbiol.* **33**: 89-94.
897. Redmond, D. L., and Kotcher, E. (1963). Cultural and serological studies on *Haemophilus vaginalis. J. Gen. Microbiol.* **33**: 77-87.
898. Redys, J. J., Parzick, A. B., and Borman, E. K. (1963). Detection of group A streptococci in throat cultures by immunofluorescence. *Public Health Rept.* **78**: 222-226.
899. Redys, J. J., Ross, M. R., and Borman, E. K. (1960). Inhibition of common-antigen fluorescence in grouping streptococci by the fluorescent antibody method. *J. Bacteriol* **80**: 823-829.
900. Reimers, E. (1965). On fluorescence microscopic demonstrable antigen of enteropathogenic *Escherichia coli.* (German) *Z. Kinderheilk.* **93**: 85-90.
901. Rhim, J. S., Jordan, L. E., and Mayor, H. D. (1962). Cytochemical, fluorescent-antibody, and electron microscopic studies on the growth of Reovirus (ECHO 12) in tissue culture. *Virology* **17**: 342-355.
902. Richardson, M., and Holt, J. N. (1964). Multiplication of *Brucella* in cultured lymphoid and nonlymphoid cells, *J. Bacteriol.* **88**: 1163-1168.
903. Ridley, A. (1963). Localization of gamma-globulin in experimental encephalomyelitis by the fluorescent antibody technique. *Z. Immunitaetsforsch.* **125**: 173-190.
904. Riggs, J. L. (1965). Application of fluorescent antibody techniques to viral infections. *Ind. Med. Surg.* **34**: 269-277.
905. Riggs, J. L., and Brown, G. C. (1962). Differentiation of active and passive poliomyelitis antibodies in human sera by indirect immunofluorescence. *J. Immunol.* **89**: 868-873.
906. Riggs, J. L., and Brown, G. C. (1962). Application of direct and indirect immunofluorescence for identification of enteroviruses and titrating their antibodies. *Proc. Soc. Exptl. Biol. Med.* **110**: 833-837.
907. Riggs, J. L., Loh, P. C., and Eveland, W. C. (1960). A simple fractionation method for preparation of fluorescein-labeled gamma globulin. *Proc. Soc. Exptl. Biol. Med.* **105**: 655-658.
908. Riggs, J. L., Seiwald, R. J., Burckhalter, J. H., Downs, C. M., and Metcalf, T. G. (1958). Isothiocyanate compounds as fluorescent labeling agents for immune serum. *Am. J. Pathol.* **34**: 1081-1097.
909. Rinderknecht, H. (1960). A new technique for fluorescent labeling of proteins. *Experientia* **16**: 430.
910. Rinderknecht, H. (1962). Ultra-rapid fluorescent labelling of proteins. *Nature* **193**: 167-168.

911. Ristic, M., Oppermann, J., Sibinovic, S., and Phillips, T. N. (1964). Equine piroplasmosis—a mixed strain of *Piroplasma caballi* and *Piroplasma equi* isolated in Florida and studied by the fluorescent-antibody technique. *Am. J. Vet. Res.* **25**: 15-23.

912. Ristic, M., and Sibinovic, S. (1964). Equine babesiosis: Diagnosis by a precipitation in gel and by a one-step fluorescent antibody-inhibition test. *Am. J. Vet. Res.* **25**: 1519-1526.

913. Ristic, M., and White, F. H. (1960). Detection of an *Anaplasma marginale* antibody complex formed *in vivo*. *Science* **131**: 987-988.

914. Ristic, M., White, F. H., and Sanders, D. A. (1957). Detection of *Anaplasma marginale* by means of fluorescein-labeled antibody. *Am. J. Vet. Res.* **18**: 924-928.

915. Ritz, H. L. (1963). Localization of *Nocardia* in dental plaque by immunofluorescence. *Proc. Soc. Exptl. Biol. Med.* **113**: 925-929.

916. Roberts, D. St. C. (1957). Studies on the antigenic structure of the eye using the fluorescent antibody technique. *Brit. J. Ophthalmol.* **41**: 338-347.

917. Roberts, J. A. (1963). Histopathogenesis of mousepox. III. Ectromelia virulence. *Brit. J. Exptl. Pathol.* **44**: 465-472.

918. Rodriguez, J., and Deinhardt, F. (1960). Preparation of a semipermanent mounting medium for fluorescent antibody studies. *Virology* **12**: 316-317.

919. Rodriguez, J. E., and Henle, W. (1964). Studies on persistent infections of tissue cultures. V. The initial stages of infection of L(MCN) cells by Newcastle disease virus. *J. Exptl. Med.* **119**: 895-921.

920. Romano, A. H., and Geason, D. J. (1964). Pattern of sheath synthesis in *Sphaerotilus natans*. *J. Bacteriol.* **88**: 1145-1150.

921. Rosenau, W., Moon, H. D., and McIvor, B. C. (1962). Localization of antibody to tissue culture cells by fluorescent antibody technique. *Lab. Invest.* **11**: 199-203.

922. Ross, M. R., and Borman, E. K. (1963). Direct and indirect fluorescent-antibody techniques for the psittacosis-lymphogranuloma venereum-trachoma group of agents. *J. Bacteriol.* **85**: 851-858.

923. Rossi, F., Zaccheo, D., and Grossi, C. E. (1964). Nuovi problemi nella tecnica dell'anticorpo fluorescente e nelle sue applicazioni istochimiche. *Riv. Istochim. Norm. Patol.* **10**: 53-153.

924. Rossman, I. (1940). The deciduomal reaction in the rhesus monkey. I. The epithelial proliferation. *Am. J. Anat.* **66**: 277-365.

925. Rotta, J., Karakawa, W. W., and Krause, R. M. (1965). Isolation of L forms from group A streptococci exposed to bacitracin. *J. Bacteriol.* **89**: 1581-1585.

926. Rotter, J., Alami, S. Y., and Kelly, F. C. (1964). Evidence for antibody-free staphylococcus-fibrinogen reactions. *J. Bacteriol.* **88**: 1810-1811.

927. Rotter, K., and Mayersbach, H. (1959). Versuche zum Nachweis

von Gewebsantikorpern bei Tuberkulose mittels immunohisto-logischer Methoden. *Schweiz. Z. Allgem. Pathol. Bakteriol.* **22**: 732-741.

928. Rowe, W. P., and Baum, S. G. (1964). Evidence for a possible genetic hybrid between adenovirus type 7 and SV40 viruses. *Proc. Natl. Acad. Sci. U.S.* **52**: 1340-1347.

929. Rubenstein, H. S., Fine, J., and Coons, A. H. (1962). Localization of endotoxin in the walls of the peripheral vascular system during lethal endotoxemia. *Proc. Soc. Exptl. Biol. Med.* **111**: 458-467.

930. Runge, W. J. (1966). A recording microfluorospectrophotometer. *Science* **151**: 1499-1506.

931. Sabin, A. B., and Messore, G. (1961). Fluorescent antibody technique in the study of fixed tissues from patients with encephalitis. *In* "Encephalitides" (L. van Bogaert, *et al.,* eds.), pp. 621-626. Elsevier, Amsterdam.

932. Sachs, L., and Fogel, M. (1960). Polyoma virus synthesis in tumor cells as measured by fluorescent antibody technique. *Virology* **11**: 722-736.

933. Sack, R. B., and Barua, D. (1964). The fluorescent antibody technique in the diagnosis of cholera. *Indian J. Med. Res.* **52**: 848-854.

934. Sadun, E. H. (1963). Seminar on immunity to parasitic helminths. VII. Fluorescent antibody technique for helminth infections. *Exptl. Parasitol.* **13**: 72-82.

935. Sadun, E. H., Anderson, R. I., Dewitt, W. B., and Jachowski, L. A. (1963). Serologic reactions to *Schistosoma mansoni.* II. Quantitative studies in human patients treated with stibophen. *Am. J. Hyg.* **77**: 146-149.

936. Sadun, E. H., Anderson, R. I., and Williams, J. S. (1961). Fluorescent antibody test for the laboratory diagnosis of schistosomiasis in humans by using dried blood smears on filter paper. *Exptl. Parasitol.* **11**: 117-120.

937. Sadun, E. H., Anderson, R. I., and Williams, J. S. (1962). Fluorescent antibody test for the serological diagnosis of trichinosis. *Exptl. Parasitol.* **12**: 423-433.

938. Sadun, E. H., Anderson, R. I., and Williams, J. S. (1962). The nature of fluorescent antibody reactions in infections and artificial immunizations with *Schistosoma mansoni. Bull. World Health Organ.* **27**: 151-159.

939. Sadun, E. H., and Bruce, J. I. (1964). Resistance induced in rats by previous exposure to and by vaccination with fresh homogenates of *Schistosoma mansoni. Exptl. Parasitol.* **15**: 32-43.

940. Sadun, E. H., Duxbury, R. E., Williams, J. S., and Anderson, R. I. (1963). Fluorescent antibody test for the serodiagnosis of African and American trypanosomiasis in man. *J. Parasitol.* **49**: 385-388.

941. Sadun, E. H., Williams, J. S., and Anderson, R. I. (1960). Fluorescent antibody technic for serodiagnosis of schistosomiasis in humans. *Proc. Soc. Exptl. Biol. Med.* **105**: 289-291.

942. Sainte-Marie, G. (1962). A paraffin embedding technique for studies employing immunofluorescence. *J. Histochem. Cytochem.* **10**: 250-256.

943. Sainte-Marie, G. (1963). Antigen penetration into the thymus. *J. Immunol.* **91**: 840-845.

944. Sainte-Marie, G., and Coons, A. H. (1964). Studies on antibody production. X. Mode of formation of plasmacytes in cell transfer experiments. *J. Exptl. Med.* **119**: 743-760.

945. Saliou, P. (1964). Diagnostic serologique du paludisme humain par l'immuno-fluorescence. M.D. thesis. Faculty of Medicine, University of Lyons, France.

946. Salmon, J., Lambotte, R., and Smoliar, V. (1962). Etude par immunofluorescence de la secretion du liquide amniotique humain. *Arch. Intern. Physiol. Biochim.* **70**: 731-734.

947. Sambrook, J. F., McClain, M. E., Easterbrook, K. B., and McAuslan, B. R. (1965). A mutant of rabbitpox virus defective at different stages of its multiplication in the three cell types. *Virology* **26**: 738-745.

948. Sanders, V., and Ritts, R. E., Jr. (1965). Ventricular localization of bound gamma globulin in idiopathic disease of the myocardium. *J. Am. Med. Assoc.* **194**: 59-61.

949. Saslaw, M. S., Jablon, J. M., and Mazzarella, J. A. (1963). Prevention of initial attacks of rheumatic fever. *Public Health Rept.* **78**: 207-221.

950. Scarpa, B. (1963). Immunofluorescent reaction in the diagnosis of diphtheria. II. Practical applications. (Italian) *Rass. Med. Sarda* **65**: 693-697.

951. Schaeffer, M., Orsi, E. V., and Widelock, D. (1964). Applications of immunofluorescence in public health virology. *Bacteriol. Rev.* **28**: 402-408.

952. Schaffer, J., Lewis, V., Nelson, J., and Walcher, D. (1963). Antepartum survey for enteropathogenic *Escherichia coli*. *Am. J. Diseases Children* **106**: 170-173.

953. Schamschula, R. G. (1964). The application of the fluorescent antibody technique to the detection of *Candida albicans* in oral pathological material. *Australian J. Exptl. Biol. Med. Sci.* **42**: 173-180.

954. Schiebe, O., and Eder, M. (1956). Lichtelektrische emissionsmessing akradin-orange-fluorochromierter gewebeschnitte. *Acta Histochem.* **3**: 6-18.

955. Schiller, A. A., Schayer, R. W., and Hess, E. L. (1953). Fluorescein-conjugated bovine albumin. Physical and biological properties. *J. Gen. Physiol.* **36**: 489-506.

956. Schmidt, E. L., and Bankole, R. O. (1962). Detection of *Aspergillus flavus* in soil by immunofluorescent staining. *Science* **136**: 776.

957. Schmidt, J. (1964). Studies on the fluorescent serological demonstration of *Staphylococcus aureus*. (German) *Zentr. Bakteriol. Parasitenk., Abt. I. Orig.* **195**: 190-201.

958. Schmidt, W. C. (1952). Group A streptococcus polysaccharide: Studies on its preparation, chemical composition and cellular localization after intravenous injection into mice. *J. Exptl. Med.* **95**: 105-118.

959. Schramm, G., and Rottger, B. (1959). Untersuchungen uber das Tabakmosaic virus mit fluoreszierenden Antikorpern. *Z. Naturforsch.* **14b**: 510-515.

960. Schroeder, W. F., and Ristic, M. (1965). Anaplasmosis. 18. An analysis of autoantigens in infected and normal bovine erythrocytes. *Am. J. Vet. Res.* **26**: 679-682.

961. Scott, D. G. (1960). Immuno-histochemical studies of connective tissue: the use of contrasting fluorescent protein tracers in the comparison of two antisera. *Immunology* **3**: 226-236.

962. Scott, E. G., and Holloway, W. J. (1963). Identification of group A streptococci in throat cultures by the fluorescent antibody technique. *Delaware State Med. J.* **35**: 34-36.

963. Seegal, B. C., Andres, G. A., Hsu, K. C., and Zabriskie, J. B. (1965). Studies on the pathogenesis of acute and progressive glomerulonephritis in man by immunofluorescein and immunoferritin techniques. *Federation Proc.* **24**: 100-108.

964. Sell, S. H. W., Cheatham, W. J., Young, B., and Welch, K. (1963). *Hemophilus influenzae* in respiratory infections. I. Typing by immunofluorescent techniques. *Am. J. Diseases Children* **105**: 466-469.

965. Sell, S. H. W., Sanders, R. S., and Cheatham, W. J. (1963). *Hemophilus influenzae* in respiratory infections. II. Specific serological antibodies identified by agglutination and immunofluorescent techniques. *Am. J. Diseases Children* **105**: 470-474.

966. Serbezov, V., Ognanov, D., Matova, E., Alexandrov, E., Makaveyeva, E., and Nedeltseva, N. (1965). Detection of ornithosis virus by the fluorescent antibody method, using convalescent anti-virus abortion sheep sera. *J. Hyg., Epidemiol., Microbiol., Immunol.* (*Prague*) **9**: 253-255.

967. Sercarz, E. E., and Coons, A. H. (1963). The absence of antibody-producing cells during unresponsiveness to BSA in the mouse. *J. Immunol.* **90**: 478-491.

968. Shapiro, L. H., and Lentz, J. W. (1963). Fluorescent antibody technic in diagnosis of gonorrhea in females. *Obstet. Gynecol.* **21**: 435-437.

969. Sharma, N. N., and Foster, J. W. (1963). Serology of *Eimeria tenella* oocysts with rabbit serum. *J. Parasitol.* **49**: 943-946.

970. Shaughnessy, H. J., Lesko, M., Dorigan, F., Forster, G. F., Morrissey, R. A., and Kessner, D. M. (1962). An extensive community outbreak of diarrhea due to enteropathogenic *Escherichia coli* 0111:B4. II. A comparative study of fluorescent antibody identification and standard bacteriologic methods. *Am. J. Hyg.* **76**: 44-51.

971. Shaw, J. J., and Voller, A. (1963). Preliminary fluorescent antibody

studies on *Endotrypanum schaudinni. Trans. Roy. Soc. Trop. Med. Hyg.* **57**: 232-233.

972. Shaw, J. J., and Voller, A. (1964). The detection of circulating antibody to kala-azar by means of immunofluorescent techniques. *Trans. Roy. Soc. Trop. Med. Hyg.* **58**: 349-352.

973. Shedden, W. I., and Emery, J. L. (1965). Immunofluorescent evidence of respiratory syncytial virus infection in cases of giant cell bronchiolitis in children. *J. Pathol. Bacteriol.* **89**: 343-347.

974. Shein, H. M., and Levinthal, J. D. (1962). Fluorescent antibody and complement fixation tests for detection of SV40 virus in cell cultures. *Virology* **17**: 595-597.

975. Sheinin, R., and Quinn, P. A. (1965). Effect of polyoma virus on the replicative mechanism of mouse embryo cells. *Virology* **26**: 73-84.

976. Sheldon, W. H. (1953). Leptospiral antigen demonstrated by the fluorescent antibody technic in human muscle lesions of *Leptospira icterohemorrhagiae. Proc. Soc. Exptl. Biol. Med.* **84**: 165-167.

977. Shepard, C. C., and Goldwasser, R. A. (1960). Fluorescent antibody staining as a means of detecting Rocky Mountain spotted fever infection in individual ticks. *Am. J. Hyg.* **72**: 120-129.

978. Shepard, C. C., and Kirsh, D. (1961). Fluorescent antibody stainability and other consequences of the disruption of mycobacteria. *Proc. Soc. Exptl. Biol. Med.* **106**: 685-691.

979. Sherris, J. C. (1963). Some recent advances in diagnostic medical bacteriology. *Ann. Rev. Microbiol.* **17**: 565-592.

980. Shi-Gie, H., and Pogodina, V. V. (1964). Use of fluorescent antibody technique in studies on Far-East tick-borne encephalitis in mice, hamsters and pigs. *Acta Virol.* **8**: 22-29.

981. Shimazaki, M., Ueda, G., Ito, M., Mukobayashi, M., and Shirakawa, J. (1962). Staining of the thyroid gland with fluorescein conjugated antithyroglobulin. Examination on the several sorts of fixatives and methods of preparing sections. *Wakayama Med. Rept.* **7**: 13-21.

982. Shiokawa, Y., Yamada, S., and Shibayama, H. (1963). Studies on rheumatic fever with immunofluorescent method. *Japan. Heart J.* **4**: 407-416.

983. Siddiqui, W. A., and Balamuth, W. (1966). Serological comparison of selected parasitic and free-living amoebae *in vitro,* using diffusion-precipitation and fluorescent antibody technics. *J. Protozool.* **13**: 175-182.

984. Silva, M. E., and Kaplan, W. (1965). Specific fluorescein-labeled antiglobulins for the yeast form of *Paracoccidioides brasiliensis. Am. J. Trop. Med. Hyg.* **14**: 290-294.

985. Silverstein, A. M. (1957). Contrasting fluorescent labels for two antibodies. *J. Histochem. Cytochem.* **5**: 94-95.

986. Sinha, R. C. (1965). Sequential infection and distribution of wound-

tumor virus in the internal organs of a vector after ingestion of virus. *Virology* **26**: 673-686.

987. Sinha, R. C., and Reddy, D. V. (1964). Improved fluorescent smear technique and its application in detecting virus antigens in an insect vector. *Virology* **24**: 626-634.

988. Sinha, R. C., Reddy, D. V., and Black, L. M. (1964). Survival of insect vectors after examination of hemolymph to detect virus antigens with fluorescent antibody. *Virology* **24**: 666-667.

989. Slack, J. M., Spears, R. G., Snodgrass, W. G., and Kuchler, R. J., (1955). Studies with microaerophilic actinomycetes. II. Serological groups as determined by the reciprocal agglutinin adsorption technique. *J. Bacteriol.* **70**: 400-404.

990. Slack, J. M., Winger, A., and Moore, D. W. (1961). Serological grouping of actinomyces by means of fluorescent antibodies. *J. Bacteriol.* **82**: 54-65.

991. Slotnick, I. J., Mertz, J. A., and Dougherty, M. (1964). Fluorescent antibody detection of human occurrence of an unclassified bacterial group causing endocarditis. *J. Infect. Diseases* **114**: 503-505.

992. Slotnick, V. B., and Rosanoff, E. I. (1963). Localization of varicella virus in tissue culture. *Virology* **19**: 589-592.

993. Smith, C. W., Marshall, J. D., Jr., and Eveland, W. C. (1959). Use of contrasting fluorescent dye as counterstain in fixed tissue preparations. *Proc. Soc. Exptl. Biol. Med.* **102**: 179-181.

994. Smith, C. W., Marshall, J. D., Jr., and Eveland, W. C. (1960). Identification of *Listeria monocytogenes* by the fluorescent antibody technic. *Proc. Soc. Exptl. Biol. Med.* **103**: 842-845.

995. Smith, C. W., Metzger, J. F., and Hoggan, M. D. (1962). Immunofluorescence as applied to pathology. *Am. J. Clin. Pathol.* **38**: 26-42.

996. Smith, M. L., Carski, T. R., and Griffin, C. W. (1962). Modification of fluorescent antibody procedures employing tetramethylrhodamine isothiocyanate. *J. Bacteriol.* **83**: 1358-1359.

997. Smith, T. B. (1965). Clinical application of immunofluorescence. I. Grouping beta-hemolytic streptococci. *J. Bacteriol.* **89**: 198-204.

998. Smithies, L. K., and Olson, C. (1964). Correlation of immunofluorescence and infectivity in the developing bovine cutaneous papilloma. *Cancer Res.* **24**: 674-681.

999. Sobeslavsky, O., Syrucek, L., Bruckova, M., and Abrahamovic, M. (1965). The etiological role of *Mycoplasma pneumoniae* in otitis media in children. *Pediatrics* **35**: 652-657.

1000. Sodeman, W. A., Jr., and Jeffery, G. M. (1964). Immunofluorescent staining of sporozoites of *Plasmodium gallinaceum*. *J. Parasitol.* **50**: 477-478.

1001. Sodeman, W. A., Jr., and Jeffery, G. M. (1965). Immunofluorescent studies of *Plasmodium berghei*: A "natural" antibody in white mice. *Am. J. Trop. Med. Hyg.* **14**: 187-190.

1002. Sokol, F., Hana, L., and Albrecht, P. (1961). Fluorescent antibody method. Quantitative determination of 1-dimethylamino-naphthalene-5-sulphonic acid and protein in labelled γ-globulin. *Folia Microbiol. (Prague)* **6**: 145-150.

1003. Sokol, F., Hulka, A., and Albrecht, P. (1962). Fluorescent antibody method. Conjugation of fluorescein-isothiocyanate with immune γ-globulin. *Folia Microbiol. (Prague)* **7**: 155-161.

1004. Sokolov, N. N., and Parfanovich, M. I. (1964). Character of the accumulation and localization of specific antigen and nucleic acids in the course of vaccinia virus infection of tissue culture as revealed by fluorescence microscopy. *Acta Virol.* **8**: 30-37.

1005. Sokolov, N. N., Parfanovich, M. I., and Mekler, L. B. (1963). On the nature of tickborne encephalitis virus. II. A comparative study of nucleic acids and specific antigen in cells from brains of white mice infected with tick-borne encephalitis virus by fluorescence microscopy. *Acta Virol.* **7**: 217-224.

1006. Solomon, A., Fahey, J. L., and Malmgren, R. A. (1963). Immunohistologic localization of gamma-1-macroglobulins, Beta-2A-myeloma proteins and Bence-Jones proteins. *Blood* **21**: 403-423.

1007. Sommerville, R. G., and MacFarlane, P. S. (1964). The rapid diagnosis of virus infections by immunofluorescent techniques applied to blood leucocytes. *Lancet* **I**: 911-912.

1008. Sonea, S., and de Repentigny, J. (1960). Observations sur les couleurs de la fluorescence primaire des microorganismes. *Can. J. Microbiol.* **6**: 519-528.

1009. Southam, C. M., Shipkey, F. H., Babcock, V. I., Bailey, R., and Erlandson, R. A. (1964). Virus biographies. I. Growth of West Nile and Guaroa viruses in tissue culture. *J. Bacteriol.* **88**: 187-199.

1010. Spendlove, R. S., and Lennette, E. H. (1962). A simplified immunofluorescent plaque method. *J. Immunol.* **89**: 106-112.

1011. Spendlove, R. S., Lennette, E. H., Knight, C. O., and Chin, J. O. (1963). Development of viral antigen and infectious virus in HeLa cells infected with reovirus. *J. Immunol.* **90**: 548-553.

1012. Spink, W. W. (1962). The young investigator and his fluorescent antibody. *J. Am. Med. Assoc.* **181**: 889-891.

1013. Stadtsbaeder, S., Tellier-Verheyden, N., and Weber, M. (1964). Serologic diagnosis of toxoplasmosis by immunofluorescence. (French) *Acta Clin. Belg.* **19**: 161-166.

1014. Stair, E. L., Rhodes, M. B., Aiken, J. M., Underdahl, N. R., and Young, G. A. (1963). A hog cholera virus-fluorescent antibody system. Its potential use in study of embryonic infection. *Proc. Soc. Exptl. Biol. Med.* **113**: 656-660.

1015. Starin, W. A., and Dack, G. M. (1923). Agglutination studies of *Clostridium botulinum*. *J. Infect. Diseases* **33**: 169-183.

1016. Steblay, R. W. (1962). Localization in human kidney of antibodies formed in sheep against human placenta. *J. Immunol.* **88**: 434-442.

1017. Steiner, R. F., and Edelhoch, H. (1962). Fluorescent protein conjugates. *Chem. Rev.* **62**: 457-483.

1018. Stevens, R. W., Boylan, J., and Memoli, A. J. (1967). A note on the fluorescent treponemal antibody-absorption (FTA-ABS) test. *Am. J. Clin. Pathol.* **47**: 408-409.

1019. Strauss, A. J. L., Seegal, B. E., Hsu, K. C., Burkholder, P. M., Nastuk, W. L., and Osserman, K. (1960). Immunofluorescence demonstration of muscle binding complement-fixing serum globulin fraction in myasthenia gravis. *Proc. Soc. Exptl. Biol. Med.* **105**: 184-191.

1020. Stulberg, C. S., Zuelzer, W. W., Nolke, A. C., and Thompson, A. L. (1955). *Escherichia coli* 127:B, a pathogenic strain causing infantile diarrhea. I. Epidemiology and bacteriology of a prolonged outbreak in a premature nursery. *Am. J. Diseases Children* **90**: 125-134.

1021. Sulzer, A. J. (1965). Indirect fluorescent antibody tests for parasitic diseases. I. Preparation of a stable antigen from larvae of *Trichinella spiralis. J. Parasitol.* **51**: 717-721.

1022. Suter, L. S., and Ulrich, E. W. (1964). "H", "O", and fluorescent antibody titers in salmonellosis. *Am. J. Gastroenterol.* **42**: 626-632.

1023. Suzuki, K., Luto, T., and Fujita, J. (1965). Serological diagnosis of toxoplasmosis by the indirect immunofluorescent staining. *Natl. Inst. Animal Health Quart.* **5**: 73-85.

1024. Swift, H., and Rasch, E. (1956). Microphotometry with visible light. *In* "Physical Techniques in Biological Research" (G. Oster and A. W. Pollister, eds.), Vol. 3, pp. 353-400. Academic Press, New York.

1025. Sydiskis, R. J., and Schultz, I. (1965). Herpes simplex skin infection in mice. *J. Infect. Diseases* **115**: 237-246.

1026. Szanto, J. (1965). Passaging in chick embryos of Newcastle disease virus from persistently infected HeLa cell cultures. *Acta Virol.* **9**: 47-54.

1027. Szanto, J., Albrecht, P., and Vilcek, J. (1963). Investigations on latent infection in the HeLa cell—Newcastle disease virus system. *Acta Virol.* **7**: 297-307.

1028. Szulman, A. E. (1960). The histological distribution of blood group substances A and B in man. *J. Exptl. Med.* **111**: 785-800.

1029. Taffs, L. F., and Voller, A. (1962). Fluorescent antibody studies *in vitro* on *Ascaris suum* Goeze, 1782. *J. Helminthol.* **36**: 339-346.

1030. Taffs, L. F., and Voller, A. (1963). *In vitro* fluorescent antibody studies on *Ascaris lumbricoides* and *Ascaris suum. Trans. Roy. Soc. Soc. Trop. Med. Hyg.* **57**: 353-358.

1031. Taffs, L. F., and Voller, A. (1964). Fluorescent antibody staining of *Ascaris suum* larvae in the liver and lung of an infected guinea-pig by means of the freeze-substitution technique. *Ann. Trop. Med. Parasitol.* **58**: 414-419.

1032. Takeda, H., Yamada, M. A., and Aoyama, Y. (1965). Demonstration of RNA synthesis caused by Japanese encephalitis virus infection in PS(Y-15) cells with the aid of chromomycin A-3. *Japan. J. Med. Sci. Biol.* **18**: 111-120.

1033. Takeuchi, I. (1963). Immunochemical and immunohistochemical studies on the development of the cellular slime mold *Dictyostelium mucoroides. Develop. Biol.* **8**: 1-26.

1034. Takumi, K., Takebayashi, I., Takeuchi, H., Ikeda, H., and Toshioka, N. (1966). The use of lyophilized parasites in indirect fluorescent antibody technique for detection of *Toxoplasma* antibody. *Japan. J. Microbiol.* **10**: 189-191.

1035. Talal, N., and Bunim, J. J. (1964). The development of malignant lymphoma in the course of Sjogren's syndrome. *Am. J. Med.* **36**: 529-540.

1036. Tanaka, N., and Leduc, E. H. (1956). A study of the cellular distribution of Forssman antigen in various species. *J. Immunol.* **77**: 198-212.

1037. Tanaka, N., Nishimura, T., Tada, T., and Okabayashi, A. (1964). Autoimmune phenomenon occurred in the course of prolonged stimulation of heterologous protein. *Japan. J. Exptl. Med.* **34**: 53-57.

1038. Tanaka, N., Yamaguchi, H., Nishimura, T., and Yoshiyuki, T. (1960). Histochemical studies on experimental typhoid by means of fluorescein-labeled antibody. III. Demonstration of gamma globulin or antibody in the typhoid granuloma. *Japan. J. Microbiol.* **4**: 433-449.

1039. Taylor, A. H. (1934). Reflection-factors of various materials for visible and ultraviolet radiation. *J. Opt. Soc. Am.* **24**: 192-193.

1040. Taylor, C. E. D., and Heimer, G. V. (1964). Rapid diagnosis of Sonne dysentery by means of immunofluorescence. *Brit. Med. J.* **II**: 165-166.

1041. Taylor, C. E. D., Heimer, G. V., Lea, D. J., and Tomlinson, A. J. H. (1964). A comparison of a fluorescent antibody technique with a cultural method in the detection of infections with *Shigella sonnei. J. Clin. Pathol.* **17**: 225-230.

1042. Tengerdy, B. P. (1963). Quantitative immunofluorescein titration of human and bovine gamma globulins. *Anal. Chem.* **35**: 1084-1086.

1043. Tevethia, S. S., Katz, M., and Rapp, F. (1965). New surface antigen in cells transformed by simian papovavirus SV40. *Proc. Soc. Exptl. Biol. Med.* **119**: 896-901.

1044. Thivolet, J., Grospiron, D., and Murat, M. (1960). Utilization of immunofluorescence for the diagnosis of syphilis (preliminary note) (French). *Rev. Hyg. Med. Soc.* **8**: 501-509.

1045. Thivolet, J., Sohier, R., Picard, M., and Blanc, G. (1963). Use of the immunofluorescence method in the diagnosis of lung diseases caused by Eaton's mycoplasma. (French). *Ann. Inst. Pasteur* **105**: 749-756.

1046. Thomas, J. B., Sikes, R. K., and Ricker, A. S. (1963). Evaluation of indirect fluorescent antibody technique for detection of rabies antibody in human sera. *J. Immunol.* **91**: 721-723.

1047. Thomason, B. M. (1965). Rapid detection of typhoid carriers by means of fluorescent antibody techniques. *Bull. World Health Organ.* **33**: 681-685.

1048. Thomason, B. M., and Cherry, W. B. (1963). Immunofluorescence techniques in the diagnosis of infections due to enteropathogenic *Escherichia coli. Rev. Latinoam. Microbiol.* **6**: 63-76.

1049. Thomason, B. M., Cherry, W. B., Davis, B. R., and Pomales-Lebron, A. (1961). Rapid presumptive identification of enteropathogenic *Escherichia coli* in faecal smears by means of fluorescent antibody. I. Preparation and testing of reagents. *Bull. World Health Organ.* **25**: 137-152.

1050. Thomason, B. M., Cherry, W. B., and Edwards, P. R. (1959). Staining bacterial smears with fluorescent antibody. VI. Identification of *Salmonellae* in fecal specimens. *J. Bacteriol.* **77**: 478-486.

1051. Thomason, B. M., Cherry, W. B., and Moody, M. D. (1957). Staining bacterial smears with fluorescent antibody. III. Antigenic analysis of *Salmonella typhosa* by means of fluorescent antibody and agglutination reactions. *J. Bacteriol.* **74**: 525-532.

1052. Thomason, B. M., Cherry, W. B., and Pomales-Lebron, A. (1961). Rapid presumptive identification of enteropathogenic *Escherichia coli* in faecal smears by means of fluorescent antibody. II. Use of various types of swabs for collection and preservation of faecal specimens. *Bull. World Health Organ.* **25**: 153-158.

1053. Thomason, B. M., Cowart, G. S., and Cherry, W. B. (1965). Current status of immunofluorescence techniques for rapid detection of shigellae in fecal specimens. *Appl. Microbiol.* **13**: 605-613.

1054. Thomason, B. M., Moody, M. D., and Goldman, M. (1956). Staining bacterial smears with fluorescent antibody. II. Rapid detection of varying numbers of *Malleomyces pseudomallei* in contaminated materials and infected animals. *J. Bacteriol.* **72**: 362-367.

1055. Thorpe, E. (1965). An immunocytochemical study with *Fasciola hepatica. Parasitology* **55**: 209-214.

1056. Tobie, J. E. (1958). Certain technical aspect of fluorescence microscopy and the Coons fluorescent antibody technique. *J. Histochem. Cytochem.* **6**: 271-277.

1057. Tobie, J. E. (1964). Detection of malaria antibodies—immunodiagnosis. *Am. J. Trop. Med. Hyg.* **13**: Suppl., 195-203.

1058. Tobie, J. E., and Coatney, G. R. (1961). Fluorescent antibody staining of human malaria parasites. *Exptl. Parasitol.* **11**: 128-132.

1059. Tobie, J. E., and Coatney, G. R. (1964). The antibody response in volunteers with cynomolgi malaria infections. *Am. J. Trop. Med. Hyg.* **13**: 786-789.

1060. Tobie, J. E., Kuvin, S. F., Contacos, P. G., Coatney, G. R., and Evans, C. B. (1962). Fluorescent antibody studies on cross reactions between human and simian malaria in normal volunteers. *Am. J. Trop. Med. Hyg.* **11**: 589-596.

1061. Tokarevich, K. N., Krasnik, F. I., and Goldin, R. B. (1963). The use of fluorescent antibody technique in serological diagnosis of ornithosis. *Acta Virol.* **7**: 478.

1062. Tokumaru, T. (1962). A kinetic study on the labeling of serum globulin with fluorescein isothiocyanate by means of the gel filtration technique. *J. Immunol.* **89**: 195-203.

1063. Tonomura, K., and Tanabe, O. (1964). Localization of cell-bound alpha-amylase in *Aspergillus oryzae* demonstrated by fluorescent-antibody technique. *J. Bacteriol.* **87**: 226-227.

1064. Toussaint, A. J. (1966). Improvement of the soluble antigen fluorescent-antibody procedure. *Exptl. Parasitol.* **19**: 71-76.

1065. Toussaint, A. J., and Anderson, R. J. (1965). Soluble antigen fluorescent-antibody technique. *Appl. Microbiol.* **13**: 552-558.

1066. Toussaint, A. J., Tarrant, C. J., and Anderson, R. I. (1965). An indirect fluorescent antibody technique using soluble antigens for serodiagnosis of *Trypanosoma cruzi* infection. *Proc. Soc. Exptl. Biol. Med.* **120**: 783-785.

1067. Trabulsi, L. R., and Camargo, M. E. (1965). Comparative study between immunofluorescence and coproculture in the diagnosis of intestinal infections by enteropathogenic *Escherichia coli*. *Rev. Inst. Med. Trop. Sao Paulo* **7**: 65-71.

1068. Truant, J. P., Hadley, I. K., and Boyd, T. T. (1965). A comparison of the immunofluorescence technique with conventional methods for the identification of Group A beta hemolytic streptococci. *Henry Ford Hosp. Med. Bull.* **13**: 357-375.

1069. Tsunematsu, Y., Shiori, K., and Kusano, N. (1964). Three cases of lymphadenopathia toxoplasmotica. *Japan. J. Exptl. Med.* **34**: 216-230.

1070. Tucker, C. B., Cameron, G. M., Buchanan, R. L., Dillon, A., and Grayson, J. H. (1962). An evaluation of the Kolmer Reiter protein and fluorescent treponemal antibody tests. *Public Health Rept.* **77**: 1089-1094.

1071. Tully, J. G. (1965). Biochemical, morphological, and serological characterization of mycoplasma of murine origin. *J. Infect. Diseases* **115**: 171-185.

1072. Tyndall, R. L., Vidrine, J. G., Teeter, E., Upton, A. C., Harris, W. W., and Fink, M. A. (1965). Cytopathogenic effects in a cell culture infected with a murine leukemia virus. *Proc. Soc. Exptl. Biol. Med.* **119**: 186-189.

1073. Uchida, Y., and Kimura, S. J. (1965). Fluorescent antibody localization of herpes simplex virus in the conjunctiva. *Arch. Ophthalmol.* **73**: 413-419.

1074. Uehleke, H. (1958). Neue Moglichkeiten zur Herstellung fluoreszenzmarkierter Proteine. *Z. Naturforsch.* **13b**: 722-724.

1075. Uehleke, H. (1959). Untersuchungen mit fluoreszenz-markierten antikorpern. IV. Die Markierung von Antikorpern mit Sulfochloriden fluoreszierender Farbstoffe. *Schweiz. Z. Allgem. Pathol. Bakteriol.* **22**: 724-729.

1076. Urso, P., and Gengozian, N. (1964). Immunofluorescent detection of proliferating human antibody-forming cells. *Nature* **203**: 1391-1392.

1077. Urso, P., and Makinodan, T. (1963). The roles of cellular division and maturation in the formation of precipitating antibody. *J. Immunol.* **90**: 897-907.

1078. Vainio, T., Saxen, L., and Toivonen, S. (1963). Viral susceptibility and embryonic differentiation. II. Immunofluorescence studies of viral infection in the developing mouse kidney *in vitro*. *Acta Pathol. Microbiol. Scand.* **58**: 205-211.

1079. Vainio, T., Saxen, L., and Toivonen, S. (1963). Viral susceptibility and embryonic differentiation. III. Correlation between an inductive tissue interaction and the onset of viral resistance. *J. Natl. Cancer Inst.* **31**: 1533-1547.

1080. Van der Veen, J., and Van Nunen, M. C. J. (1963). Role of *Mycoplasma pneumoniae* in acute respiratory disease in a military population. *Am. J. Hyg.* **78**: 293-301.

1081. Van Nunen, M. C. J., and Van der Veen, J. (1965). Examination for toxoplasmosis by the fluorescent antibody technique. *Trop. Geograph. Med.* **17**: 246-253.

1082. Vassalli, P., and McCluskey, R. T. (1964). The pathogenic role of fibrin deposition in immunologically induced glomerulonephritis. *Ann. N.Y. Acad. Sci.* **116**: 1052-1062.

1083. Vassalli, P., and McCluskey, R. T. (1964). The pathogenic role of the coagulation process in rabbit Masugi nephritis. *Am. J. Pathol.* **45**: 653-677.

1084. Vazquez, J. J. (1958). Immunocytochemical study of plasma cells in multiple myeloma. *J. Lab. Clin. Med.* **51**: 271-275.

1085. Vazquez, J. J., and Dixon, F. J. (1956). Immunohistochemical analysis of amyloid by the fluorescence technique. *J. Exptl. Med.* **104**: 727-736.

1086. Vazquez, J. J., and Dixon, F. J. (1957). Immunohistochemical study of lesions in rheumatic fever, systemic lupus erythematosis, and rheumatoid arthritis. *Lab. Invest.* **6**: 205-217.

1087. Villella, R. L., Halling, L. W., and Biegeleisen, J. Z., Jr. (1963). A case of listeriosis of the newborn with fluorescent antibody histologic studies. *Am. J. Clin. Pathol.* **40**: 151-156.

1088. Vogel, R. A., and Padula, J. F. (1958). Indirect staining reaction with fluorescent antibody for detection of antibodies to pathogenic fungi. *Proc. Soc. Exptl. Biol. Med.* **98**: 135-139.

1089. Vogt, P. K. (1965). A heterogeneity of Rous sarcoma virus revealed by selectively resistant chick embryo cells. *Virology* **25**: 237-247.

1090. Vogt, P. K., and Luykx, N. (1963). Observations on the surface of cells infected with Rous sarcoma virus. *Virology* **20**: 75-87.

1091. Voller, A. (1962). Fluorescent antibody studies on malaria parasites. *Bull. World Health Organ.* **27**: 283-287.

1092. Voller, A. (1964). Comments on the detection of malaria antibodies. *Am. J. Trop. Med. Hyg.* **13**: 204-208.

1093. Voller, A. (1964). Fluorescent antibody methods and their use in malaria research. *Bull. World Health Organ.* **30**: 343-354.

1094. Voller, A., and Bray, R. S. (1962). Fluorescent antibody staining as a measure of malarial antibody. *Proc. Soc. Exptl. Biol. Med.* **110**: 907-910.

1095. Voller, A., and Toffs, L. F. (1963). Fluorescent-antibody staining of exoerythrocytic stages of *Plasmodium gallinaceum. Trans. Roy. Soc. Trop. Med. Hyg.* **57**: 32-33.

1096. Voller, A., and Wilson, H. (1964). Immunological aspects of a population under prophylaxis against malaria. *Brit. Med. J.* **5408**: 551-552.

1097. Vozza, R., and Balducci, D. (1961). The technique of fluorescent antibodies in ophthalmology. A study of herpes simplex and vaccine keratoconjunctivitis and human trachomatous infection. *Am. J. Ophthalmol.* **52**: 72-77.

1098. Wagner, M. (1964). Studien mit fluoreszierenden Antikorpern an wachsunden Bakterien. I. Die Neubildung bei Zellwand bei *Diplococcus pneumoniae. Zentr. Bakteriol. Parasitenk., Abt. I. Orig.* **195**: 87-94.

1099. Waksman, B. H., and Bocking, D. (1953). Study with fluorescent antibody of fate of intradermally injected proteins in rabbits. *Proc. Soc. Exptl. Biol. Med.* **82**: 738-742.

1100. Walker, R. V. (1962). Studies on the immune response of guinea pigs to the envelope substance of *Pasteurella pestis.* I. Immunogenicity and persistence of large doses of Fraction I in guinea pigs observed with fluorescent antibody. *J. Immunol.* **88**: 153-163.

1101. Walker, R. V. (1962). Studies on the immune response of guinea pigs to the envelope substance of *Pasteurella pestis.* II. Fluorescent antibody studies of cellular and tissue response in mice and guinea pigs to large doses of Fraction I. *J. Immunol.* **88**: 164-173.

1102. Walker, R. V. (1962). Studies on the immune response of guinea pigs to the envelope substance of *Pasteurella pestis.* III. Immunounresponsiveness to high concentrations of Fraction I in oil. *J. Immunol.* **88**: 174-183.

1103. Wallnerova, Z., and Albrecht, P. (1964). Detection of Tahyna virus in tissue cultures by the fluorescent antibody technique. *Acta Virol.* **8**: 474.

1104. Walton, B. C., Benchoff, B. M., and Brooks, W. H. (1966). Comparison of the indirect fluorescent antibody test and methylene blue dye test for detection of antibodies to *Toxoplasma gondii. Am. J. Trop. Med. Hyg.* **15**: 149-152.

1105. Wanebo, H. J., and Clarkson, B. D. (1965). Essential macroglobulinemia. Report of a case including immunofluorescent and electron microscopic studies. *Ann. Internal Med.* [N.S.] **62**: 1025-1045.

1106. Watson, B. K. (1952). Fate of mumps virus in the embryonated egg as determined by specific staining with fluorescein-labelled immune serum. *J. Exptl. Med.* **96**: 653-664.

1107. Watson, B. K. (1952). Distribution of mumps virus in tissue cultures as determined by fluorescein-labeled antiserum. *Proc. Soc. Exptl. Biol. Med.* **79**: 222-224.

1108. Watson, B. K., and Coons, A. H. (1954). Studies of influenza virus infection in the chick embryo using fluorescent antibody. *J. Exptl. Med.* **99**: 419-428.

1109. Weber, G. (1952). Polarization of the fluorescence of macromolecules. II. Fluorescent conjugates of ovalbumin and bovine serum albumin. *Biochem. J.* **51**: 155-167.

1110. Webster, R. G., Laver, W. G., and Fozekas, de St. Groth, S. (1962). Methods in immunochemistry of viruses. 3. Simple techniques for labelling antibodies with ^{131}I and ^{35}S. *Australian J. Exptl. Biol.* **40**: 321-328.

1111. Weiler, E. (1956). Antigenic differences between normal hamster kidney and stilboestrol induced kidney carcinoma: Histological demonstration by means of fluorescing antibodies. *Brit. J. Cancer* **10**: 560-563.

1112. Weiser, R. S., and Laxson, C. (1962). The fate of fluorescein-labeled soluble antigen-antibody complex in the mouse. *J. Infect. Diseases* **111**: 55-58.

1113. Weitz, B. (1963). The specificity of trypanosomal antigens by immunofluorescence. *J. Gen. Microbiol.* **32**: 145-149.

1114. Weller, T. H., and Coons, A. H. (1954). Fluorescent antibody studies with agents of varicella and herpes zoster propagated *in vitro*. *Proc. Soc. Exptl. Biol. Med.* **86**: 789-794.

1115. Wells, A. F., Miller, C. E., and Nadel, M. K. (1966). Rapid fluorescein and protein assay method for fluorescent-antibody conjugates. *Appl. Microbiol.* **14**: 271-275.

1116. Wells, H. (1964). The use of immunofluorescent techniques as a diagnostic aid in rheumatic heart diseases. *Virginia Med. Monthly* **91**: 516-518.

1117. Wertz, R. K., and Adams, W. R. (1963). Presence of viral antigen in inclusion bodies formed in Ehrlich ascites tumor cells infected with Newcastle disease virus. *Yale J. Biol. Med.* **36**: 234-240.

1118. Wheelock, E. F., and Tamm, I. (1961). Enumeration of cell-infecting particles of Newcastle disease virus by the fluorescent antibody technique. *J. Exptl. Med.* **113**: 301-316.

1119. Wheelock, E. F., and Tamm, I., (1961). Effect of multiplicity of infection on Newcastle disease virus-HeLa cell interaction. *J. Exptl. Med.* **113**: 317-338.

1120. Whitaker, J., Nelson, J. D., and Fink, C. W. (1961). The fluorescent anti-toxin test for the immediate diagnosis of diphtheria. *Pediatrics* **27**: 214-218.

1121. Whitaker, J., Page, R. H., Stulberg, C. S., and Zuelzer, W. W. (1958). Rapid identification of enteropathogenic *Escherichia coli* 0127:B$_8$ by the fluorescent antibody technique. *J. Diseases Children* **95**: 1-8.

1122. Whitaker, J., Zuelzer, W., Robinson, A. R., and Evans, M. (1959). The use of the fluorescent antibody technique for the demonstration of erythrocyte antigens. *J. Lab. Clin. Med.* **54**: 282-283.

1123. White, J. D., and McGavran, M. H. (1965). Identification of *Pasteurella tularensis* by immunofluorescence. *J. Am. Med. Assoc.* **194**: 294-296.

1124. White, L. A., and Kellogg, D. S., Jr. (1965). *Neisseria gonorrhoeae* identification in direct smears by a fluorescent antibody-counterstain method. *Appl. Microbiol.* **13**: 171-174.
1125. White, R. G. (1958). Antibody production by single cells. *Nature* **182**: 1383-1384.
1126. White, R. G. (1960). Fluorescent antibody technique. In "Tools of Biological Research" (H. J. B. Atkins, ed.), Vol. II, pp. 89-104. Thomas, Springfield, Illinois.
1127. White, R. G. (1963). The applications of fluorescent antibody techniques in bacteriology and virology. *Proc. Roy. Soc. Med.* **56**: 474-478.
1128. White, R. G., Coons, A. H., and Connolly, J. M. (1955). Studies on antibody production. III. The alum granuloma. *J. Exptl. Med.* **102**: 73-82.
1129. White, R. G., Coons, A. H., and Connolly, J. M. (1955). Studies on antibody production. IV. The role of a wax fraction of *Mycobacterium tuberculosis* in adjuvant emulsions on the production of antibody to egg albumin. *J. Exptl. Med.* **102**: 83-104.
1130. Wiktor, T. J., Fernandes, M. V., and Koprowski, H. (1964). Cultivation of rabies virus in human diploid cell strain WI-38. *J. Immunol.* **93**: 353-366.
1131. Wilkinson, A. E. (1963). The fluorescent treponemal antibody test in the serological diagnosis of syphilis. *Proc. Roy. Soc. Med.* **56**: 478-481.
1132. Williams, J. S., Duxbury, R. E., Anderson, R. L., and Sadun, E. H. (1963). Fluorescent antibody reactions in *Trypanosoma rhodesiense* and *T. gambiense* in experimental animals. *J. Parasitol.* **49**: 380-384.
1133. Williamson, A. P., and Blattner, R. J. (1965). Immunofluorescence of Newcastle disease virus in paraffin embedded tissues of early chick embryos. *Proc. Soc. Exptl. Biol. Med.* **118**: 576-580.
1134. Wilsnack, R. E., and Rowe, W. P. (1964). Immunofluorescent studies of the histopathogenesis of lymphocytic choriomeningitis virus infection. *J. Exptl. Med.* **120**: 829-840.
1135. Winter, C. L., and Moody, M. D. (1959). Rapid identification of *Pasteurella pestis* with fluorescent antibody. I. Production of specific antiserum with whole cell *Pasteurella pestis* antigen. *J. Infect. Diseases* **104**: 274-280.
1136. Winter, C. L., and Moody, M. D. (1959). Rapid identification of *Pasteurella pestis* with fluorescent antibody. II. Specific identification of *Pasteurella pestis* in dried smears. *J. Infect. Disease* **104**: 281-287.
1137. Witmer, R. (1955). Antibody formation in rabbit eye studied with fluorescein-labeled antibody. *Arch. Ophthalmol.* **53**: 811-816.
1138. Wolfe, J. D., and Cameron, G. M. (1959). Fluorescent antibody techniques versus cultural methods as a routine procedure for finding beta-hemolytic streptococci in throat cultures. *Public Health Lab.* **17**: 76-82.

1139. Wolfe, M. D., Cameron, G. M., and West, M. E. (1960). Further observations on the fluorescent antibody technique as a procedure for detecting Group A streptococci in throat cultures. *Public Health Lab.* **18**: 120-126.

1140. Wolpert, L., and O'Neill, C. H. (1962). Dynamics of the membrane of *Amoeba proteus* studied with labelled specific antibody. *Nature* **196**: 1261-1266.

1141. Wood, B. T., Thompson, S. H., and Goldstein, G. (1965). Fluorescent antibody staining. III. Preparation of fluorescein-isothiocyanate-labeled antibodies. *J. Immunol.* **95**: 225-229.

1142. Wood, R. M. (1964). Identification of viruses. *Intern. Ophthalmol. Clin.* **4**: 301-310.

1143. Woolf, N. (1961). The distribution of fibrin within the aortic intima. *Am. J. Pathol.* **39**: 521-532.

1144. Yager, R. H., Spertzel, R. O., Jaeger, R. F., and Tigertt, W. D. (1960). Domestic fowl-source of high titer *P. tularensis* serum for the fluorescent antibody technic. *Proc. Soc. Exptl. Biol. Med.* **105**: 651-654.

1145. Yamaguchi, B. T., Jr., Adriano, S., and Braunstein, H. (1963). *Histoplasma capsulatum* in the pulmonary primary complex: Immunohistochemical demonstration. *Am. J. Pathol.* **43**: 713-719.

1146. Yobs, A. R., Brown, L., and Hunter, E. F. (1964). Fluorescent antibody technique in early syphilis. *Arch. Pathol.* **77**: 220-225.

1147. Young, M. R. (1961). Principles and technique of fluorescence microscopy. *Quart. J. Microscop. Sci.* **102**: 419-450.

1148. Zak, K., and Veznik, Z. (1963). The possibility of detecting *Brucella* antigens by means of fluorescent antibodies in gynecology. (German) *Zentr. Gynaekol.* **85**: 1058-1063.

1149. Zaman, V. (1965). The application of fluorescent antibody test to *Balantidium coli. Trans. Roy. Soc. Trop. Med. Hyg.* **59**: 80-82.

1150. Zaman, V. (1965). The application of fluorescent-antibody test to cysts of *Entamoeba invadens. Experientia* **27**: 357-359.

1151. Zardi, O. (1963). Fluorescent antibodies in the diagnosis of toxoplasmosis. (Italian) *Nuovi Ann. Igiene Microbiol.* **14**: 585-612.

1152. Zhdanov, V. M., Azadova, N. B., and Uryvayev, L. V. (1965). Topography of synthesis of S and V antigens of Sendai virus. *J. Immunol.* **94**: 658-661.

1153. Zinner, D. D., Jablon, J. M., Aran, A. P., and Saslaw, M. S. (1965). Experimental caries induced in animals by streptococci of human origin. *Proc. Soc. Exptl. Biol. Med.* **118**: 766-770.

1154. Zinner, D.D., Jablon, J.M., Haddox, C.H., Jr., Aran, A., and Saslaw, M.S. (1965). Use of fluorescent-antibody technique to identify experimental hamster and rat strains of cariogenic streptococci. *J. Dental Res.* **44**: 471-475.

1155. Zwann, J., and Van Dam, A.F. (1961). Rapid separation of fluorescent antisera and unconjugated dye. *Acta Histochem.* **11**: 306-308.

AUTHOR INDEX

Numbers in parentheses are reference numbers and indicate that an author's work is referred to, although his name is not cited in the text. Numbers in italics show the page on which the complete reference is listed.

Picard, M., 184 (1045), *265*
Piekarski, G., 89 (222), 186 (222), *210*
Pier, A. C., 185 (847), *252*
Pierce, G. B., 143 (732), 189 (732), *245*
Pierce, W. A., Jr., 185 (262), *213*
Pillot, J., 184 (848), *252*
Pina, A., 186 (58), *200*
Pine, L., 185 (849), *252*
Piomelli, S., 189 (850), *252*
Pirie, E., 186 (176), *207*
Pital, A., 149, *253*
Pittman, B., 83, 95 (428), 181, 185 (749), *201, 224, 246, 253*
Pittman, F. E., 190 (853), *253*
Plowright, W., 188 (632), *238*
Poetschke, G., 88 (856), 183 (855), 185 (854, 856), *253*
Pogodina, V. V., 187 (980), *261*
Pollard, L. W., 97, 99 (706), 104 (706), 126 (706), 127 (706), 131 (706), 177, *243*
Pollister, A. W., 84, *253*
Pomales-Lebron, A., 88 (1049), 184 (136, 1049, 1052), *205, 266*
Pomeroy, B. S., 188 (34), *198*
Ponten, J., 103 (551), 137 (551), *232*
Pope, J. H., 187 (859, 860), *253*
Popper, H., 89 (18), 186 (18), 189 (160, 829, 830, 831), *197, 206, 251*
Porath, J., 103 (861), *253*
Porter, D. D., 188 (863), *253*
Porter, B. M., 185 (862), *253*
Potter, J. L., 109 (9), 116 (9), *196*
Pratesi, V., 184 (744, 754), *245, 246*
Pressman, D., 5, 10, 30, 83, 92 (724), 93, 170, 189 (383, 448, 450, 451, 452, 453, 454, 456, 716, 724), 190 (383, 455, 864), *221, 225, 226, 243, 244, 253*
Preston, J. A., 185 (865), *254*
Price, G. R., 58, 59, 68, 175, *254*
Prince, A. M., 90 (869), 187 (868), 188 (869), *254*
Pringsheim, P., 20
Prochazka, O., 184 (325), *217*

Procknow, J. J., 88 (870), 140 (870), 185 (870), *254*
Proietti, A. M., 186 (194), *208*
Pruzansky, J. J., 189 (837), *252*
Puhvel, S. M., 184 (871), *254*
Purcell, R. H., 184 (760), *246*

Quan, S. F., 184 (473, 872), *227, 254*
Quinn, L. Y., 184 (407), *223*
Quinn, P. A., 187 (975), *261*
Quock, C., 184 (402), *223*

Rabin, E. R., 187 (425), 188 (873), *224, 254*
Rabson, A. S., 187 (810), *250*
Radke, M. G., 186 (874), *254*
Radley, J. A., 20
Rado, J. P., 187 (875), *254*
Raffel, S., 96, 189 (891), *255*
Rahman, A. N., 144 (876), *254*
Randall, R. J., 123, *240*
Rapp, F., 187 (161, 559, 726, 881, 877, 878, 879, 880, 882, 883, 884, 885, 887, 1043), 188 (100), *202, 206, 233, 244, 254, 255*
Rappaport, B. Z., 179, 189 (887), 190 (886, 887), *255*
Rasch, E., 84 (1024), *264*
Raskin, J., 188 (890), 189 (889), *255*
Rasmussen, L. E., 187 (883), *255*
Rathova, V., 187 (70), *200*
Rauch, H. C., 185 (892), 189 (891), *255*
Rauscher, F. J., 133 (312), 189 (310, 312), *216, 217*
Ravetta, M., 187 (807), *250*
Rawson, A. J., 190 (893), *255*
Ray, C. G., 88 (870), 140 (870), 185 (870), *254*
Ray, H. N., 186 (761), *247*
Reda, I. M., 188 (894), *256*
Reddy, D. V., 188 (987, 988), *262*
Redetzki, H. M., 10, 127 (895), 137, *256*
Redmond, D. L., 184 (896, 897), *256*

SUBJECT INDEX